Dementia: management of behavioural and psychological symptoms

Edited by

Clive Ballard and John O'Brien

Institute for the Health of the Elderly
Wolfson Research Centre
Newcastle General Hospital
Newcastle upon Tyne

Ian James and Alan Swann

Centre for the Health of the Elderly
Newcastle General Hospital
Newcastle upon Tyne

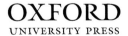

OXFORD

UNIVERSITY PRESS

*This book has been printed digitally and produced in a standard specification
in order to ensure its continuing availability*

OXFORD
UNIVERSITY PRESS

Great Clarendon Street, Oxford OX2 6DP

Oxford University Press is a department of the University of Oxford.
It furthers the University's objective of excellence in research, scholarship,
and education by publishing worldwide in

Oxford New York

Auckland Cape Town Dar es Salaam Hong Kong Karachi
Kuala Lumpur Madrid Melbourne Mexico City Nairobi
New Delhi Shanghai Taipei Toronto
With offices in
Argentina Austria Brazil Chile Czech Republic France Greece
Guatemala Hungary Italy Japan South Korea Poland Portugal
Singapore Switzerland Thailand Turkey Ukraine Vietnam

Oxford is a registered trade mark of Oxford University Press
in the UK and in certain other countries

Published in the United States
by Oxford University Press Inc., New York

ISBN 0-19-263175-6

Antony Rowe Ltd., Eastbourne

Foreword

Alzheimer's disease and other dementias have been defined by their cognitive and neuro-psychological characteristics. Memory decline is the core feature of most of these disorders, many of which also have impairment of visual spatial skills, language and executive functions. The emphasis on cognitive abnormalities as central to defining the dementia syndromes has led to an under-emphasis on the behavioural and neuro-psychiatric symptoms associated with these diseases. The lack of clinical studies and research on the behavioural and psychological symptoms of dementia (BPSD) is unfortunate given the distress produced by these symptoms in the patients, the exaggeration of carer burden they produce and the significant life consequences related to them, such as nursing home placement. *Dementia: management of behavioural and psychological symptoms*, by Clive Ballard, John O'Brien, Ian James and Alan Swann, is part of a growing attempt to redress the imbalance and to provide information relevant to BPSD. The authors are eminently qualified to lead the reader through this complex area.

In the past decade there has been a rapid growth in our understanding of the neuro-psychiatric manifestations of dementing disorders. New measurement methodology has evolved which allows semi-quantification of behavioural abnormalities. Both cross-sectional and longitudinal studies have documented the high frequency of behavioural disturbances among patients with dementias. Behavioural changes may be the harbinger of the onset of a dementing disorder in an elderly individual and many BPSD worsen as the diseases progress. The clinical features of the neuropsychiatric disorders occurring in dementia syndromes are described in the current volume in chapters individually addressing psychosis, depression, wandering and restlessness, aggression, and other BPSD.

The majority of care for dementia patients is provided by family carers. They are usually the first to detect changes in cognition and behaviour. They provide most of the support and care for the patient during the course of the illness and they frequently suffer tremendous guilt if nursing home placement becomes required. The burden of caregiving manifests itself in depression, physical illness, excessive substance use and occasional outbursts directed at the family member. This book addresses these important issues in chapters describing depression and burden in dementia carers, training carers in behavioural management skills, managing carers' psychological needs and working with professional carers in nursing home environments.

The first response to a carer's report of a behavioural disturbance often is to prescribe a psychotropic agent and this has led to the use of medication as the primary intervention for BPSD. This is unfortunate since many patients respond to environmental changes. Our currently available medications often have only modest efficacy and psychotropic medications produce many adverse side effects in the elderly. Thus, use of non-pharmacological interventions to reduce behavioural disturbances, while not exposing the patient to the risk of psychotropic medication, is critically important in the management of behavioural disturbance in dementia patients. This book does an unusually good job of providing highly relevant and useful information on non-pharmacological management of dementia. Chapters address psychological therapies in dementia, cognitive therapy formulations and interventions for treating distress in dementia, training carers in behavioural management skills, and other non-pharmacological approaches.

Use of non-pharmacological interventions will reduce behavioural disturbances in many patients but others will require pharmacological management. In many cases, clinicians are forced to use psychotropic agents developed for treatment of behavioural syndromes in non-demented patients. Thus, antipsychotics have typically been imported from their use in schizophrenia, antidepressants from their application in idiopathic depressive disorders and anti-agitation agents from their original use in patients with mania and bipolar disorders. Recently, psychotropic agents have been specifically studied in dementia populations with patients exhibiting behavioural disturbances. This is a great step forward in terms of developing pharmacotherapy for dementia patients that is evidence-based. Dr O'Brien and Dr Ballard provide a comprehensive assessment of the effects and side effects of psychotropic medications used to reduce behavioural disturbances in dementia patients. Separate chapters discuss the side effects of psychotropic medications, pharmacological treatment of psychosis, pharmacotherapy of depression, pharmacological management of agitation, aggression and restlessness, and management of other behavioural and psychological symptoms in dementia. The final chapter in this book outlines an integrated treatment approach comprising accurate diagnosis and characterization, collaboration with family and/or professional carers, intervention with non-pharmacological strategies, and appropriate use and monitoring of psychopharmacological interventions.

This volume will prove to be useful for all clinicians involved in providing care for dementia patients manifesting behavioural changes. Understanding of the information provided and implementation of the recommendations will result in an improved quality of life for both patients and carers.

Jeffrey L. Cummings, MD
Augustus S. Rose Professor of Neurology
Professor of Psychiatry and Biobehavioral Sciences
Director, UCLA Alzheimer's Disease Center, Los Angeles, CA
July, 2000

Contents

1 Background—behavioural and psychological symptoms in dementia

Dementia is a syndrome characterized by cognitive and non-cognitive symptoms. Traditionally it is the cognitive impairments which have been the main focus of attention, although over the last 15 years the importance of non-cognitive symptoms has become increasingly recognized. Their pronounced and diverse impact is discussed in the relevant chapters dealing with the respective individual symptoms. There are several clinically distinct categories of frequent and troublesome non-cognitive symptoms. The International Psychogeriatric Association grouped them together under the umbrella term 'behavioural and psychological symptoms in dementia' or BPSD (Finkel *et al.* 1996). This has been very successful in highlighting this as an important clinical and research topic, although it has perhaps in some studies encouraged disparate symptoms to be grouped together.

It is important that the nature of the term is clearly understood. The key symptoms include agitation (describing a cluster of related symptoms including anxiety, irritability and motor restlessness, often leading to behaviours such as pacing, wandering, aggression, shouting and night-time disturbance), psychosis (referring to three main categories of symptom: (i) hallucinations, usually visual; (ii) delusions, which are usually simple ideas pertaining to theft or being talked about; and (iii) delusional misidentification, which includes the Capgras delusion as well as misidentification of television and mirror images) and mood disorders (mainly depression and anxiety, although hypomania does sometimes occur). Other symptoms which can be important include sexual disinhibition, eating problems and abnormal vocalizations (shouting, screaming and demanding attention).

Why are BPSD seen in patients with dementia?

There are many reasons why a patient with dementia may develop BPSD. Some are related to the dementia whilst others are specific to it. Dementia-related causes include pain, concurrent physical problems (constipation, sensory impairments and infections) and concurrent psychiatric symptoms (BPSD symptoms co-occur more frequently than explained by chance). Dementia-specific causes include reactions to the patient's interaction with his physical and social environment and how this is affected by cognitive deficit. The specific associations of individual BPSD symptoms are discussed in the respective chapters. BPSD may emerge as a primary feature of a dementia syndrome, although in the majority of cases an explanation will be found in an examination of the patient's interactions with his environment.

Assessment

Because BPSD may have many different aetiologies, a full and careful assessment of possible physical, psychological and environmental factors is essential. Since not all BPSD necessarily require treatment, it is important to determine whether the symptoms are causing significant distress or risk to the patient, carers and others. If a prompt intervention is not imperative, it is usually advisable to review severity and impact over a period of weeks. These themes are developed further in the individual chapters.

Management

A detailed evaluation of the literature is presented in the relevant chapters. In general, several principles should be borne in mind. Many symptoms are not severely distressing and they are frequently self-limiting. Assuming that no reversible physical cause for the BPSD has been identified, for minor problems the clinician can reassure carers that the behaviours are often self-limiting and likely to resolve. Often the assessment itself is effective as a treatment. As, for most BPSD symptoms, there are few adequate data to inform practice, we recommend a structured sequential approach to management, where if an intervention is clearly necessary, psychosocial interventions should in the majority of instances be applied before pharmacological treatment.

Summary

The current brief chapter serves as an introduction and to highlight several key principles. Much more detailed accounts of the individual BPSD symptoms and approaches to management are given in the subsequent chapters.

REFERENCE

Finkel, S. I., Costa de Silva, J., Cohen, G., Miller, S. and Sartorius, N. (1996). Behavioral and psychological signs and symptoms of dementia: a consensus statement on current knowledge and implications for research and treatment. *International Journal of Pychogeriatrics*, **8**, 497–500.

2 Identification and measurement of behavioural and psychological symptoms in dementia

Introduction

There are two key questions: (i) Why do we need standardized rating scales? and (ii) Why can scales that have been developed to measure mood and psychosis in the absence of cognitive impairment not serve the same purpose in the assessment of behavioural and psychological symptoms in dementia (BPSD)?

The first question is best addressed by comparing some of the studies that evaluated the prevalence of BPSD from case-note reviews or clinical interviews with those that utilized a standardized schedule. For psychosis, for example, reported frequencies are 60–70% in clinical cohorts assessed using a standardized scale, but only 30% in studies using case-note information or clinical interviewing (Ballard and Oyebode 1995). This dramatic under-reporting of symptoms is also seen for other BPSD unless standardized methodologies are adopted (Ballard *et al.* 1996a). There are several probable reasons for this under-reporting, related to the fact that information is mainly acquired from a caregiver or informant who may fail to recall mild to moderate symptoms unless asked very specific questions.

The second question is more difficult. Certainly several key behaviours such as agitation are uncommon other than amongst people with dementia, and as such have not been the subject of well-developed rating scales. Other BPSD occurring in people with dementia are superficially similar to symptoms arising in the context of functional psychiatric disorders, for example depression and psychosis. However, the phenomenology of psychosis in dementia is very different from that of either schizophrenia or paraphrenia, and specific rating schedules are required. Depression appears to be rather more similar, although it may tend to be milder, more likely to spontaneously resolve within a few months (Ballard *et al.* 1996b) and less likely to respond to antidepressant therapy (Winblad *et al.* 2000). Despite the generally similar symptom profiles, scales devised for measuring depression, such as the Hamilton rating scale for depression and the Geriatric Depression Scale, have been rather unreliable for assessing depression in the presence of dementia (Burke *et al.* 1989, Lichtenberg *et al.* 1992). It is hence clear that specific scales are required to assess BPSD.

Developing specific scales

Even people with very mild dementia frequently under-report symptoms (Ballard *et al.* 1991). This does not, however, mean that the information obtained from the patient is not useful, as when a patient does describe a symptom, it is usually present and often significant (Ballard *et al.* 1991). A good example of a scale specifically developed to assess a BPSD symptom that combines patient and informant interview is the Cornell Depression Scale (Alexopolous *et al.* 1988). The majority of instruments, however, rely upon information from a caregiver or informant. This is not ideal, but generally works well for someone who lives with a caregiver or has frequent visits. It may be rather less satisfactory for people who have less frequent contact with an informant, or who live in a care facility environment where staff members may not have the same detailed knowledge of a patient as a family caregiver. Generally, standardized informant assessments can still be valuable in care settings, although it is important to speak to a person's key worker or to a member of staff that has frequent contact with the individual. We would also recommend a short general conversation about the person with dementia prior to commencing the formal BPSD assessment, to confirm that the staff member has a good knowledge of this particular resident. One of the standard BPSD rating scales, the Neuropsychiatric Inventory (NPI), has a separate version for use with care staff (Cummings 1997).

The main alternative approaches are to use direct observation from a professional member of staff, such as a nurse or doctor. The Neurobehaviour Rating Scale (Levin *et al.* 1987) is an instrument developed as a clinician assessment within the clinic, and has the advantage of skilled observation, but the disadvantage of a short period of evaluation in an unfamiliar setting. In general, direct observation is too time-consuming to be a feasible method of assessment in clinical practice or in most research studies. Particularly if direct observation is combined with video recording, it can, however, be a very powerful technique for checking concurrent and inter-rater reliability.

What scales to use

In general, informant scales can be divided into: (i) comprehensive scales covering a spectrum of BPSD symptoms; (ii) summary scales covering the important symptom areas; or (iii) specific scales developed to give a detailed profile of a particular category or cluster of BPSD. Scales covering specific BPSD are described in the relevant chapters focusing upon these symptoms. Comprehensive scales include the Present Behavioural Examination (PBE) (Hope and Fairburn 1992), and its derivative, the Manchester and Oxford Universities Scale for the Psychopathological Assessment of Dementia (MOUSPAD) (Allen *et al.* 1996). The PBE is an excellent instrument, which provides detailed information regarding a broad spectrum of BPSD symptoms. Whilst it is probably the gold standard, it takes a considerable amount of time to complete and is certainly not feasible within routine clinical practice. It is probably the instrument of choice within a research setting, if the main focus of the study is BPSD symptoms, if there are few additional assessment instruments to be completed and if the evaluation is not repeated too often. The instrument has been used, for example, to produce a detailed longitudinal profile of BPSD symptoms as part of a comprehensive MRC study in Oxford, UK. The length of the interview may be a problem if BPSD symptoms are being assessed as part of a larger evaluation, as the time taken to complete the total assessment may reduce participation or be beyond the available staff resources. The MOUSPAD, although slightly shorter, does not evaluate mood symptoms and probably has no real advantages over the PBE.

There are a number of briefer assessments based upon an informant interview which provide a broad assessment of the key BPSD symptoms. The NPI, the BEHAV-AD and the Behaviour Rating Scale for dementia (BRSD) all provide a measure of severity as well as determining whether a symptom is present or absent (Reisberg *et al.* 1987, Cummings *et al.* 1994, Tariot *et al.* 1995) and are therefore suitable for measuring change in the context of a therapeutic intervention. All can be completed within about 15–20 min and are therefore useful in both research and clinical settings. The authors strongly recommend that one of these schedules should be routinely used. The items from the NPI, the BEHAV-AD and the BRSD are shown in Figs 2.1, 2.2 and 2.3, respectively.

The NPI has 12 sub-scales, 10 covering BPSD and two measuring neurovegatative symptoms. Each sub-scale has an 'entry question'. If this is answered positively, the full sub-scale is completed; if not, the interviewer moves on to the next symptom cluster. This has the advantage of considerably speeding up the interview and avoids irritating informants when no or few BPSD symptoms are present. A panel of experts agreed that the scale had good content validity (Cummings 1997), and the instrument has good test–retest (Cummings 1997) as well as good inter-rater reliability (Cummings *et al.* 1994, Cummings 1997). The scale also has good concurrent validity with the BEHAV-AD (Cummings 1997). The frequency and severity of symptoms over the month prior to interview are determined and multiplied to produce a measure of severity, which, although useful, is a non-linear scale, with implications for statistical analysis. A useful carer distress scale has been developed as an adjunct (Cummings 1997, Kaufer *et al.* 1998). The NPI has been widely used, with the advantage that there is now a considerable body of normative data for different dementia groups.

The BEHAV-AD (Reisberg *et al.* 1987, 1996) has 25 items covering seven domains: delusions, hallucinations, activity disturbances, aggressiveness, diurnal rhythm disturbances, affective disturbances and anxieties/phobias. Symptoms are assessed by informant interview covering a defined time period, usually 1 month. Each

Description of the NPI

The NPI consists of 12 behavioural areas:

delusions	apathy
hallucinations	disinhibition
agitation	irritability
depression	aberrant motor behaviour
anxiety	night-time behaviours
euphoria	appetite and eating disorders

Frequency is rated as
1   occasional (less than once per week)
2   often (about once per week)
3   frequent (several times a week but less than every day)
4   very frequent (daily or essentially continuously present)

Severity is rated as
1   mild (produce little distress in the patient)
2   moderate (more disturbing to the patient but can be redirected by the caregiver)
3   severe (very disturbing to the patient and difficult to redirect)

Distress is scored as
0   no distress
1   minimal
2   mild
3   moderate
4   moderately severe
5   very severe or extreme

For each domain there are four scores: frequency, severity, total (frequency × severity) and caregiver distress. The total possible score is 144 (i.e. a maximum of 4 in the frequency rating × 3 in the severity rating × 12 remaining domains). This relates to changes, usually over the 4 weeks prior to completion.

Fig. 2.1   Neuropsychiatric Inventory (NPI). Source: Cummings *et al.* (1994). © JL Cummings, 1994; the Neuropsychiatric Inventory is a copyrighted instrument and permission to use it in a commercial study must be negotiated with copyright owner Jeffrey Cummings, MD, Reed Neurological Research Center, UCLA School of Medicine, 710 Westwood Plaza, Los Angeles, California, USA, 90095–1769.

symptom is rated on a four-point severity scale and an overall global rating of severity is also recorded. No ratings of frequency are made. The scale has been very widely used in clinical and treatment studies, and the inter-rater reliability has been confirmed by two independent groups in three samples (Patterson *et al.* 1990, Sclan *et al.* 1996). The BEHAV-AD has good concurrent validity with the NPI (Cummings 1997).

More recently, the Consortium to Establish a Registry for Alzheimer's Disease (CERAD) group has developed the BRSD. This is a 51-item scale, developed by expert consensus, which has been broken down into eight factors. The scale measures the presence or absence of BPSD symptoms over the month prior to the interview and since the onset of the dementia. The frequency of symptoms over the previous month is determined for 46 of the items. The scale has excellent inter-rater reliability (Tariot *et al.* 1995), but has not yet been used as widely as the NPI or BEHAV-AD.

Part 1: Symptomatolgy

Assessment interval: Specific:_____ weeks

Total score:_____

a. Paranoid and delusional ideation

1. 'People are stealing things' delusion
- 0 = not present
- 1 = delusion that people are hiding objects
- 2 = delusion that people are coming into the home and hiding objects or stealing objects
- 3 = talking and listening to people coming into the home

2. 'One's house is not one's home' delusion
- 0 = not present
- 1 = conviction that the place in which one is residing is not one's home (e.g. packing to go home; complaints, while at home, of 'take me home')
- 2 = attempt to leave domicilliary to go home
- 3 = violence in response to attempts to forcibly restrict exit

3. 'Spouse (or other caregiver) is an impostor' delusion
- 0 = not present
- 1 = conviction that spouse (or other caregiver) is an impostor
- 2 = anger towards spouse (or other caregiver) for being an impostor
- 3 = violence towards spouse (or other caregiver) for being an impostor

4. 'Delusion of abandonment' (e.g. to an institution)
- 0 = not present
- 1 = suspicion of caregiver plotting abandoment or institutionalization (e.g. on telephone)
- 2 = accusation of a conspiracy to abandon or institutionalize
- 3 = accusation of impending or immediate desertion or institutionalization

5. 'Delusion of infidelity'
- 0 = not present
- 1 = conviction that spouse and/or children and/or other caregivers are unfaithful
- 2 = anger towards spouse, relative or other caregiver for supposed infidelity

6. 'Suspiciousness/paranoia' (other than above)
- 0 = not present
- 1 = suspicious (e.g. hiding objects that he/she later may be unable to locate)
- 2 = paranoid (i.e. fixed conviction with respect to suspicions and/or anger as a result of suspicions)
- 3 = violence as a result of suspicions

Unspecified?

Describe

7. Delusions (other than above)
- 0 = not present
- 1 = delusional
- 2 = verbal or emotional manifestations as a result of delusions
- 3 = physical actions or violence as a result of delusions

Unspecified

Fig. 2.2   Continued

b. Hallucinations

8. Visual hallucinations
0 =   not present
1 =   vague; not clearly defined
2 =   clearly defined hallucinations of objects or
        persons (e.g. sees other people at the table)
3 =   verbal or physical actions or emotional
        responses to the hallucinations

9. Auditory hallucinations
0 =   not present
1 =   vague; not clearly defined
2 =   clearly defined
3 =   verbal or physical actions or emotional
        responses to the hallucinations

10. Olfactory hallucinations
0 =   not present
1 =   vague; not clearly defined
2 =   clearly defined
3 =   verbal or physical actions or emotional
        responses to the hallucinations

11. Haptic hallucinations
0 =   not present
1 =   vague; not clearly defined
2 =   clearly defined
3 =   verbal or physical actions or emotional
        responses to the hallucinations

12. Other hallucinations
0 =   not present
1 =   vague; not clearly defined
2 =   clearly defined
3 =   verbal or physical actions or emotional
        responses to the hallucinations
Unspecified?
Describe

c. Activity disturbances

13. Wandering: away from home or caregiver
0 =   not present
1 =   somewhat, but not sufficient to necessitate restraint
2 =   sufficient to require restraint
3 =   verbal or physical actions or emotional
        responses to attemtps to prevent wandering

14. Purposeless activity (cognitive abulia)
0 =   not present
1 =   repetitive, purposeless activity (e.g. opening and
        closing pocketbook, packing and unpacking
        clothing, repeatedly putting on and removing
        clothing, opening and closing drawers, insistent
        repeating of demands or questions)
2 =   pacing or other purposeless activity sufficient
        to require restraint
3 =   abrasions or physical harm resulting from
        purposeless activity

15. Inappropriate activity
0 =   not present
1 =   inappropriate activities (e.g. storing and hiding
        objects in inappropriate places, such as throwing
        clothing in wastebasket or putting empty plates
        in the oven; inappropriate sexual behaviour, such
        as inappropriate exposure)
2 =   present and sufficient to require restraint
3 =   present, sufficient to require restraint, and
        accompanied by anger or violence when restraint
        is used

Fig. 2.2   Continued

d. Aggressiveness

16. Verbal outbursts
0 = not present
1 = present (including unaccustomed use of foul or abusive language)
2 = present and accompanied by anger
3 = present, accompanied by anger, and clearly directed at other persons

17. Phsysical threats and/or violence
0 = not present
1 = threatening behaviour
2 = physical violence
3 = physical violence accompanied by vehemence

18. Agitation (other than above)
0 = not present
1 = present
2 = present with emotional component
3 = present with emotional and physical component
Unspecified?
Describe

e. Diurnal rhythm disturbances

19. Day/night disturbance
0 = not present
1 = repetitive wakenings during night
2 = 50–75% of former sleep cycle at night
3 = complete disturbance of diurnal rhythm (i.e. <50% of former sleep cycle at night)

f. Affective disturbance

20. Tearfulness
0 = not present
1 = present
2 = present and accompanied by clear affective component
3 = present and accompanied by affective and physical component (e.g. 'wrings hands' or other gestures)

21. Depressed mood: other
0 = not present
1 = present (e.g. occasional statement 'I wish I were dead', without clear affective concomitants)
2 = present with clear concomitants (e.g. thoughts of death)
3 = present with emotional and physical component (e.g. suicide gestures)
Unspecified?
Describe

g. Anxieties and phobias

22. Anxiety regarding upcoming events (Godot syndrome)
0 = not present
1 = present: repeated queries and/or other activities regarding upcoming appointments and/or events
2 = present and disturbing to caregivers
3 = present and intolerable to caregivers

23. Other anxieties
0 = not present
1 = present
2 = present and disturbing to caregivers
3 = present and intolerable to caregivers
Unspecified?
Describe

Fig. 2.2 Continued

24. Fear of being left alone
 0 = not present
 1 = present: vocalized fear of being alone
 2 = vocalized and sufficient to require specific action
   on part of caregiver
 3 = vocalized and sufficient to require patient to be
   accompanied at all times
25. Other phobias
 0 = not present
 1 = present
 2 = present and of sufficient magnitude to require
   specific action on part of caregiver
 3 = present and sufficient to prevent patient
   activities
Unspecified?
Describe

Part 2: Global rating

With respect to the above symptoms, they are of sufficient magnitude as to be:
 0 = not at all troubling to the caregiver or dangerous
   to the patient
 1 = mildly troubling to the caregive or dangerous to
   the patient
 2 = moderately troubling to the caregiver or
   dangerous to the patient
 3 = severely troubling or intolerable to the caregiver
   or dangerous to the patient

Fig. 2.2 BEHAVE-AD. Source: Reisberg *et al.* (1987).
(By Permission Resiberg B, Auer S.R. and Monteiro I.M. (1996) Behavioural Pathology in
Alzheimer's disease rating scale (BEHAV-AD). In International Psychogeriatrics **8** (supp. 2)
169–180)

Although all of these scales have achieved excellent inter-rater reliability, these
reliability evaluations have been undertaken for raters who have been through a
formal training procedure. It is therefore very important that these training
procedures are followed for any centre wishing to use these instruments, as inter-
rater reliability cannot be assumed in different settings. This is facilitated for the
NPI by the availability of an educational pack and training video.

There are several other summary scales such as the Alzheimer Assessment Scale
non-cognitive portion, the Caretaker Obstreperous Behaviour Rating Assessment
(Drachman *et al.* 1992), the Gottfries–Brane–Steen Scale (Gottfries *et al.* 1982)
and the Clifton Assessment Procedure for the Elderly (Pattie 1981). Some of these
have the advantage of combining some evaluation of activities of daily living
(ADL) and cognition with an assessment of BPSD. However, purely as a measure
of BPSD, none of these scales is as comprehensive as the NPI, BEHAV-AD or
BRSD, and the recommendation of the authors would be to use one of these three
scales in combination with separate instruments for ADL and cognition.

Code

Has {S} *said* that {S} feels anxious, worried, tense or fearful? (For example, has   A
{S} expressed worry or fear about being left alone? Has {S} said {S} is anxious or
afraid of certain situations?) If so, describe.

Has {S} shown *physical signs* of anxiety, worry, tension, or fear? (For example, is   A
{S} easily startled?
Does {S} appear nervous? Does {S} have a tense or worried facial expression?) If
so, describe.

Has {S} appeared sad or 'blue' or depressed?   A
Has {S} expressed feelings of hopelessness or pessimism?   A
Has {S} cried within the past month?   A
Has {S} said that {S} feels guilty? (For example, has {S} blamed {S's} self for   A
things {S} did in the past?) If yes, describe nature and extent of guilt.

Has {S} expressed feelings of poof self-esteem? For example, has {S} said that {S}   A
feels like a failure or that {S} feels worthless? *This item is intended to reflect global
loss of self-esteem rather than simply a concern over loss of, for example, a particular
ability.*

Has {S} said {S} feels life is not worth living? Or has {S} expressed a wish to die or   A
done something that suggested {S} was considering suicide? If yes, specify what {S}
said or did.

If yes or a rating of 8, ask: Has {S} ever made a suicide attempt? *Include any suicidal* (0) no
gestures in rating this probe.

(1) yes
(9) n/a

Have there been times when {S} doesn't enjoy the things {S} does as much as {S}   B
used to before {S's} dementia began? This item refers to any specific loss of enjoyment so long as {S} actually engages in the activity in question. {S} need not be an
active participant in this activity; {S} need only be present.

Do you find {S} sometimes can't seem to get started on things {S} used to do before   B
{S's} dementia began, even though {S} is capable of doing them? (For example, do
you find {S} won't start a task or pastime on {S's} own, but with a little encourage-
ment {S} goes ahead and carries it out?) *This item refers to any failure to initiate
activities, so long as the activities are those which {S} is still capable of carrying out
when given the opportunity.*

Has {S} seemed tired or lacking in energy   A
Was {S's} sleeping pattern in the past month different from the way it was before   B
{S's} dementia began? (For example, does {S} sleep more or less than {S} used to?
Does {S} sleep at a different time of day than {S} used to?). If yes, describe change.

Has {S} had difficulty falling asleep or remaining asleep? If yes, describe.   A
Has {S's} appetite during the past month changed from the way it was before {S's}   B
dementia began? (For example, at meal times does {S's} desire to eat seem different?) (1) increased
'Appetite' refers to {S's} response to food when it is presented in the usual manner. (2) decreased
If yes, circle either increased or decreased appetite, according to informant's
judgment.

In the past month, has {S} gained or lost weight without intending to?   B
If yes, circle amount gained or lost. gained up to 5 lbs
gained more than 5 lbs
lost up to 5 lbs
lost more than 5 lbs

Has {S} had physical complaints that seemed out of proportion to {S's} actual   A
physical problems?
In the past month, has {S's} sexual interest been different from the way it was before   B
{S's} dementia began? If yes, describe.
Has {S} shown sudden changes in {S's} emotions? (For example does {S} go from   A
laughter to tears quickly?)
Have there been times when {S} was agitated or upset? *This item refers to <u>observable</u>*   A
*signs of emotional distress, such as verbal comments, facial expressions or gestures. It
is the <u>emotional</u> components that distinguish this item from item 24.*
Have there been times when {S} was easily irritated or annoyed?   A

Fig. 2.3 Continued

Code

Has {S} been uncooperative? (For example, does {S} refuse to accept appropriate   A
help? Does {S} insist on doing things {S's} own way?)

Has {S} been threatening or verbally abusive towards others?   A

Has {S} been physically aggressive towards people or things? (For example, has   A
{S} shoved or physically attacked people or thrown or broken objecs?)

Has {S} seemed restless or overactive? (For example does {S} fidget or pace? Does   A
{S} finger things or seem unable to sit still?) *When the overactive behaviour is
associated with emotional agitation that is rated in item 19, it should not be rated
here also.*

Has {S} done things that seem to have no clear purpose or a confused purpose?   A
(For example, does {S} open and close drawers? Does {S} put things in
inappropriate places? Does {S} hoard things or rummage through things?) *If {S's}
bevaiour shows a high level of motor activity rather than confusion or lack or purpose,
it should be rated under item 24.*

Has there been a particular time of day during which {S} seemed more confused   B
than at other times?   (1) daytime
  (2) evening (6.00 pm
to bedtime)
  (3) night

Has {S} wandered or tried to wander for no apparent reason? *'Wandering' includes*   A
wandering away from one's residence or caregiver, as well as within the residence. If yes,
describe incidents.

Has {S} tried to leave home or get away from whoever was taking care of {S} with   A
an apparent purpose or destination in mind? If yes, describe incidents.

Has {S} done socially inappropriate things? (For example, does {S} make vulgar   A
remarks? Does {S} talk excessively to strangers? Has {S} sexually exposed {S's} self
or done other things such as making gestures of touching people inappropriately?)
*This item is intended to reflect a loss of propriety, not simply confusion. If inappropriate
behaviour can be rated under a more specific item, such as abusive behaviour (item 22)
or aggressive behaviour (item 23), it should not be rated here.*

Does {S} tend to say the same things repeatedly? *This item refers to repetitive*   A
statements, including questions, phrases, demands, etc.

Does {S} withdraw from social situations? (For example, does {S} avoid groups of   A
people or prefer to be alone? Does {S} avoid participating in activities with others?)

Does {S} seek out more visual or physical contact? Does {S} follow you about and   B
seem to want to be in the same room with you?)

Has {S} misidentified people? (For example, has {S} confused one familiar person   A
with another, or has {S} thought that a familiar person was a stranger?) *'Misidentification' means an actual belief that one person was another, not simply a
misnaming or failure to remember who someone is, and it refers to someone actually
seen by {S}.*

Has {S} looked at {S's}-self in a mirror and not recognised {S's}-self?   A

Has {S} misidentified things? Has {S} though common things were something else?   A
(For example, has {S} said that a pillow was a person or that a light bulb was a
fire?) If yes, describe.

Has {S} done or said anything that suggests {S} believes people are harming,
threatening or taking advantage of {S} in some way? (For example, with no good
reason has {S} thought things have been given away or stolen; has {S} thought {S}
was mischarged or over charged for purchase; has {S} seemed suspicious or wary?)   A
If yes, ask: if you try to correct {S}, will {S} accept the truth?   (1) yes
  (2) no
  (9) n/a

Has {S} done or said anything that suggests {S} thinks {S's} spouse is unfaithful?   A
If yes, ask: If you try to correct {S}, will {S} accept the truth?   (1) yes
  (2) no
  (9) n/a

Fig. 2.3 Continued

	Code
Has {S} done or said anything that suggests {S} thinks {S's} spouse or caregiver is plotting to abandon {S}?	A
If yes, ask: If you try to correct {S}, will {S} accept the truth?	(1) yes
	(2) no
	(9) n/a
Has {S} done or said anything that suggests {S} thinks {S's} spouse or caregiver is an impostor?	A
If yes, ask: If you try to correct {S}, will {S} accept the truth?	(1) yes
	(2) no
	(9) n/a
Has {S} done or said anything that suggests {S} thinks that characters on television are real? (For example, has {S} talked to them, acted as if they could hear or see {S} or said that they were friends or neighbours?)	A
If yes, ask: If you try to corect {S}, will {S} accept the truth?	(1) yes
	(2) no
	(9) n/a
Has {S} done or said anything that suggest {S} believes that there are people in or around the house beyond those who are actually there?	A
If yes, ask: If you try to correct {S}, will {S} accept the truth?	(1) yes
	(2) no
	(9) n/a
Has {S} done or said anything that suggests {S} believes that a dead person is still alive, even though {S} used to know they were dead? *Do not rate memory problems. If {S} simply cannot remember whether a particular person has died, it should not be rated a mistaken belief.*	A
If yes, ask: If you try to correct {S}, will {S} accept the truth?	(1) yes
	(2) no
	(9) n/a
Has {S} done or said anything that suggests {S} thinks where {S} lives is not really {S's} home, even though {S} used to consider it home?	A
If yes, ask: If you try to correct {S}, will {S} accept the truth?	(1) yes
	(2) no
	(9) n/a
Has {S} heard voices or sounds when there was no sound? If yes, describe.	A
If yes, rate for clarity.	vague, 0; clear, 1
Has {S} seen things or people that were not there? If yes, describe.	A
If yes, rate for clarity.	vague, 0; clear, 1
Before we stop, I want to be sure we've covered all of {S's} problems, except, of course, for those related to memory loss. Has {S} done anything else in the past month that seemed strange or created difficulties? Has {S} said anything that suggests {S} have some unusual ideas or beliefs that I haven't asked you about? *If response concerns purely cognitive symptoms, do not rate. If response contains behaviours that can be rated under other items, do so. Any behaviour that is rated here should be described. Indicate the most frequently occurring problem and rate it.*	A

Fig. 2.3 CERAD Behavioural Rating Scale. {S} is the subject. **Code A**: 0, has not occurred since illness began; 1, has occurred on 1–2 days in past month; 2, has occurred on 3–8 days in past month (up to twice per week); 3, has occurred on 9–15 days in past month; 4, has occurred on 16 days or more in past month; 8, has occurred since illness began, but not in past month; 9, unable to rate. **Code B:** 0, has not occurred since illness began; 1, has occurred in past month; 8, has occurred since illness began, but not in the past month; 9, unable to rate. Source: Tariot *et al.* (1995). (By Permission Tariot P.N., Mack J.L., Patterson M.B., *et al.* (1995) The Behavior Rating Scale for Dementia for the Consortium to Establish a Registry for Alzheimer's Disease (CERAD). In American Journal of Psychiatry **152** 1349–59) The Behaviour Rating Scale for Dementia for the Consortium to Establish a Registry for Alzheimer's Disease (CERAD). Tariot P. N., Mack J. L., Patterson M. B., Edland S. D., Weiner M. F., Fillenbaum G., Blazina L., Terri L., Rubin E., Mortimer J., and Stern Y. *American Journal of Psychiatry* (1995) **152**, 1349–1359. Reprinted with permission.

REFERENCES

Alexopoulos, G. S., Abrams, R. C., Young, R. C. and Shamoian, C. A. (1988). Cornell Scale for Depression in Dementia. *Biological Psychiatry*, **23**, 271–84.

Allen, N. H. P., Gordon, S., Hope, T. and Burns, A. (1996). Manchester and Oxford Universities Scale for the Psychopathological Assessment of Dementia. *British Journal of Psychiatry*, **169**, 293–307.

Ballard, C. G. and Oyebode, F. (1995). Psychotic symptoms in patients with dementia. *International Journal of Geriatric Psychiatry*, **10**, 743–752.

Ballard, C. G., Mohan, R., Handy, S., Bannister, C. and Todd, N. (1991). Information reliability in dementia sufferers. *International Journal of Geriatric Psychiatry*, **6**, 313–16.

Ballard, C. G., Harrison, R., Lowery, K. and McKeith, I. (1996a). Non-cognitive symptoms in Lewy body dementia. In *Dementia with Lewy Bodies* (Perry, R. H, McKeith, I. G. Perry, E. K., eds), pp. 000–000. Cambridge University Press, Cambridge.

Ballard, C. G., Patel, A., Solis, M., Lowe, K. and Wilcock, G. (1996b). A one year follow up study of depression in dementia sufferers. *British Journal of Psychiatry*, **68**, 287–91.

Burke, W. J., Houston, M. J., Poust, S. T. and Roccaforte, W. H. (1989). Use of the Geriatric Depression Scale in dementia of the Alzheimer type. *Journal of the American Geriatrics Society*, **37**, 856–60.

Cummings, J. L. (1997). The Neuropsychiatric Inventory: assessing psychopathology in dementia patients. *Neurology*, **48** (Suppl. 6), s10–s16.

Cummings, J. L., Mega, M., Gray, K., Rosenberg-Thomspon, S. and Gombien, T. (1994). The Neuropsychiatric Inventory: comprehensive assessment of psychopathology in dementia. *Neurology*, **44**, 2308–14.

Drachman, D. S., Swearer, J. M., O'Donnell, B F., Mitchell, A.L. and Maloon, A. (1992). The Caretaker Obstreperous Behavior Rating Assessment (COBRA) scale. *Journal of the American Geriatrics Society*, **40**, 463–80.

Gottfries, C. G., Braine, G., Guilberg, B. and Steen, G. (1982). A new rating scale for dementia symptoms. *Archives of Gerontology and Geriatrics*, **1**, 311–30.

Hope, T. and Fairburn, C. G. (1992). The Present Behavioural Examination (PBE): the development of an interview to measure current behavioural abnormalities. *Psychological Medicine*, **22**, 223–30.

Kaufer, D. I., Cummings, J. L., Christine, D., Bray, T., Castellon, S., Masterman, D., MacMillan, A., Ketchel, P. and Dekosky, S. T. (1998) Assessing the impact of neuropsychiatric symptoms in Alzheimer's disease: the Neuropsychiatric Inventory Caregiver Distress Scale. *Journal of the American Geriatrics Society*, **46**, 210–15.

Levin, H. S., High, W. M., Goethe, K. E., Sisson, R. A. and Overall, T. E. (1987). The Neuro-Behavioral Rating Scale: assessment of sequalae of head injury by the clinician. *Journal of Neurology, Neurosurgery and Psychiatry*, **50**, 183–93.

Lichtenberg, P. A., Steiner, D. A., Marcopulos, B. A. and Tabscott, J. A. (1992). Comparison of the Hamilton Depression Rating Scale and the Geriatric Depression Scale: detection of depression in dementia patients. *Psychological Reports*, **70**, 515–21.

Patterson, M. B., Schnell, M. H., Martin, R. J., Mendez, M. F. and Smyth, K. A. (1990). Assessment of behavioral and affective symptoms in Alzheimer's disease. *Journal of Geriatric Psychiatry and Neurology*, **3**, 21–30.

Pattie, A. H. (1981). A survey version of the Clifton Assessment Procedures for the Elderly (CAPE). *British Journal of Clinical Psychology*, **20**, 173–8.

Reisberg, B., Auer, S. R. and Monteiro, I. M. (1996). Behavioural Pathology in Alzheimer's disease (BEHAV-AD) rating scale. *International Psychogeriatrics*, **8** (Suppl. 2), 169–80.

Reisberg, B., Borenstein, J., Salob, S. P., Ferris, S. H., Franssen, E. and Georgotas, A. (1987). Behavioral symptoms in Alzheimer's disease: phenomenology and treatment. *Journal of Clinical Psychiatry*, **48** (Suppl. 5), 9–15.

Scian, S. G., Saillon, A., Franssen, E., Hugonot-Diener, L. and Saillon, A. (1996). The Behavioral Pathology in Alzheimer's Disease Rating Scale (BEHAV-AD): reliability and analysis of symptom category scores. *International Journal of Geriatric Psychiatry*, **11**, 819–30.

Tariot, P. N., Mack, J. L., Patterson, M. B., Edland, S. D., Weiner, M. F., Fillenbaum, G., Blazina, L., Terri, L., Rubin, E., Mortimer, J. and Stern, Y. (1995). The Behavior Rating Scale for Dementia of the Consortium to Establish a Registry for Alzheimer's Disease. *American Journal of Psychiatry*, **152**, 1349–57.

Winblad, B., Ballard, C. and O'Brien, J. (2000). Clinical trials in Alzheimer's disease. *Science Press*. In press.

3 Psychosis in dementia

Introduction

The current chapter covers the definition and measurement of psychotic symptoms in the context of dementia and the impact upon dementia sufferers and their caregivers. The frequency, natural course and associations of psychosis are described. A summary of the main points is given at the end of the chapter. The text deals with the occurrence of psychotic symptoms in the common late-onset dementias, Alzheimer's disease (AD), vascular dementia (VaD) and dementia with Lewy bodies (DLB). Issues relating to psychosis arising in people with pre-senile dementia, or other specific conditions such as Pick's disease and Huntington's chorea are not discussed, largely because there is so little literature covering these areas.

The objective of the current chapter is to give a detailed background and understanding of the nature of psychosis in people with dementia, to aid consideration of management approaches.

Classification of psychosis

Within the context of dementia, Burns *et al.* (1990) classified psychosis into three main categories: delusions, hallucinations and delusional misidentification. Delusions were defined as false, unshakable ideas or beliefs that are held with extraordinary conviction and subjective certainty. They also had to be reiterated on at least two occasions more than 1 week apart; this latter stipulation was designed to minimize overlap with confabulation and delirium. Hallucinations were described as precepts in the absence of a stimulus, and had to be directly reported either by the patient or indirectly via an informant to be classified as a psychotic presentation (i.e. they could not be inferred from observed behaviours). Delusional misidentification included:

- Capgras syndrome (the belief that a person, object or environment has been replaced by a double or replica);
- delusional misidentification of visual images (whereby figures on television or in photographs are thought to exist in the real environment);

- delusional misidentification of mirror images (one's reflection is perceived as the image of a separate person); and
- the phantom boarder delusion (believing that strangers are living in, or visiting the house).

This theoretical classification system is supported by empirical evidence from a principal components analysis of a detailed list of individual symptoms (Ballard *et al.* 1995b).

Although, broadly speaking, hallucinations, delusions and delusional mis-identification also occur in functional psychoses, there are important differences. Two of the predominant forms of delusional misidentification in dementia, mis-identification of mirror images and misidentification of television images, are, for example, exclusively seen in organic disorders. In addition, the most common forms of hallucinations are visual, in contrast to functional psychosis where auditory hallucinations predominate. Diagnosing delusions in the presence of dementia can also be difficult. The majority of delusional beliefs are simple, and the types of complex elaborate delusional symptom seen in functional psychosis are extremely rare and are confined to a small number of people in the early stages of the dementia process (Burns *et al.* 1990). The crux of the issue is to be able to distinguish people who make confabulations or assumptions which can be entirely explained as a result of impairments in higher cognitive functions, from those who are experiencing delu-sions. For example, does a person who does not remember leaving a handbag else-where, and suggests that someone may have stolen it, have a delusion? This is where the standard operationalized definition of a delusion, and the additions made by Burns *et al.* (1990), are particularly helpful. A delusion has to be an unshakeable belief; hence, in the example given, if an alternative explanation is put to the person that they may have forgotten their handbag and they accept this as a plausible expla-nation, they are not experiencing a delusion. The additional stipulation by Burns *et al.*, that a delusion must be repeated, is helpful in distinguishing delusions from confabulation. In the example given, if a person had made a one-off suggestion that a handbag had been stolen, even if held with conviction this would be a confabula-tion. If similar beliefs were reiterated over a period of time, they would be delusional.

Psychotic beliefs are usually simple and it is rare for them to be incorporated into a delusional system. The most common individual symptoms are delusions of reference (the belief that other people are talking about the person), delusions of theft or possessions being hidden, and the phantom boarder delusion. Visual hallu-cinations are also common. Figure 3.1 displays the prevalence of individual symptoms in a cohort of people with dementia.

The majority of people with dementia experiencing psychotic symptoms have more than one symptom concurrently, with more than half experiencing symptoms more than once a week and a quarter experiencing them on a daily basis. This is shown in Fig. 3.2. The more frequent the symptoms, the more likely people are to

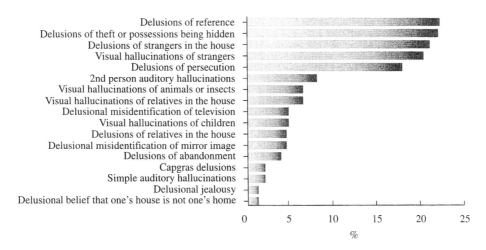

Symptoms occurring in 1 patient – delusion of partition, delusion of sexual interference, auditory hallucination of a relative, Fregoli syndrome, olfactory hallucination, erotomania, musical hallucination, visual hallucination of a complex scene, misidentification of an object and 3rd person auditory hallucination.

Fig. 3.1 Rank order of psychotic symptoms (per cent prevalence for whole sample displayed). From Ballard *et al.* (1995b). © John Wiley & Sons Limited. Reproduced with permission.

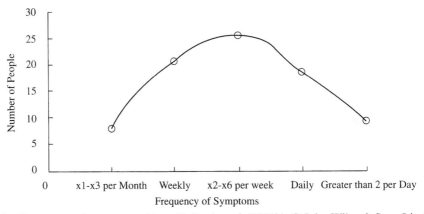

Fig. 3.2 Frequency of symptoms. From Ballard *et al.* (1995b). © John Wiley & Sons Limited. Reproduced with permission.

be distressed by them, and the less likely they are to have any insight into their psychotic nature (Ballard *et al.* 1995b).

Assessment tools

As it can be difficult to identify psychotic symptoms, and as informants tend to under-report individual symptoms from a general question, a standardized informant interview can be helpful. This is well illustrated in the research literature, where the frequency of identified psychotic symptoms is doubled in studies using structured assessment methods (Ballard 1995b). Many of these tools are brief and suitable for use in clinical practice by a range of healthcare professionals. The schedules available include the BEHAVE-AD (Reisberg *et al.* 1987), the CUSPAD (Devanand *et al.* 1992), the Burns' symptom checklist (Ballard *et al.* 1995b), the MOUSEPAD (Allen *et al.* 1996), the PBE (Hope and Fairburn *et al.* 1992) and the NPI (Cummings *et al.* 1994). The BEHAVE-AD and the NPI are widely used and well validated, with the NPI having the advantage of a more comprehensive list of psychotic symptoms, together with a section rating carer distress. Both schedules collate information regarding other behavioural disturbances. The 59-item MOUSEPAD (Allen *et al.* 1996) assesses the psychopathological and behavioural changes associated with dementia, in a more comprehensive schedule, but takes longer to administer and has been less widely used. Other studies have utilized operationalized diagnostic criteria such as those of Burns *et al.* (1990), DSM IIIR or DSM IV, either as the main evaluation tool or in combination with a standardized schedule. The latter is the preferable method as it facilitates comprehensive symptom detection and evaluation, whilst minimizing false-positive diagnoses. The BEHAV-AD and NPI each take 15–20 min to administer. Rating scales for BPSD are discussed in more detail in Chapter 2.

Impact of psychosis

Psychotic symptoms in dementia can be unpleasant for the sufferers, with a third of people experiencing these symptoms feeling marked distress (Gilley *et al.* 1991, Ballard *et al.* 1995b). Distress tends to occur in the people with the greatest number of different symptoms, who are experiencing them on at least a daily basis (Ballard *et al.* 1995b). In addition, psychoses are amongst the symptoms that carers find most problematic (Rabins *et al.* 1982), and there is some evidence to suggest a possible association with psychiatric morbidity amongst caregivers (Donaldson *et al.* 1998). To compound the situation further, psychosis often occurs in conjunction with behavioural disturbances such as aggression or agitation (Rockwell *et al.* 1994). It is therefore not surprising that a number of studies (Steele *et al.* 1990, Haupt *et al.* 1996) have reported an association between psychotic symptoms and admission to residential or nursing home care.

Dementia patients with psychosis, particularly those experiencing visual hallucinations, have a two- to three-fold accelerated rate of cognitive decline (Drevets and Rubin 1989, Rosen and Zubenko 1991, Förstl *et al.* 1993, Chui *et al.* 1994). Further work needs to determine whether psychotic symptoms are indicative of a more virulent dementia process, whether they have a direct action upon the rate of decline or whether the course of the illness is detrimentally influenced iatrogenically with antipsychotic prescriptions (McShane *et al.* 1997).

Prevalence, incidence and natural course of psychotic symptoms

Alzheimer's disease

Prevalence

The current review only incorporates data from prospective studies utilizing standardized methodology. Table 3.1 indicates the cross-sectional prevalence rates of psychosis in a variety of settings with a mean prevalence of 44% in clinical samples (hallucinations: overall, 21%; auditory, 7%; visual, 14%; delusions, 32%; delusional misidentification, 30%). People in research samples had lower overall prevalence of psychosis (mean 37%), possibly explained by selection biases, with research cohorts including younger, less impaired patients. The mean prevalence of psychosis in community studies is 23% (Gilley et al. 1991, Skoog 1993, Hope et al. 1997), indicating that the presence of psychotic symptoms may increase the likelihood of referral to specialist services. There is a paucity of reports from nursing homes (Rovner et al. 1986, Chandler and Chandler 1988, Morriss et al. 1990, Cohen et al. 1998, Ballard et al. 1999), a particular problem given the large number of dementia patients cared for in these environments. This gap in our knowledge is rather paradoxical given that psychosis is a common precipitant of admission to residential or nursing home care. The two largest studies suggest that psychosis is seen in more than a quarter of these residents.

Over the course of the illness, the cumulative prevalence of psychosis is much higher, probably exceeding 80% (Allen and Burns 1995, Ballard et al. 1997).

Incidence and resolution

Knowledge regarding the natural course of psychosis in AD is important, but has been a rather neglected area. Annual incidence rates for psychosis range from 1% to 5% (Liston 1979, Cummings et al. 1987, Burns et al. 1990, Chen et al. 1991, Flynn et al. 1991, Jeste et al. 1992), in the initial studies conducted in the late 1980s and early 1990s, whereas in a more recent report the annual incidence was 46% (Ballard et al. 1997). The diversity probably reflects the different methodologies adopted within individual studies. For example, although all studies used a standardized assessment at baseline, most used case-note review to provide follow-up details (Cummings et al. 1987, Burns et al. 1990). At the other extreme, Ballard et al. (1997) conducted monthly interviews for 1 year. Fewer studies have investigated the annual incidence of delusions (range 30–47%) or hallucinations (range 10–20%), although the findings are more consistent (McShane et al. 1995, 1996, Ballard et al. 1997, 1998).

Ballard et al. (1997, 1998b) and McShane et al. (1995) reported annual resolution rates of 43% and 65%, respectively, with approximately 50% of symptoms spontaneously resolving over 3 months, an observation consistent with the extremely high

Table 3.1 Prevalence of psychotic symptoms in dementia sufferers: a summary of standardized studies

Study and year	N	Diagnosis	Associations reported	Prevalence (%)					
				delusion	hallucination	auditory hallucination	visual hallucination	general psychosis	delusional misidentification
(a) Hospital settings									
Hirono et al. (1998)*	228	AD		52	11	6	3	52	
Gilley et al. (1997)*	270	AD		47	41				
Ballard et al. (1995b)	124	AD, DLB, VaD		48		13	35	67	29 (36)
Binetti et al. (1995)	99	AD, VaD		24					11
Burns et al. (1990)	178	AD		16		10	13		
Cooper et al. (1990)*	677	AD		26	17				
Devanand et al. (1992)	91	AD				1	4		
Sultzer et al. (1993)	56	AD, VaD						36	
Ballard et al. (1991)	66	AD		29	22				
Ballinger et al. (1982)**	100				34				
Jost et al. (1997)*	100	AD						45	
Ballard et al. (1997)	87							47	
Mega et al. (1996)*	50	AD		22	10	4	14		
Haupt et al. (1996)	78	AD		33	15	4	20		
Cummings et al. (1987)	45	AD, VaD		33	16				
Mortimer et al. (1992)*	65	AD		28					
Holroyd and Sheldon-Keller et al. (1995)	98	AD					18		
Jeste et al. (1992)	107	AD		35		1.9	12		
Flynn et al. (1991)	33	AD, VaD						69	
McShane et al. (1995)	41	AD					32		
Migliorelli et al. (1995)	103	AD						37	
Förstl et al. (1994)	56			16	23	13	18		
Chui et al. (1994)	135	AD		12	13				25
mean				31 (n = 686)	21 (n = 371)	9 (n = 62)	14 (n = 144)	44 (n = 167)	30 (n = 97)
(b) Nursing homes									
Morriss et al. (1990)	84	AD and VaD		35				39	
Rovner et al. (1986)	50	AD and VaD						13	
Chandler and Chandler (1988)	65	AD and VaD							
mean				35 (n = 29)				24 (n = 28)	

(c) Community

	n		mean					
Hope et al. (1997)	97	AD and VaD					37	
Skoog (1993)	147	AD and VaD					14	
Gilley et al. (1991)	230	AD	5	29	17	19		11
mean			5 (n = 8)	29 (n = 67)	19 (n = 39)	19 (n = 44)	23 (n = 57)	11 (n = 26)

(d) Research clinics

	n							
Lopez et al. (1996)*	40	AD	33		5	15	43	
Drevets and Rubin (1989)	82	AD					27	34
Förstl et al. (1993)	50	AD	43	34	16	32		30
Deutsch et al. (1991)*	181	AD	44	24	10	19		
Rosen and Zubenko (1991)	32	AD	34	31	16	22	47	
Patterson et al. (1990)	34	AD	38	18	6	15		
Lopez et al. (1991)*	113	AD	71	76	24	53	15	
Rubin et al. (1988)*	110	AD		25	10	15	56	23
Zubenko et al. (1991)	27	AD					48	
mean			49 (n = 219)	39 (n = 190)	13 (n = 73)	26 (n = 145)	36 (n = 146)	28 (n = 96)

AD, Alzheimer's disease; DLB, dementia with Lewy bodies; VaD, vascular dementia.

*presented summary data from Ballard & Walker (2000)

**presented summary data from Ballard & Oyebode (1995)

(Ballard C, Gray, Ayre. Revue Neurologique (Paris) 1999 and © Masson Editeur) placebo response rates in treatment studies (Ballard & O'Brian 1999). The people at greatest risk of psychoses lasting for >3 months were those who had already experienced ≥3 months of psychotic symptoms at the time of the baseline assessment (Ballard *et al.* 1997). Conversely, an earlier study (Rosen and Zubenko 1991) suggested that only 2% of dementia patients recovered from their psychosis each year. Clearly, further work is needed to inform planning and management decisions.

The consistency of symptom profiles over time is also important. Haupt *et al.* (1996) illustrated, with a short but very detailed follow-up study, that the profile of psychotic symptoms remained consistent over a period of 3 weeks. There have been few longer-term studies, although McShane *et al.* (1997) suggested that there were two longitudinal syndromes. In their report, patients who initially had symptoms of sadness developed aggression later on in the dementia, whereas those who experienced persecutory ideas tended to become restless in the later stages of follow up. It is an interesting notion that, at a later stage of the dementia when people have more severe cognitive impairments, some of the symptoms they experience may be 'behavioural correlates' of psychiatric syndromes. This needs to be examined in further studies but may have important implications for treatment.

Clinical associations

Putative clinical associations of psychosis in AD have been considered in >20 standardized studies. Positive associations have been reported with female gender (four studies), male gender (one study), extrapyramidal symptoms (three studies), older age (seven studies), later onset of dementia (three studies), more severe cognitive impairment (five studies) and greater duration of illness (three studies), although none of these variables have been identified as significant associations in >50% of studies (Table 3.2 shows the studies that have examined clinical associations).

The association with more severe cognitive impairment has been more robust for visual hallucinations than for delusions or psychosis overall. Studies that have examined the relationship between the severity of cognitive impairments and psychosis using a categorical approach have perhaps thrown a little more light on the subject. Whilst both visual hallucinations and delusions are relatively uncommon amongst people with mild AD (Ballard *et al.* 1991, 1999, Jeste *et al.* 1992), the prevalence of delusions appears to peak in people with AD of moderate severity, whereas visual hallucinations are even more prevalent amongst those with severe dementia. This perhaps indicates that a certain level of cognitive processing may be necessary in order to generate a delusional belief.

Perhaps most importantly, impaired visual acuity has been identified as a consistent association of visual hallucinations (Ballard *et al.* 1995a, Holroyd 1995, McShane *et al.* 1995, Chapman *et al.* 1999), with a positive relationship demonstrated in all of the studies. The report of Chapman *et al.* (1999) indicates that none of the individuals with normal visual acuity experienced visual hallucinations, and provided some anecdotal evidence that referral to an optician was associated with improvement. In addition, it appeared that cataracts were the most important indi-

Table 3.2 Prevalence of psychotic symptoms in Alzheimer's disease

	Study and year	Setting	N	Diagnosis (probable)	Positive psychotic associations reported
1	Hirono et al. (1998)*	hospital	228	AD	✓
2	Gilley et al. (1997)*	out-patients	270	AD	✓
3	Ballard et al. (1995a)	hospital	124	AD and DLB	✓
4	Binetti et al.(1995)	hospital	99	AD and VaD	✓
5	Burns et al. (1990)	hospital	178	AD	✓
7	Cooper et al. (1991)*	hospital	677	AD	✓
8	Devanand et al. (1992)	hospital	91	AD	✓
15	Haupt et al. (1996)	out-patients	78	AD	✓
16	Cummings et al. (1987)	out-patients	45	AD and VaD	✓
17	Mortimer et al. (1992)*	out-patients	65	AD	✓
18	Holroyd and Sheldon-Keller et al. (1995)	out-patients	98	AD	✓
19	Jeste et al. (1992)	out-patients	107	AD	✓
20	Flynn et al. (1991)	out-patients	33	AD and VaD	✓
21	McShane et al. (1995)	clinic	41	AD	✓
22	Migliorelli et al. (1995)*	clinic	103	AD	✓
24	Chui et al. (1994)	clinic	135	AD	✓
29	Skoog (1993)	community	147	AD and VaD	✓
30	Gilley (1991)	community	230	AD	✓
32	Drevets and Rubin (1989)	research	82	AD	✓
33	Förstl et al. (1993)	research	50	AD	✓
35	Rosen and Rubenko (1991)	research	32	AD	✓
36	Patterson et al. (1990)*	research	34	AD	✓
37	Lopez et al. (1991)*	research	113	AD	✓

AD, Alzheimer's disease; DLB, dementia with Lewy bodies; VaD, vascular dementia.

* presented data from Ballard & Walker (1999)

vidual eye pathology. The association is particularly convincing given the presence of a similar relationship between visual hallucinations and impaired visual acuity amongst elderly people without cognitive impairment in Charles–Bonnet syndrome (Teunisse et al. 1996). There is also preliminary evidence to suggest a possible relationship between the severity of visuospatial impairments on cognitive testing and the occurrence of visual hallucinations (Ayre et al. 2000, Ballard et al. 1999). Although this requires further study, it suggests the possibility that impairments at a variety of levels of the visual pathway may predispose to visual hallucinations in people with dementia.

No robust clinical associations of delusions or delusional misidentification have been identified. Ballard et al. (1995a) suggested that delusions may be linked to deafness in dementia sufferers, but this has not been investigated by other groups.

Biological and experimental correlates of psychosis

Work in this area is still at a very preliminary stage. Several groups have reported that calcification of basal ganglia may be important in the genesis of delusions in some patients (Burns *et al.* 1990), possibly through 'deficient sensory gating' mechanisms. Zubenko *et al.* (1991) reported a link between psychotic symptoms and a reduction of 5-hydroxytryptamine, with relative preservation of norepinephrine, but did not identify any associations with dopaminergic parameters. Förstl *et al.* (1994) suggested that patients with delusional misidentification and those with hallucinations had significantly more neurons in the parahippocampal gyrus, but fewer in the dorsal Raphé nucleus, whilst patients presenting with delusions had fewer neurons in the hippocampus (CA1). Parallel studies investigating visual hallucinations in DLB have indicated an association with cholinergic loss and relative preservation of 5-hydroxytryptamine in the temporal cortex (Perry *et al.* 1993), particularly in the visual association areas. Neuroimaging studies using CT (Binetti *et al.* 1995) and SPECT (Kotrla *et al.* 1995) techniques have reported that increased atrophy or reduced blood flow of the frontal lobe areas might be important in patients with delusions. A further study did not find any link between plasma homovanillic acid and psychotic features (Sweet *et al.* 1997), although the same group did identify a weak but significant link between psychosis and a D3 receptor polymorphism (Sweet *et al.* 1998).

Animal work has indicated that occlusion of visual fields results in spontaneous firing of neurons in the visual association areas (Recanzone *et al.* 1992). Although there is no parallel human work, taken in conjunction with the work of Perry *et al.* (1993) demonstrating a relationship between visual hallucinations and cholinergic deficits in visual association areas, this is consistent with the hypothesis stated previously that insults at a variety of levels of the visual system may precipitate visual hallucinations and suggests possible mechanisms.

Gray (1982) has proposed a 'comparator' model to explain the occurrence of psychosis in schizophrenia, arguing that the hippocampus plays a key role in the system. Gray suggests that the 'comparator' continually monitors sensory data from the outside world and compares this with expected perceptual configurations. If discrepancies are identified, a control process then alters the internal working model of the world to accommodate the mismatches. Amongst dementia sufferers, particularly if they also have sensory impairments, this comparator function is put under particularly severe stress, trying to maintain a temporally correct representation of the outside world. This model provides a theoretical role for the hippocampus in the geneses of delusions. A number of psychological assessment paradigms have been utilized to study some of the functions of this comparator system in schizophrenia, and to evaluate related constricts such as a 'jump-to-conclusions style of thinking'. Although these paradigms would be too complex to transfer directly to the study of psychosis in dementia, development of the simpler tests to assess these psychological processes may give us a better understanding of the psychological constricts underlying delusional thinking in the context of dementia.

The literature is very inconsistent. It does appear, however, that delusions and hallucinations may have a different biological basis. In addition, there is no direct evidence supporting a link between psychosis and abnormal dopaminergic function, giving very little theoretical support to the use of neuroleptic agents for the treatment of these symptoms.

Psychosis in other common late-onset dementias

Retrospective studies of neuropathologically confirmed cases suggested that visual hallucinations are a key diagnostic feature of DLB, with a prevalence of 60% in psychiatric samples and 20% in cohorts from neurology settings (Ballard *et al.* 1996). Prospective studies have confirmed the high prevalence (>80% in psychiatric clinics), whilst all reports confirm a significantly higher prevalence of visual hallucinations in DLB compared with AD (Ballard *et al.* 1996, 1998b, 1999, Galasko *et al.* 1996, McShane *et al.* 1996, Weiner *et al.* 1996). There may also be phenomenological differences between DLB and AD. DLB patients are more likely to experience accompanying auditory hallucinations (Ballard *et al.* 1996, 1999), experience their hallucinations more frequently during an average week (Ballard *et al.* 1995b), are more distressed by their psychosis (Ballard *et al.* 1995b) and experience greater persistence of their psychotic symptoms, especially visual hallucinations (McShane *et al.* 1995, Ballard *et al.* 1997, 1998). The persistence and severity of the symptoms are a particular problem given the limited treatment options, because of the severe neuroleptic sensitivity reactions experienced by many DLB patients (McKeith *et al.* 1992), which occur even with the newer atypical agents (Ballard *et al.* 1998a).

Other psychotic symptoms including delusions (mean prevalence: 68% in psychiatry settings, 39% in neurology settings (Ballard *et al.* 1996)), auditory hallucinations (mean prevalence 27% (Ballard *et al.* 1996)) and delusional misidentification (mean prevalence 38% (Ballard *et al.* 1999)) are also significantly more common in DLB sufferers. The majority of work examining the associations of psychosis in these patients has focused upon the post-mortem neurochemistry, suggesting a link between visual hallucinations and the severity of cholinergic deficit in the temporal cortex, particularly if serotonergic function is relatively preserved (Perry *et al.* 1993).

Psychosis in VaD has received far less attention. A number of small clinical studies have, however, examined rates. The mean prevalence of psychosis is 37% (delusions, 19–50%; visual hallucinations, 14–60%; delusional misidentification, 19–30%; Birkett *et al.* 1972, Berrios and Brook 1985, Rovner *et al.* 1986, Chandler and Chandler 1988, Cummings *et al.* 1987, Morriss *et al.* 1990, Ballard *et al.* 1991, 1995b, Flynn *et al.* 1991, Binetti *et al.* 1993, Corey-Bloom *et al.* 1993, Sultzer *et al.* 1993), with few differences from AD. Associations have not been studied, but given the focal nature of lesions in VaD, they may offer important information regarding the regions of interest.

Psychosis in the nursing home

Residential and nursing homes form an integral part of the care network for individuals with dementia, particularly during the later stages of the disease process

(Bannister *et al.* 1998) or when concurrent psychiatric morbidity or behavioural problems arise (Steele *et al.* 1990). The increase in the elderly population inevitably means a progressive increase in the number of people with dementia well into the twenty first century, and a corresponding increase in the need for residential and nursing home places. The changes in population demographic, together with the influence of political changes, have already had a marked impact upon places in care facilities in the UK, with a six-fold increase in the private sector care provisions over the last 14 years (Royal College of Physicians 1997). Understanding the mental health needs of these people is particularly important given that they provide essential care to a large group of very vulnerable individuals with complex physical and mental health needs and limited ability to comment upon the care which they receive (Brooker 1995). Residents of these facilities are frequently physically frail, with a very high risk of fall-related injuries (Thappa *et al.* 1995) and many are taking psychotropic medication (Furniss *et al.* 1998), often inappropriately (McGrath and Jackson 1996), and commonly with adverse effects (Tune *et al.* 1991).

Although there are relatively few studies examining this area, it appears that more than a quarter of residents living in these care settings experience psychotic symptoms (Cohen *et al.* 1998, Ballard *et al.* 1999). These are residents for whom providing good quality care is particularly difficult (Wilcocks *et al.* 1997), and few receive input from specialist healthcare services (Burns *et al.* 1993). This is clearly an area where a great deal of additional work needs to be focused, and is discussed in more detail in Chapter 20.

Summary

Common symptoms

- visual hallucinations (usually complete representations of people or animals);
- delusions, e.g. theft or the false belief that one is being talked about (delusions of reference);
- delusional misidentification, e.g. a false belief that strangers are visiting or living in the house, believing that images on the television are real or that one's mirror image represents somebody else.

Assessment

- brief standardized informant interviews using scales such as the BEHAVE-AD and NPI can be valuable.

Impact of psychosis

- sometimes, but not invariably distressing for people experiencing these symptoms;
- can create considerable management problems for caregivers;

- may precipitate admission to residential or nursing home care;
- may be associated with more rapid progression of cognitive impairments.

Frequency

- Psychotic symptoms are present in ≤50% of people with AD from cross sectional hospital based studies, and as many as 80% in longitudinal evaluations.
- Psychosis is also common in people with dementia residing in care facilities (>25%).
- Psychosis is less common amongst people with mild dementia and people with dementia living in the community who have not been referred to specialist services.

Important associations of psychosis

- People with visual impairment and those with more severe cognitive impairment are at high risk of visual hallucinations.
- People with dementia of moderate severity are at highest risk of experiencing delusions.
- Although psychoses are common in all late-onset dementias, they are particularly prevalent in DLB.

Biological correlates

- Delusions and visual hallucinations probably have a different biological basis.
- There is very little evidence to support a dopaminergic theory of psychosis in dementia.

Diagnostic conundrums

(1) *Mrs X believes that her purse has been stolen. On enquiry, she acknowledges that it is possible that she may have just left it in her room.* As the idea is not unshakeable, this is not a delusional belief.

(2) *Mrs X believes that her handbag has been stolen from her room. She is absolutely convinced that this is the case despite plausible alternatives. She has, however, only expressed this belief on one occasion and does not express it again, although she does say later in the week that she sees children in the corner of her room.* Part of the definition of a delusion requires it to be repeated on at least two occasions 1 week apart, so this does not meet these criteria and should probably be considered as a confabulation. If the second psychotic symptom was also a false and unshakeable belief, relating to a similar theme, such as the theft of an alternative object, or people trying to hide things; this would constitute a delusion.

(3) *Mr X bends over and is picking at the carpet. When asked what he is doing, he does not reply. When asked if he can see anything on the carpet, again he does not*

reply. One possible explanation for the behaviour in which Mr X is engaged might be related to a visually perceived phenomenon. It is, however, also possible that he is interested in the pattern on the carpet, has poor eyesight and therefore may be misperceiving an actual pattern or object on the carpet, or may be engaged in some form of repetitive motor behaviour. It therefore cannot be assumed without a clear verbal report (either directly from the person with dementia, or indirectly from an informant who has received a verbal report from the person) that a visual hallucination has occurred.

(4) *Mr X fails to recognize his wife and asks who she is. Later, the sister-in-law visits, and he asks her if she is his wife.* Whilst Mr X is clearly having difficulties in identifying familiar people, which can be a very distressing experience for the family and difficult for the person with dementia, as described there is no clear evidence in these circumstances that this is a delusional belief. In order for this to constitute a delusional misidentification, there would have to be clear delusional element, i.e. a false unshakeable belief that is not purely understood in terms of deficits in higher cognitive function. It must therefore extend beyond just a failure of recognition. Hence if Mr X believed that his wife had been replaced by an impostor, had been changed into someone else or that somebody had taken his wife away from him, these would constitute delusional beliefs. This is true of any form of Capgras-type delusional misidentification: whether it is of an object or a person, there must be a delusional elaboration.

Examples of commonly experienced psychotic phenomena

- **Delusions of reference**—usually the belief that somebody is being talked about. This is generally simple and not part of the delusional system. It will be a recurrent and unshakeable belief.

- **Delusions of theft**—a belief that one's possessions are being hidden or stolen. Again it is usually simple and not part of a perceived complex plot. Whilst the basic idea may have its basis in a memory deficit, i.e. not remembering that an object has been left in a particular place, the belief is nevertheless unshakeable and will be repeated frequently.

- **Phantom boarder delusions**—a belief that people are visiting or living in the house. These beliefs are sometimes secondary to visual hallucinations of strangers in the house, but may appear as a delusional belief without any abnormal perceptions.

- **Visual hallucinations**—these are usually of people (strangers, family members or children) but may be of animals or objects or, on occasions, of complex scenes. They are usually of complete figures which tend to move but rarely speak.

- **Delusions of persecution**—beliefs that somebody else means harm to somebody. Again, these are usually simple, and must be unshakeable and repeated in order to be considered delusional.

- **Auditory hallucinations**—third-person auditory hallucinations, i.e. hearing two people talking about you, is extremely uncommon. Most auditory hallucinations are either second-person, hearing someone talking directly to you, or are simple auditory hallucinations such as noises.

- **Delusional misidentification of television images**—this is the belief that people on the television are actually existing in real space. An example of this might be somebody who becomes extremely frightened when a gunshot is fired on the television, expressing the belief that someone is firing a gun in the room. A similar delusional misidentification sometimes occurs with photographs or newspapers where pictures are believed to be real people.

- **Delusional misidentification of a mirror image**—this delusional misidentification occurs when somebody looks in the mirror and believes the mirror image is of somebody else. It is not just the failure to recognize one's own image but is associated with delusional elaboration such as the idea that the image is a separate person who has come to visit or that there are people living behind the mirror.

- **Delusions of abandonment**—this is the belief that someone is going to be abandoned, deserted or thrown out of their home. This would not include the belief that the family want to place someone in a residential home, if it is not an unshakeable belief or has some basis in fact. It is, however, delusional if it is completely unshakeable, cannot be understood as an exaggeration of the truth and is repeated on several occasions.

- **Capgras delusions**—these are delusional misidentifications where a person or object is believed to have been replaced. Examples of these beliefs might include a marital partner being thought to be replaced by an impostor, objects or furniture in the house believed to have been replaced by very similar but not quite identical furniture or, on occasions, the belief that one's whole house has been replaced and is not one's own home. There is a clear delusional element to these beliefs and they are not just the failure to recognize a person or familiar object.

- **Delusional jealousy**—the belief that one's partner is having an affair. Again this has to be an unshakeable belief which is repeated on numerous occasions. Somebody might, for example, believe that every day when their wife was going out shopping they are having a liaison with a lover, and may seek evidence that this is occurring. They would have no doubt that this is the only explanation for what is happening. Occasionally these beliefs might be secondary to visual hallucinations of people in the house, but more commonly they are delusional in the absence of hallucinatory experiences.

REFERENCES

Allen, N. H. P. and Burns, A. (1995). The noncognitive features of dementia. *Reviews in Clinical Gerontology*, **5**, 57–75.

Allen, N. H. P., Gordon, S., Hope, T. and Burns, A. (1996) Manchester and Oxford Universities Scale for the Psychological Assessment of Dementia (MOUSEPAD). *British Journal of Psychiatry*, **169**, 293–307.

Ayre, G. A., Sahgal, A., McKeith, I., Ballard, C., Lowery, K., Pincock, C. P., Walker, M. and Wesnes, K. (2000). Distinct profiles of neuropsychological impairment in dementia with Lewy bodies and Alzheimer's disease. *Neurology*. In press.

Ballard, C. G., Chithiramohan, R. N., Bannister, C., Handy, S. and Todd, N. (1991). Paranoid features in the elderly with dementia. *International Journal of Geriatric Psychiatry*, **6**, 155–7.

Ballard, C., Bannister, C., Graham C., Oyebode, F. and Wilcock, G. (1995a). Associations of psychotic symptoms in dementia sufferers. *British Journal of Psychiatry*, **167**, 537–40.

Ballard, C. G., Saad, K., Patel, A., Gahir, M., Solis, M., Coope, B. and Wilcock ,G. (1995b). The prevalence and phenomenology of psychotic symptoms in dementia sufferers. *International Journal of Geriatric Psychiatry*, **10**, 477–85.

Ballard, C., Lowery, K., Harrison, R. and McKeith, I. G. (1996). Noncognitive symptoms in Lewy body dementia. In *Dementia with Lewy Bodies* (Perry, R., McKeith, I. G. and Perry, E. K., eds), pp. 000–000. Cambridge University Press, Cambridge.

Ballard, C. G. and O'Brien J. (1999). Pharmacological Treatment of Behavioural and Psychological Signs in Alzheimer's Disease. How good is the evidence for current pharmacological treatment? *British Medical Journal*, **319**, 138–139.

Ballard C. G. and Oyebode R., (1995). Psychotic symptions in patients with dementia. *International Journal of Geriatric Psychiatry*, **6**, 313–216.

Ballard C. G. and Walker M. P., (1999). Neuropsychiatric Aspects of Alzheima's disease. Current Psychiatry Reports **1**, 49–60.

Ballard, C., O'Brien, J., Coope, B., Fairbairn, A., Abid, F. and Wilcock, G. (1997). A prospective study of psychotic symptoms in dementia sufferers: psychosis in dementia. *International Psychogeriatrics*; **9**, 57–64.

Ballard, C., McKeith, I., Grace, J. and Holmes, C. (1998a). Neuroleptic sensitivity in dementia with Lewy bodies and Alzheimer's disease. *Lancet*, **351**, 1032–3.

Ballard, C. G., O'Brien, J., Lowery, K., Ayre, G. A., Harrison, R., Perry, R., Ince, P., Neill, D. and McKeith, I. G. (1998b). A prospective study of dementia with Lewy bodies. *Age and Ageing*, **27**, 631–6.

Ballard, C., Lana, M., Reichelt, K., Bannister, C., Mynt, P., Potkins, D., O'Brien, J. and Swann, A. (1999). Behavioural and psychological symptoms amongst dementia sufferers in residential and nursing home care (abstract). Proceedings of the International Psychogeriatric Association Conference, Vancouver, August 1999.

Bannister, C., Ballard, C., Lana, M., Fairbairn, A. and Wilcock, G. (1998). Placement of dementia sufferers in residential and nursing home care. *Age and Ageing*, **27**, 189–93.

Berrios, G. E. and Brook, P. (1985). Delusions and the psychopathology of the elderly with dementia. *Acta Psychiatrica Scandinavica*, **72**, 296–301.

Binetti, G., Bianchetti, A., Padovani, A., Lenzi, G., De Leo, D. and Trabucchi M. (1993). Delusions in Alzheimer's disease and multi-infarct dementia. *Acta Neurologica Scandinavica*, **88**, 5–9.

Binetti, G., Padovani, A., Magni, E., Bianchetta, A., Scuratti, A., Lenzi, G. L. and Trabucchi, M. (1995). Delusions and dementia: clinical CT correlates. *Acta Neurologica Scandinavica*, **91**, 271–5.

Birkett, D. P. (1972). The psychiatric differentiation of senility and arteriosclerosis. *British Journal of Psychiatry*, **120**, 321–5.

Brooker, D. (1995). Looking at them looking at me. A review of observational studies into the quality of institutional care for elderly people with dementia. *Journal of Mental Health*, **4**, 145–56.

Burns, A., Jacoby, R. and Levy, R. (1990). Psychiatric phenomena in Alzheimer's. *British Journal of Psychiatry*, **157**, 72–96.

Burns, B. J., Wagner, H. R., Taibe, J. F., Magaziner, J., Permutt, T. and Landermen, L. R. (1993). Mental health service use by the elderly in nursing homes: another perspective. *American Journal of Public Health*, **83**, 331–7.

Chandler, J. D. and Chandler, J. E. (1988). The prevalence of neuropsychiatric disorders in a nursing home population. *Journal of Geriatric Psychiatry and Neurology*, **1**, 71–6.

Chapman, F., Dickinson, J., McKeith, I. and Ballard, C. G. (1990). Visual acuity and visual hallucinations in Alzheimer's disease. *American Journal of Psychiatry*, **156**, 1983–1985.

Chen, J. Y., Stern, Y., Sano, M. and Mayeux, R. (1991). Cumulative risks of developing extrapyramidal signs, psychosis or myoclonnus in the course of Alzheimer's disease. *Archives of Neurology*, **48**, 1141–3.

Chui, H. C., Lyness, S. A., Sobel, E. and Schneider, L. S. (1994). Extrapyramidal signs and psychiatric symptoms predict faster cognitive decline in Alzheimer's disease. *Archives of Neurology*, **51**, 676–81.

Cohen, C. I., Hyland, K. and Magai, C. (1998). Inter-racial and intra-racial differences in neuropsychiatric symptoms, sociodemography and treatment among nursing home patients with dementia. *Gerontologist*, **38**, 355–61.

Corey-Bloom, J., Galasko, D., Hofstetter, R., Jackson, J. E. and Thal, L. J. (1993). Clinical features distinguishing large cohorts with possible AD, probable AD, and mixed dementia. *Journal of the American Geriatrics Society*, **41**, 31–7.

Cummings, J. L., Miller, B., Hill, M. A. and Neshkes, R. (1987). Neuropsychiatric aspects of multi-infarct dementia and dementia of the Alzheimer type. *Archives of Neurology*, **44**, 389–93.

Cummings, J. L., Mega, M., Gray, K., Rosenberg-Thompson, S., Carusi, D. A. and Gornbein, J. (1994). The Neuropsychiatric Inventory: comprehensive assessment of psychopathology in dementia. *Neurology*, **44**, 2308–14.

Devanand, D. P., Miller, L., Richards, M., Marder, K., Bell, K., Mayeux, R. and Stern, Y. (1992). The Columbia University Scale for Psychopathology in Alzheimer's Disease. *Archives of Neurology*, **49**, 371–6.

Donaldson, C., Tarrier, N. and Burns, A. (1998). Determinants of carer stress in Alzheimer's disease. *International Journal of Geriatric Psychiatry*, **13**, 248–56.

Drevets, W. C. and Rubin, E. H. (1989). Psychotic symptoms and the longitudinal course of senile dementia of the Alzheimer type. *Biological Psychiatry*, **25**, 39–48.

Flynn, G. G., Cummings, J. L. and Gorbein, J. (1991). Delusions in dementia syndromes: investigation of behavioural and neuropsychological correlates. *Journal of Neuropsychiatry and Clinical Neurosciences*, **3**, 364–70.

Förstl, H., Besthorn, C., Geiger-Kabisch, C., Sattel, H. and Schreiter-Gasser, U. (1993). Psychotic features and the course of Alzheimer's disease: relationship to cognitive electro-encephalographic and computerised tomography. *Acta Psychiatrica Scandinavica*, **87**, 395–9.

Förstl, H., Burns, A., Levy, R. and Cairns, N. (1994). Neuropathological correlates of psychotic phenomena in confirmed Alzheimer's disease. *British Journal of Psychiatry*, **165**, 53–9.

Furniss, L., Lloyd Craig, S. K. and Burns, A. (1998). Medication use in nursing homes for the elderly. *International Journal of Geriatric Psychiatry*, **13**, 433–9.

Galasko, D., Katzman, R., Salmon, D. P. and Hansen, L. (1996). Clinical and neuropathological findings in Lewy body dementias. *Brain and Cognition*, **31**, 166–75.

Gilley, D. W., Whalen, M. E., Wilson, R. S. and Bennett, D. A. (1991). Hallucinations and associated factors in Alzheimer's disease. *Journal of Neuropsychiatry*, **3**, 371–6.

Gray, J. A. (1982). *The Neuropsychology of Anxiety*. Oxford University Press, Oxford.

Haupt, M., Romero, B. and Kurz, A. (1996). Psychotic symptoms in Alzheimer's disease: results from a two year longitudinal study. *International Journal of Geriatric Psychiatry*, **Vol II**, 965–72.

Holroyd, S. and Sheldon-Keller, A. (1995). A study of visual hallucinations in Alzheimer's disease. *American Journal of Geriatric Psychiatry*, **3**, 198–205.

Hope, T. and Fairburn, C. G. (1992). The Present Behavioural Examination: the development of an interview to measure current behavioural abnormalities. *Psychological Medicine*, **22**, 223–30.

Hope, T., Keene, J., Fairburn, C., McShane, R. and Jacoby, R. (1997). Behavioural changes in dementia. 2: Are there behavioural syndromes? *International Journal of Geriatric Psychiatry*, **12**, 1074–8.

Jeste, D. V., Wragg, R. E., Salmon, D. P., Harris, M J. and Thal, L. J. (1992). Cognitive deficits of patients with Alzheimer's disease with and without delusions. *American Journal of Psychiatry*, **149**, 184–9.

Kotrla, K. J., Chacko, R. C., Harper, R. G., Jhingran, S. and Doody, R. (1995). SPECT findings on psychosis in Alzheimer's disease. *American Journal of Psychiatry*, **152**, 1470–75.

Liston, E. H. (1979). Clinical findings in pre-senile dementia. *Journal of Nervous Mental Disorders*, **167**, 337–42.

McGrath, A. M. and Jackson, G. A. (1996). Survey of prescribing in residents of nursing homes in Glasgow. *British Medical Journal*, **314**, 611–12.

McKeith, I. G., Fairbairn, A., Perry, R., Thompson, P. and Perry, E. (1992). Neuroleptic sensitivity in patients with senile dementia of Lewy body type. *British Medical Journal*, **305**, 673–8.

McShane, R., Gedling, K., Reading, M., McDonald, B., Esiri, M. M. and Hopt, T. (1995). Prospective study of relations between cortical Lewy bodies, poor eyesight, and hallucinations in Alzheimer's disease. *Journal of Neurology, Neurosurgery, and Psychiatry*, **59**, 185–8.

McShane, R., Keene, J., Gedling, K. and Hope, T. (1996). Hallucinations, cortical Lewy body pathology, cognitive function and neuroleptic use in dementia. In *Dementia with Lewy Bodies* (Perry, R. H., McKeith, I. G. and Perry, E. K., eds), pp. 000–000. Cambridge University Press, Cambridge.

McShane, R., Keene, J., Gedling, K., Fairburn, C., Jacoby, R. and Hope, T. (1997). Do neuroleptic drugs hasten cognitive decline in dementia?: prospective study with necropsy follow-up. *British Medical Journal*, **314**, 266–70.

Morriss, R. K., Rovner, B. W., Folstein, M. F. and German, P. S. (1990). Delusions in newly admitted residents of nursing homes. *American Journal of Psychiatry*, **147**, 299–302.

Perry, E. K., Marshall, E., Thompson, P., McKeith, I. G., Collerton, D., Fairburn, A. F., Ferrier, I. N., Irving, D. and Perry, R. H. (1993). Monoaminergic activities in dementia with Lewy bodies: relation to hallucinations and extrapyramidal features. *Journal of Neural Transmission* (Parkinson's Disease and Dementia Section), **6**, 167–77.

Rabins, P. V., Mace, N. L. and Lucas, M. J. (1982). The impact of dementia on the family. *Journal of the American Medical Society*, **248**, 333–5.

Recanzone, G. H., Merzenich, M. and Jenkins, W. M. (1992). Topographic reorganisation of the hand representation in cortical area 36 of owl monkeys trained in a frequency discrimination task. *Journal of Neurophysiology*, **5**, 1031–56.

Reisberg, G., Borenstein, J., Salob, S., Ferris, S. H., Franssen, E. and Georgotas, A. (1987). Behavioural symptoms in Alzheimer's disease: phenomenology and treatment. *Journal of Clinical Psychiatry*, **47**, 9–15.

Rockwell, E., Jackson, E., Vilke, G. and Jeste, D. V. (1994). A study of delusions in a large cohort of Alzheimer's disease patients. *American Journal of Psychiatry*, **2**, 157–64.

Rosen, J. and Zubenko, G. S. (1991). Emergence of psychosis and depression in the longitudinal evaluation of Alzheimer's disease. *Biological Psychiatry*, **29**, 2224–32.

Rovner, B. W., Kajonck, S., Filipp, L., Lucas, M. J. and Folstein, M. F. (1986). The prevalence of mental illness in a community nursing home. *American Journal of Psychiatry*, **143**, 1446–9.

Royal College of Physicians. (1997). *Medicine for Older People*. Royal College of Physicians, London.

Skoog, I. (1993). The prevalence of psychotic, depressive, and anxiety syndromes in demented and non-demented 85 year olds. *International Journal of Geriatric Psychiatry*, **8**, 247–53.

Steele, C., Rovner, B., Chase, G. A. and Folstein, M. (1990). Psychiatric symptoms and nursing home placement of patients with Alzheimer's disease. *American Journal of Psychiatry*, **147**, 1049–51.

Sultzer, D. L., Levin, H. S., Mahler, M. E., High W.M. and Cummings, J. L. (1993). A comparison of psychiatric symptoms in vascular dementia and Alzheimer's disease. *American Journal of Psychiatry*, **150**, 1806–12.

Sweet, R. A., Pollock, B. G., Mulsant , B. H., Rosen, J., Lo, K. H., Yao, J. K., Hentcleff, R. A. and Mazumadar, S. (1997). Association of plasma homovanillic acid with behavioural symptoms in patients diagnosed with dementia: a preliminary report. *Biological Psychiatry*, **42**, 1016–23.

Sweet, R. A., Nimgaonkar, V. L., Kamboh, M. I., Lopez, O. L., Zhang, F. and DeKosky, S. T. (1998). Dopamine receptor genetic variation, psychosis, and aggression in Alzheimer disease. *Archives of Neurology*, **55**, 1335–40.

Teunisse, R. J., Cruysberg, J. R., Hoefnagels, W. H., Verbeek, A. L. and Zitman, F. G. (1996). Visual hallucinations in psychologically normal people: Charles Bonnet's syndrome. *Lancet*, **347**, 794–7.

Thapa, P. B., Gideon, P., Fought, R. L. and Ray ,W. A. (1995). Psychotropic drugs and risk of recurrent falls in ambulatory nursing home residents. *American Journal of Epidemiology*, **142**, 202–11.

Tune, L. E., Steele, C. and Cooper, T. (1991). Neuroleptic drugs in the management of behavioural symptoms of Alzheimer's disease. *Psychiatric Clinics of North America*, **14**, 353–73.

Weiner, W. F., Risser, R. C., Cullum, C. M., Honig, L., White, C., III, Speciale, S. and Rosenberg, R. N. (1996). Alzheimer's disease and its Lewy body variant: a clinical analysis of post-mortem verified cases. *American Journal of Psychiatry*, **153**, 1269–73.

Zubenko, G. S., Moossy, J., Marinez, A. J., Rao, G., Classen, D., Rosen, J. and Kopp, U. (1991). Neuropathological and neurochemical correlates of psychosis in primary dementia. *Archives of Neurology*; **48**, 19–624.

4 Depression

Introduction

Depression and dementia are the two most common psychiatric disorders in the elderly, so it is not surprising that they often co-exist. The prevalence of dementia is usually quoted as 5% among those aged >65 years, while the corresponding prevalence of major depression is 1–3%. However, approximately 10–20% of patients with Alzheimer's disease (Burns *et al.* 1990) and probably a higher proportion of those with vascular dementia, also suffer from depression (Newman 1999), demonstrating that the two co-exist more often than would be expected on the basis of chance. It is important to realize that the relationship between depression and dementia is complex and that differential diagnosis is not always straightforward. Depression in the absence of dementia can still be associated with cognitive impairments which are sometimes misdiagnosed as dementia (so-called 'pseudodementia') (Wells 1979). Depression may occur during a dementing illness, which is the main focus of this chapter. Finally, in the absence of a co-existent depression, particular signs and symptoms of dementia (such as apathy, agitation or sleep disturbance) can be wrongly diagnosed as signifying the presence of a depressive illness.

Depression is a potentially reversible and disabling condition; it causes distress for patients, is associated with carer stress and carries an adverse prognosis with regard to morbidity and mortality. Kales *et al.* (1999) showed that demented patients with co-existing depression used significantly more psychiatric in-patient days than demented patients without depression. Depression may be associated with other behavioural disturbances, particularly aggression (Lyketsos *et al.* 1999) and it may be that the identification and successful treatment of depression in dementia may be a means of preventing and managing subsequent physically aggressive behaviour (McShane *et al.* 1998). As such, the accurate recognition of depression in patients with dementia is clearly important and all those involved in the care of patients with dementia should have an understanding of how to assess depressive symptoms and make an accurate diagnosis of depression in someone with cognitive impairment.

Classification of depression

Terminology can be confusing, because the word 'depression' can be used in a lay sense to mean normal transient sadness, as a means of describing the symptom of depressed mood and as a term defining a psychiatric illness with a characteristic clinical profile and course (e.g. a major depression). It is usually quite easy to separate the transient sadness which is a part of normal experience from patho-logical changes in mood. Transient feelings of sadness are common, usually occur in reaction to external events, are experienced by the individual and those around them as part of 'normal' experience and are not associated with other features such as sleep and appetite disturbance, feelings of self-harm or loss of interest in other activities. In contrast, clinically significant depressed mood is characterized by a feeling of low mood which differs both in quality and duration from that of normal sadness. The quality is more intense, less inclined to vary over the day and would need to be accompanied by other signs and symptoms of depression as described in Table 4.1. Duration is an important criterion, and a cut-off of 2 weeks is adopted by most of the classification systems in current use. Table 4.2 shows the *DSM-IV* criteria (APA 1994) for a major depressive episode, which are a useful guide when thinking about whether a clinically significant depression (i.e. one that requires treatment) is present. It is important to note that 'understandability' is not in itself a criterion that should be taken into account when assessing depression. In other words, it is not appropriate to feel that someone's depression is understand-able and should not be treated because their severe persistent depression associated with weight loss, diurnal mood variation and suicidal ideation follows their move

Table 4.1 Signs and symptoms of depression

- Depressed mood, or loss of interest or pleasure in nearly all activities
- Anhedonia
- Irritability
- Appetite loss (or gain)
- Weight loss (or gain)
- Sleep disturbance (early morning wakening and hypersomnia can both occur)
- Decreased energy
- Feelings of worthlessness or guilt
- Difficulty thinking, or problems concentrating
- Recurrent thoughts of death or suicidal ideation
- Agitation (e.g. inability to sit still; pacing; hand wringing)
- Retardation (e.g. slowed speech and thinking)
- Fatigue
- Irritability
- Excessive worry over physical health
- Complaints of pain
- Obsessive or compulsive behaviour
- Guilt

Table 4.2 DSM-IV criteria for major depressive episode

A. Five (or more) of the following symptoms have been present during the same 2 week period and represent a change from previous functioning; at least one of the symptoms is either (1) or (2):[a]
   (1) depressed mood most of the day, nearly every day, as indicated by either subjective report (e.g. feels sad or empty) or observation made by others (e.g. appears tearful);
   (2) markedly diminished interest or pleasure in all, or almost all, activities most of the day, nearly every day (as indicated by either subjective account or observation made by others);
   (3) significant weight loss when not dieting or weight gain (e.g. a change of more than 5% of body weight in a month), or decrease or increase in appetite nearly every day;
   (4) insomnia or hypersomnia nearly every day;
   (5) psychomotor agitation or retardation nearly every day (observable by others, not merely subjective feelings of restlessness or being slowed down);
   (6) fatigue or loss of energy nearly every day;
   (7) feelings of worthlessness or excessive or inappropriate guilt (which may be delusional) nearly every day (not merely self-reproach or guilt about being sick);
   (8) diminished ability to think or concentrate, or indecisiveness, nearly every day (either by subjective account or as observed by others);
   (9) recurrent thoughts of death (not just fear of dying), recurrent suicidal ideation without a specific plan, or a suicide attempt or a specific plan for committing suicide.
B. The symptoms do not meet criteria for a mixed episode.
C. The symptoms cause clinically significant distress or impairment in social, occupational or other important areas of functioning.
D. The symptoms are not due to the direct physiological effects of a substance (e.g. a drug of abuse, a medication) or a general medical condition (e.g. hypothyroidism).
E. The symptoms are not better accounted for by bereavement, i.e. after the loss of a loved one, the symptoms persist for longer than 2 months or are characterized by marked functional impairment, morbid preoccupation with worthlessness, suicidal ideation, psychotic symptoms or psychomotor retardation.

[a] Note: do not include symptoms that are clearly due to a general medical condition, or mood-incongruent delusions or hallucinations.
American Psychiatric Association. *Diagnostic and Statistical Manual of Mental Disorders* (Fourth edition). Washington DC. American Psychiatric Association. (1994) Reprinted with permission from *Diagnostic and Statistical Manual of Mental Disorders* (Fourth edition). Copyright 1994 American Psychiatric Association.

away from family into residential care. It is the symptoms, not the cause, which respond to treatment. It should also be noted from the criteria that other features important in making the diagnoses are that the signs and symptoms cause clinically significant distress or impairment in functioning and are not due to substance abuse or a general medical condition. For these purposes, the presence of dementia does not constitute a medical condition known to cause low mood. In summary, therefore, in thinking about mood disturbances in patients with dementia, it is important to ask the following questions:

(1) For how long has the period of low mood been present? Is it persistent and different in quality from the normal experience of sadness?

(2) Is it associated with other signs and symptoms of a depressive illness (Table 4.1)?

(3) Does the depression cause significant distress to the patient (or their carer) or is there evidence it has had a significant impact in terms of how they function?

Assessment tools

A number of assessment tools exist to both diagnose and provide some assessment of the severity depressive symptomatology. These include the Geriatric Mental State Examination (Gurland *et al.* 1976), the Hamilton Depression Rating Scale (Hamilton 1967), the Montgomery and Asberg Depression Rating Scale (Montgomery and Asberg 1979) and the self-report Geriatric Depression Scale (Yesavage *et al.* 1982). However, few have been validated in patients who are cognitively impaired. For example, although the Geriatric Depression Scale has been used in patients with dementia, there are mixed reports in the literature about whether it is or is not a valid measure of depressive symptomatology in such patients (Montorio and Izal 1996).

The Montgomery and Asberg Depression Rating Scale is widely used for the assessment of depressive symptoms and would appear to be more useful than the Hamilton Depression Rating Scale in this population, since it relies less on somatic features (such as decreased libido, sleep and appetite disturbance) which may also be part of a dementing illness in the absence of depression. However, direct validation studies are not available.

One of the few depression instruments that has been validated in people with dementia is the Cornell Depression Rating Scale (Alexopoulos *et al.* 1988a,b), which relies on an interview with both the patient and a carer, with the rater being the final arbitrator if there is conflict in answer between the two. The scale is relatively simple to use and has the advantage that it allows the *DSM-IV* criteria for major depression to be applied. In clinical practice, it will rarely be appropriate to administer standardized assessments to all patients, though in certain settings some will be very useful as screening instruments for depression. In most circumstances the important point is that staff and relatives are aware of the possibility of depression complicating a dementing illness and are very alert to the signs of this. These may include increased restlessness or agitation, sleep disturbance, loss of appetite, loss of weight, increasing tearfulness or social withdrawal and apathy. If any of these features occur, then a careful search should be made for other signs and symptoms of depression as listed in Table 4.1.

Differential diagnosis

The issue of separating a depressive illness from normal sadness has been covered. Some symptoms, particularly night-time disturbance, appetite changes, apathy, loss of motivation and agitation, are all very common as part of a dementing illness and do not necessarily indicate the presence of co-existing depression. The problem then becomes how to recognize when such features are part of a depression and when they are not. One useful guide is whether there has been a change from previous functioning. A demented person who suddenly becomes agitated, or whose agitation increases significantly, is far more likely to be suffering from a depressive episode than if agitation had always been a part of the dementia. The co-existence of other features of depression is also important: an increase in agitation on its own would be unlikely to be caused by depression, though if it was also accompanied by depressed mood, tearfulness, early morning wakening and loss of appetite, then the diagnosis would be clearer. It is always important to enquire about factors such as a past history of depression or a family history of depression, both of which would increase the vulnerability to depression. Adverse life events, particularly exit events, are known to be an important cause of depression in non-demented people (Murphy 1982) and, although specific research has not addressed the issue of life events and depression in dementia, clinical experience indicates that at least those with milder degrees of impairment will remain at risk of developing depressive episodes after a major life event such as a bereavement or change in accommodation.

It is also important to rule out other general medical conditions which may cause depressive symptoms. These include a number of widely prescribed drugs, including steroids, beta-blockers, digoxin and non-steroidal anti-inflammatory drugs, and conditions such as hypothyroidism, electrolyte disturbances, infections and neoplasms (Baldwin 1997). As such, the assessment and investigation of depression occurring as part of dementing illness need to be every bit as vigorous as when depression occurs in the cognitively intact elderly.

Pseudodementia

One particular diagnostic problem is that of 'pseudodementia' (McAllister 1983; Wells 1979). This is still a widely used term and very useful both for teaching purposes and as a clinical label since it is a reminder that a depressive illness in the absence of dementia can produce deficits in cognition which can be misdiagnosed as an organic dementia. However, use of the term 'pseudodementia' has often been criticized on several grounds. Firstly, most research suggests that cognitive impairments occurring during depression are very real and not in any sense 'pseudo' or false (Abas et al. 1990, Beats et al. 1996, Dahabra et al. 1998). Secondly, although reversibility of cognitive impairment on recovery from depression is often cited as the hallmark of a 'pseudodementia', this is probably not the case. Whilst improvement in cognitive function is often seen in cognitively intact people following recovery of depression, they still remain impaired in a number of areas and so reversibility is certainly not complete (Abas et al. 1990; Dahabra et al. 1998). Finally, the term 'pseudodementia' implies a simple dichotomy between depression or dementia, whereas in fact a much more complex relationship exists. For example, it is now clear that depression is an independent risk factor for dementia (Jorm et al. 1991) and long-term follow-up studies of depressed subjects who become cognitively impaired during their depression suggests that having 'pseudodementia' puts patients at very high risk of subsequently developing a true dementia (Kral and Emery 1989).

Even accepting the term 'pseudodementia', no accurate figures exist for its prevalence, though a pooled review suggested it may be a label that should apply to 20%

Table 4.3 Clinical features that may differentiate 'pseudodementia' from dementia

- a short history
- past history of depression
- multiple complaints of cognitive deficits
- responds with 'don't know' rather than incorrect answers
- behavioural competency in daily activities in compatible severity of cognitive impairment
- absence of nocturnal confusion
- inconsistent cognitive performance
- absence of cortical signs (dysphasia, dyspraxia)

of all elderly depressed subjects. Desrosiers (1992) found that approximately 10% of cases initially diagnosed as an organic dementia were later rediagnosed as depressive dementia. Mis-diagnosis appears particularly likely in cases of early-onset (pre-senile) dementia and Nott and Fleminger (1975) could confirm the initial diagnosis of pre-senile dementia in less than half of the cases they examined (albeit retro-spectively) presenting to a psychiatric hospital. Wells (1979) proposed a number of clinical features which distinguished depressed cases from those with dementia. These are shown in Table 4.3. However, apart from the presence of memory com-plaints and behavioural competency that is incompatible with cognitive testing (for example, a very cognitively impaired patient who is able to use the telephone), few have been prospectively validated (Desrosiers 1992).

Neuropsychological performance has also been suggested as being helpful in dif-ferentiating 'pseudodementia' from dementia. Dementias, particularly Alzheimer's disease, are associated with cortical deficits such as agnosia, dyspraxia, dysphasia and dyscalculia, while 'pseudodementia' typically has a more 'subcortical' presenta-tion with psychomotor slowing, impaired concentration and impaired memory in the absence of other 'cortical' signs (Reynolds *et al.* 1988). Certainly, prospective studies have confirmed that cortical signs are associated with Alzheimer's disease rather than depression, though absolute discrimination does not appear possible, even in studies that have carefully selected clear-cut cases of depression and Alzheimer's disease. Differentiation is likely to be even more problematic when con-sidering dementias with more of a subcortical presentation such as vascular dementia, dementia with Lewy bodies, Huntington's disease and dementia associated with Parkinson's disease. Laboratory tests may also be helpful in separating dementia from depression. Whilst a detailed discussion is outwith the scope of this chapter, dementias are more likely to be associated with abnormalities on the electro-encephalogram (EEG), on structural imaging (such as computerized tomography (CT) and magnetic resonance imaging (MRI)) and on functional imaging (such as perfusion single photon emission tomography (SPECT) scanning, which looks at blood flow) than depression. These changes have been best characterized for Alzheimer's disease which is associated with slowing of the EEG (Besthorn *et al.* 1997), generalized atrophy on CT (Burns *et al.* 1991, Forstl *et al.* 1995), hippocampal atrophy on MRI (Jack *et al.* 1989, O'Brien 1995, Barber *et al.* 1999a) and temporo-parietal hypoperfusion on SPECT scanning (O'Brien *et al.* 1992). O'Brien *et al.* (1997) showed that hippocampal atrophy on MRI could separate those with Alzheimer's disease and those with depression with an accuracy of about 90%. In clinical practice, a combination of careful history taking, detailed mental and cognitive state examination and physical examination with appropriate investigations will be needed to inform diagnosis properly.

Prevalence and incidence of depression in dementia

Published studies on the prevalence of depression in Alzheimer's disease, the dementia that has been best studied in this regard, vary enormously so that one can find studies with rates of 0% and 87% in the literature (Burns *et al.* 1990). Much of this variation is due to differences in the way patients are selected (i.e. whether they are taken from referrals to a psychiatric unit, where the prevalence of depression may be high, or from the community, where it may be low), the assessment instruments used for depression (for example, self-report measures may be unreliable) and differences in the severity of dementia (depression is particularly hard to assess in patients with severe dementia when the only guide may be changes in vegetative features such as sleep or appetite). A balanced review would suggest a prevalence of depression of 10–20% for patients with Alzheimer's disease, about 20–30% for those with vascular dementia (Newman 1999) and higher (perhaps 40–50%) for those with Parkinson's disease (Cummings and Masterman 1999). In a mixed group of 124 patients with dementia referred to a clinical service, Ballard *et al.* (1996a) found a prevalence of depression of 25%. This is very similar to the rate reported by Burns *et al.* (1990) who found that 24% of those with Alzheimer's disease were rated as being depressed by a trained observer. Interestingly, 63% had at least one depressive symptom (confirming that depressive symptoms are a lot more common in dementia than a depressive episode) but also that 40% were rated by the carers as being depressed. This illustrates that, whilst it is always important to pay attention to what carers notice and report, they may have a tendency to over-diagnose depression. The reasons for this are unclear but are likely to be due to features of dementia (such as withdrawal and apathy) being misinterpreted as depression. The relationship between severity of intellectual decline and likelihood to have depression is inconsistent in the literature. Burns *et al.* (1990) found that those with depressive symptoms had milder degrees of cognitive impairment and less cerebral atrophy on their CT scans, though this finding has not always been replicated and some neurobiological work summarized below would suggest that depression may be expected to be more common in those with more severe illness. On current evidence it would seem most sensible to conclude that depression can occur at any stage of a dementia and so should always be considered when assessing patients.

Only a few of the studies that have investigated the longitudinal course of depression in dementia looked at incidence. Ballard *et al.* (1996b) followed 124 dementia subjects monthly for 1 year. The annual incidence was 10.6% for major depression and 29.8% for minor depression. Persistent depression (that lasting ≥6 months or longer) only occurred in 20% of those with depression and was significantly more likely to occur in those with vascular dementia as compared with other disorders. Because of the high spontaneous resolution rate of depressive episodes in those with dementia, it may be prudent when possible to wait a month or two before intervening to see if the depression spontaneously remits. Of course, such a judgement must be balanced by the severity of the depression, the length of time it has already been present and the negative impact and distress it is causing for patients and caregiver. Any indication of an intent for self-harm would indicate early treatment.

Hypomania

Hypomania, i.e. extreme elevation of mood, is much less common in demented patients than depression. Whilst cases have been described, they are generally rare and prevalence is of the order of 1–2% (Burns *et al.* 1990, Lyketsos *et al.* 1995). It can arise *de novo* in the context of a dementing illness, particularly after a vascular insult, or may present in those with longstanding bipolar illness that has become more unstable with the onset of organic brain disease. Clinically, such cases are typified by extreme elevation of mood, irritability, motor hyperactivity (pacing), sleep disturbance, appetite disturbance, increases in energy and libido and sometimes inappropriate social and sexual behaviour. Occasionally, psychotic features can occur with mood-congruent delusions ('I am the Queen') and hallucinations ('You have the power to heal others').

Biological correlates of depression

There are three main themes underlining biological investigations in depression and all of these have been examined in relation to depression occurring as part of a dementing illness:

(1) dysregulation of the hypothalamic–pituitary–adrenal (HPA) axis or hyper-cortisolaemia, which is common in depressed patients. This has been directly associated with lowering of mood (for example, depressed mood is common after oral steroid therapy) while agents that reduce blood cortisol concentrations have been shown to be antidepressant (McAllister-Williams *et al.* 1998);

(2) dysregulation of the monoamine systems, particularly the serotonergic and noradrenergic system;

(3) particular structural and functional brain changes in areas thought to be important in the regulation of mood, such as the frontal lobe (in particular the cingulate and dorsolateral prefrontal cortex) and the basal ganglia.

Several studies have investigated hypercortisolaemia in dementia (O'Brien *et al.* 1993). An often-used test, that of non-suppression of cortisol after 1 mg of oral dexamethasone (the dexamethasone suppression test) is abnormal in many cases, though reported prevalence varies from 0 to 100%. Most studies report a prevalence of 30–40% among those with Alzheimer's disease, 60 – 70% for those with vascular dementia (compared with 5% for controls) and 60 – 70% for those with depression in the absence of dementia (O'Brien *et al.* 1993). However, it is still not clear whether the hypercortisolaemia associated with dementia is associated with depression. Some studies have found a correlation (O'Brien *et al.* 1996b) whilst others have not (McKeith 1984). Whilst a relationship may exist, it is clear that hypercortisolaemia does not appear to be the sole explanation for the ocurrence of depression in dementia.

The best evidence that neurochemical systems are involved in the genesis of depression in dementia comes from post-mortem studies that have compared transmitter systems in demented patients who suffered from depression compared with those who did not. Many of these studies are problematic, both because small numbers of subjects are included and because the assessment of whether or not a demented patient was depressed was often made retrospectively from clinical notes. Zweig *et al.* (1988) found that cell loss in the locus coeruleus and dorsal raphe was greater in Alzheimer's disease patients who had suffered from depression during their life than in those who had not. Forstl *et al.* (1992) also found that there were fewer neurons in the locus coeruleus in depressed demented subjects. They found that neuronal counts in the cholinergic basal nucleus of Meynert were higher and suggested that disproportionate loss of monoaminergic compared with cholinergic neurons may be an important organic substrate of depression (Forstl *et al.* 1994). In contrast, Halliday *et al.* (1992) found no relationship between serotonergic raphe pathology and depression in their sample and Hoogendijk *et al.* (1999), although finding loss of neurons in the locus coeruleus in patients with Alzheimer's disease, found no correlation between this loss and the presence of depression during life. Chen *et al.* (1996) found that patients with Alzheimer's disease who had persistent depressive symptoms during life had significantly fewer serotonin uptake sites in temporal and frontal cortex than those without these symptoms. Overall, despite conflicting evidence, there is some support for the notion that cell loss and/or dysfunction in the serotonergic and noradrenergic systems may make demented patients vulnerable to depression.

The most consistent changes on brain scanning that have been noted in elderly depressed patients without cognitive impairments are an increase in deep white matter lesions, as visualized by MRI (these may represent areas of subtle vascular damage (Coffey *et al.* 1990, Greenwald *et al.* 1996, 1998, O'Brien *et al.* 1996a)), and frontal hypoperfusion on functional brain imaging (Goodwin *et al.* 1993). An association between white matter lesions in the frontal lobes and depressive symptoms in patients with Alzheimer's disease, dementia with Lewy bodies and vascular dementia has been reported (Barber *et al.* 1999b) and Hirono *et al.* (1998) found that, in subjects with Alzheimer's disease, bilateral superior frontal and left anterior cingulate cortex glucose metabolism was impaired in those who had depression compared with those who did not.

Possession of the apolipoprotein E4 allele is strongly associated with Alzheimer's disease and a number of studies have investigated whether genotype affects BPSD symptoms such as depression. Although Holmes *et al.* (1998) found that demented patients who possessed the E4 allele were more likely to develop depression than those without, other studies have not generally supported this view (Lyketsos *et al.* 1997, Hirono *et al.* 1999) and the relationship between genotype and the presence of depression occurring during dementia remains unclear.

Overall, findings from investigations of the HPA axis, neurochemical systems and structural and functional brain-imaging studies provide some support for the suggestion that neurobiological changes in depression in the presence of dementia are similar to those in depression in the absence of dementia. However, it is far from clear as to what the most important neurobiological change is, though the similarity of biological changes in 'organic' and 'non-organic' depression provides some rationale for the use of similar treatments in the two conditions.

Case studies

> Mr X is a nursing home resident with moderately severe dementia. Over the last 2 weeks he has shown reduced appetite and has become more agitated. Nursing staff wonder if he has become depressed. On close questioning he is cheerful and sleeps well. There are not other features of depression. Further enquiry reveals nausea and constipation.

Although newly emerging loss of appetite and agitation may be signs of a depressive illness, this was not the case in this example. Many physical conditions, even as basic as simple constipation, can also be the cause.

> Mr M, who has dementia of moderate severity, has a 2 week history of loss of appetite and agitation. He has lost 5 lb in weight, is waking early in the morning and is often noted to be tearful. He is spending much more time alone in his room and has lost interest in watching television. He is somewhat inconsistent when asked directly about his mood but does admit to feeling low and looks quite downcast most of the time. His wife, who visits three times a week, feels there has been quite a dramatic change and that he is gloomy. Although he has not previously suffered a depressive episode, he has a younger brother who has had three episodes of depression.

There is ample evidence that Mr M's symptoms are due to a superimposed depressive illness. The symptoms have been present for 2 weeks, thus just meeting criteria for a depressive episode. Given what is known about the high resolution rate of symptoms, it may be prudent to wait a short time to see if his symptoms spontaneously resolve, though in this case the depression is moderately severe and associated with some weight loss, so it is likely that treatment will need to be instigated sooner rather than later.

> Mrs Y is the carer of Mr Y, a man with mild dementia who is still living at home and functions fairly independently. Mrs Y notes that her husband is more withdrawn than normal and less interested in activities. He is less sociable and converses less than usual. She describes these problems as coming on gradually over the last 6 months. On exami-

nation, Mr Y admits to being troubled by his memory but denies being depressed or having thoughts of self-harm. His appetite is extremely good and he sleeps well. He described some lack of energy but does appear to enjoy activities in which he is involved. Mrs Y feels her husband is depressed and requests antidepressant tablets.

The symptoms noted by Mrs Y are likely to be part of the dementia rather than due to a superimposed depressive illness. The time course and pattern would support this and Mr Y has no other features suggestive of a depressive episode. However, it would be important to monitor these symptoms to ensure that they are not part of an emerging depression. A full explanation will be need to be given to Mrs Y to explain that medication will not help her husband's symptoms, which are a result of underlying brain disease and not a superimposed depressive illness.

Mr Y is a 60 year old man with a 3 month history of memory difficulties. He complains specifically about his poor memory and cannot remember (i) where he has laid things around the house or (ii) things that happened the day before. Although these memory difficulties are confirmed by his wife and by objective cognitive testing, neither he nor his wife can give any examples of major memory lapses. For example, he has never got lost and has never forgotten to take his keys with him when going out. On cognitive testing he is disorientated in time and place and has very poor attention and concentration. He performs at the level of someone with a moderate dementia, though there is no impairment of language and his constructional skills (for example, drawing a clock face) are well preserved. His poor scoring on objective testing is at variance with the lack of major problems caused by poor memory outside of hospital. He appears slowed down and on closer questioning admits to feelings of low mood and loss of pleasure and activities. He has also become increasingly anxious and has had some thoughts of self-harm. He has started waking at 4.00 a.m. and has marked diurnal variation in his mood, with it improving towards the afternoon.

This man's presentation is more compatible with a depressive 'pseudodementia' than a dementia with co-existent depression. However, he would require full investigation and active management of his depression. It would be most important to repeat and document cognitive testing which should be performed again on recovery from depression. Ultimately careful follow-up would determine the diagnosis.

REFERENCES

Abas, M. A., Sahakian, B. J. and Levy, R. (1990). Neuropsychological deficits and CT scan changes in elderly depressives. *Psychological Medicine*, **20**, 507–20.

Alexopoulos, G. S., Abrams, R. C., Young, R. C. and Shamoian, C. A. (1988a). Cornell Scale for Depression in Dementia. *Biological Psychiatry*, **23**, 271–84.

Alexopoulos, G. S., Abrams, R. C., Young, R. C. and Shamoian, C. A. (1988b). Use of the Cornell Scale in nondemented patients. *Journal of the American Geriatrics Society*, **36**, 230–36.

APA (1994). *Diagnostic and Statistical Manual of Mental Disorders*, 4th edn [*DSM-IV*]. American Psychiatric Association, Washington, DC.

Baldwin, R. (1997). Depressive illness. In *Psychiatry in the Elderly*. (Jacoby, R. and Oppenheimer, C., eds), pp. 536–573. Oxford University Press, Oxford.

Ballard, C., Bannister, C., Solis, M., Oyebode, F. and Wilcock, G. (1996a). The prevalence, associations and symptoms of depression amongst dementia sufferers. *Journal of Affective Disorders*, **36**, 135–44.

Ballard, C. G., Patel, A., Solis, M., Lowe, K. and Wilcock, G. (1996b). A one-year follow-up study of depression in dementia sufferers. *British Journal of Psychiatry*, **168**, 287–91.

Barber, R., Gholkar, A., Scheltens, P., Ballard, C., McKeith, I. G. and O'Brien, J. T. (1999a). Medial temporal lobe atrophy on MRI in dementia with Lewy bodies. *Neurology*, **52**, 1153–8.

Barber, R., Gholkar, A., McKeith, I., Perry, R., O'Brien, J., Ballard, C., Ince, P. and Scheltens, P. (1999b). White matter lesions on magnetic resonance imaging in dementia with Lewy bodies, Alzheimer's disease, vascular dementia, and normal aging. *Journal of Neurology, Neurosurgery and Psychiatry*, **67**, 66–72.

Beats, B. C., Sahakian, B. J. and Levy, R. (1996). Cognitive performance in tests sensitive to frontal lobe dysfunction in the elderly depressed. *Psychological Medicine*, **26**, 591–603.

Besthorn, C., Zerfass, R., Geiger-Kabisch, C., Sattel, H., Daniel, S., Schreiter-Gasser, U. and Forstl, H. (1997). Discrimination of Alzheimer's disease and normal aging by EEG data. *Electroencephalography and Clinical Neurophysiology*, **103**, 241–8.

Burns, A., Jacoby, R. and Levy, R. (1990). Psychiatric phenomena in Alzheimer's disease. III: Disorders of mood. *British Journal of Psychiatry*, **157**, 81–6.

Burns, A., Jacoby, R., Philpot, M. and Levy, R. (1991). Computerised tomography in Alzheimer's disease. Methods of scan analysis, comparison with normal controls, and clinical/radiological associations. *British Journal of Psychiatry*, **159**, 609–14.

Chen, C. P., Alder, J. T., Bowen, D. M., Esiri, M. M., McDonald, B., Hope, T., Jobst, K. A. and Francis, P. T. (1996). Presynaptic serotonergic markers in community-acquired cases of Alzheimer's disease: correlations with depression and neuroleptic medication. *Journal of Neurochemistry*, **66**, 1592–8.

Coffey, C. E., Figiel, G. S., Djang, W. T. and Weiner, R. D. (1990). Subcortical hyperintensity on magnetic resonance imaging: a comparison of normal and depressed elderly subjects. *American Journal of Psychiatry*, **147**, 187–9.

Cummings, J. L. and Masterman, D. L. (1999). Depression in patients with Parkinson's disease. *International Journal of Geriatric Psychiatry*, **14**, 711–18.

Dahabra, S., Ashton, C. H., Bahrainian, M., Britton, P. G., Ferrier, I. N., McAllister, V. A., Marsh, V. R. and Moor, P. B. (1998). Structural and functional abnormalities in elderly patients clinically recovered from early-and late-onset depression. *Biological Psychiatry*, **44**, 4–46.

Desrosiers (1992). Primary or depressive dementia: clinical features. *International Journal of Geriatric Psychiatry*, **7**, 629–38.

Forstl, H., Burns, A., Luthert, P., Cairns, N., Lantos, P. and Levy, R. (1992). Clinical and neuropathological correlates of depression in Alzheimer's disease. *Psychological Medicine*, **22**, 877–84.

Forstl, H., Levy, R., Burns, A., Luthert, P. and Cairns, N. (1994). Disproportionate loss of noradrenergic and cholinergic neurons as cause of depression in Alzheimer's disease—a hypothesis. *Pharmacopsychiatry*, **27**, 11–15.

Forstl, H., Zerfass, R., Geiger-Kabisch, C., Sattel, H., Besthorn, C. and Hentschel, F. (1995). Brain atrophy in normal ageing and Alzheimer's disease. Volumetric discrimination and clinical correlations. *British Journal of Psychiatry*, **167**, 739–46.

Goodwin, G. M., Austin, M. P., Dougall, N., Ross, M., Murray, C., O'Carroll, R. E., Moffoot, A., Prentice, N. and Ebmeier, K. P. (1993). State changes in brain activity shown by the uptake of 99mTc-exametazime with single photon emission tomography in major depression before and after treatment. *Journal of Affective Disorders*, **29**, 243–53.

Greenwald, B. S., Kramer-Ginsberg, E., Krishnan, R. R., Ashtari, M., Aupperle, P. M. and Patel, M. (1996). MRI signal hyperintensities in geriatric depression. *American Journal of Psychiatry*, **153**, 1212–15.

Greenwald, B. S., Kramer-Ginsberg, E., Krishnan, K. R. R., Ashtari, M., Auerbach, C. and Patel, M. (1998). Neuroanatomic localization of magnetic resonance imaging signal hyper-intensities in geriatric depression. *Stroke*, **29**, 613–17.

Gurland, B., Copeland, J., Sharpe, L. and Kelleher, M. (1976). The Geriatric Mental Status interview (GMS). *International Journal of Aging and Human Development*, **7**, 303–11.

Halliday, G. M., McCann, H. L., Pamphlett, R., Brooks, W. S., Creasey, H., McCusker, E., Cotton, R. G., Broe, G. A. and Harper, C. G. (1992). Brain stem serotonin-synthesizing neurons in Alzheimer's disease: a clinicopathological correlation. *Acta Neuropathologica*, **84**, 638–50.

Hamilton, M. (1967). Development of a rating scale for primary depressive illness. *British Journal of Social and Clinical Psychology*, **6**, 278–96.

Hirono, N., Mori, E., Ishii, K., Ikejiri, Y., Imamura, T., Shimomura, T., Hashimoto, M., Yamashita, H. and Sasaki, M. (1998). Frontal lobe hypometabolism and depression in Alzheimer's disease. *Neurology*, **50**, 380–3.

Hirono, N., Mori, E., Yasuda, M., Imamaura, T., Shimomura, T., Hashimoto, M., Tanimukai, S., Kazui, H. and Yamashita, H. (1999). Lack of effect of apolipoprotein E E4 allele on neuropsychiatric manifestations in Alzheimer's disease. *Journal of Neuropsychiatry and Clinical Neurosciences*, **11**, 66–70.

Holmes, C., Russ, C., Kirov, G., Aitchison, K. J., Powell, J. F., Collier, D. A. and Lovestone, S. (1998). Apolipoprotein E: depressive illness, depressive symptoms, and Alzheimer's disease. *Biological Psychiatry*, **43**, 159–64.

Hoogendijk, W. J., Sommer, I. E., Pool, C. W., Kamphorst, W., Hotman, M., A., Eckelenboom, P. and Swaab, D. F. (1999). Lack of association between depression and loss of neurons in the locus coeruleus in Alzheimer disease. *Archives of General Psychiatry*, **56**, 45–51.

Jack, C. R., Twomey, C. K., Zinsmeister, A. R., Sherbrough, F. W., Petersen, R. C., Ciscino, G. D. *et al.* (1989). Anterior temporal lobes and hippocampal formations: normative volumetric measurements from MR images in young adults. *Radiology*, **172**, 549–54.

Jorm, A. F., Van Duijn, C. M., Chandra, V., Fratiglioni, L., Graves, A. B., Heyman, A., Kokmen, E., Kondo, K., Mortimer, J. A. and Rocca, W. A. (1991). Psychiatric history and related exposures as risk factors for Alzheimer's disease: a collaborative re-analysis of case-control studies. EURODEM. *International Journal of Epidemiology*, **20**, 43–7.

Kales, H. C., Blow, F. C., Copeland, L. A., Bingham, R.C., Kammerer, E. E. and Mellow, A. M. (1999). Health care utilization by older patients with coexisting dementia and depression. *American Journal of Psychiatry*, **156**, 550–6.

Kral, V. A. and Emery, O. B. (1989). Long-term follow-up of depressive pseudodementia of the aged. *Canadian Journal of Psychiatry*, **34**, 445–6.

Lyketsos, C. G., Corazzini, K. and Steele, C. (1995). Mania in Alzheimer's disease. *Journal of Neuropsychiatry and Clinical Neurosciences*, **7**, 350–52.

Lyketsos, C. G., Baker, L., Warren, A. *et al.* (1997). Depression, delusions, and hallucinations in Alzheimer's disease: no relationship to apolipoprotein E genotype. *Journal of Neuropsychiatry and Clinical Neurosciences,* **9**, 64–7.

Lyketsos, C. G., Steele, C., Galik, E., Rosenblatt, A., Steinberg, M., Warren, A. and Sheppard,

J.-M. (1999). Physical aggression in dementia patients and its relationship to depression. *American Journal of Psychiatry*, **156**, 66–71.

McAllister, T. W. (1983). Overview: pseudodementia. *American Journal of Psychiatry*, **140**, 528–33.

McAllister-Williams, R. H., Ferrier, I. N. and Young, A. H. (1998). Mood and neuropsychological function in depression: the role of corticosteroids and serotonin. *Psychological Medicine*, **28**, 573–84.

McKeith, I. G. (1984). Clinical use of the DST in a psychogeriatric population. *British Journal of Psychiatry*, **145**, 389–93.

McShane, R., Keene, J., Fairburn, C., Jacoby, R. and Hope, T. (1998). Psychiatric symptoms in patients with dementia predict the later development of behavioural abnormalities. *Psychological Medicine*, **28**, 1119–27.

Montgomery, S. A. and Asberg, M. (1979). A new depression scale designed to be sensitive to change. *British Journal of Psychiatry*, **134**, 382–9.

Montorio, I. and Izal, M. (1996). The Geriatric Depression Scale: a review of its development and utility. *International Psychogeriatrics*, **8**, 103–12.

Murphy, E. (1982). Social origins of depression in old age. *British Journal of Psychiatry*, **141**, 35–142.

Newman, S. C. (1999). The prevalence of depression in Alzheimer's disease and vascular dementia in a population sample. *Journal of Affective Disorders*, **52**, 169–76.

Nott, P. N. and Fleminger, J. J. (1975). Presenile dementia: the difficulties of early diagnosis. *Acta Psychiatrica Scandinavica*, **51**, 210–17.

O'Brien, J. T. (1995). Is hippocampal atrophy on magnetic resonance imaging a marker for Alzheimer's disease? *International Journal of Geriatric Psychiatry*, **10**, 431–5.

O'Brien, J. T., Eagger, S., Syed, G. M., Sahakian, B. J. and Levy, R. (1992). A study of regional cerebral blood flow and cognitive performance in Alzheimer's disease. *Journal of Neurology, Neurosurgery and Psychiatry*, **55**, 1182–7.

O'Brien, J., Ames, D. and Schweitzer, I. (1993). HPA axis function in depression and dementia: a review. *International Journal of Geriatric Psychiatry*, **8**, 887–98.

O'Brien, J., Desmond, P., Ames, D., Schweitzer, I., Harrigan, S. and Tress, B. (1996a). A magnetic resonance imaging study of white matter lesions in depression and Alzheimer's disease. *British Journal of Psychiatry*, **168**, 477–85.

O'Brien, J. T., Ames, D., Schweitzer, I., Colman, P., Desmond, P. and Tress, B. (1996b). Clinical and magnetic resonance imaging correlates of hypothalamic–pituitary–adrenal axis function in depression and Alzheimer's disease. *British Journal of Psychiatry*, **168**, 679–87.

O'Brien, J. T., Desmond, P., Ames, D., Schweitzer, I., Chiu, E. and Tress, B. (1997). Temporal lobe magnetic resonance imaging can differentiate Alzheimer's disease from normal ageing, depression, vascular dementia and other causes of cognitive impairment. *Psychological Medicine*, **27**, 1267–75.

Reynolds, C. F. D., Hoch, C. C., Kupfer, D. J., Buysse, D. J., Houck, P. R., Stick, J. A., Campbell, D. W. *et al.* (1988). Bedside differentiation of depressive pseudodementia from dementia. *American Journal of Psychiatry*, **145**, 1099–103.

Wells, C. E. (1979). Pseudodementia. *American Journal of Psychiatry*, **136**, 895–900.

Yesavage, J. A., Brink, T. L., Rose, T. L., Lium, O., Huang, V., Adey, M. and Leirer, V. O. (1982). Development and validation of a geriatric depression screening scale: a preliminary report. *Journal of Psychiatric Research*, **17**, 37–49.

Zweig, R. M., Ross, C. A., Hedreen, J. C., Steele, C., Cardillo, J. E., Whitehouse, P. J., Folstein, M. F. and Price, D. L. (1988). The neuropathology of aminergic nuclei in Alzheimer's disease. *Annals of Neurology*, **24**, 233–42.

5 Wandering and restlessness

Introduction

The term 'wandering' is commonly used both clinically and in the literature to describe a wide range of different behavioural abnormalities. The looseness of the term is evident by the wide range of definitions used in various studies. One useful definition is 'a tendency to move about in either the seemingly aimless or disorientated fashion or in pursuit of an indefinable or unobtainable goal'. (Snyder *et al.* 1978, Stokes 1986). De Leon *et al.* (1984) suggest a putative causal mechanism by stating that 'wanderers are patients with navigational difficulties.'

The importance of wandering as a problematic behaviour is undisputed. It is poorly tolerated by carers (Rabins *et al.* 1982) and is an important cause of referral of patients to psychiatric services (Margo *et al.* 1980). It is also a prominent cause of hospital admission amongst dementia suffers (Sanford 1975) and presents problems within the general hospital environment (Allan 1994). Most available studies have focused solely on Alzheimer's disease (Teri *et al.* 1988, Burns *et al.* 1990). One study reported that patients with Alzheimer's disease were more likely to get lost outside the home than those with a vascular dementia (Ballard *et al.* 1991). Interestingly, Ballard *et al.* found no correlation between wandering and the severity of cognitive impairment in their 92 community-dwelling subjects.

Prevalence

There have been relatively few reports. Most studies include wandering together with a range of other behavioural problems. There are relatively few studies specifically devoted to this particular problem. In the Camberwell community-based studies (Burns *et al.* 1990), it was reported that the prevalence of wandering among patients with Alzheimer's disease was 90%. In a similar sample (Teri *et al.* 1988) a prevalence of 26% is quoted. Both of these studies found a strong correlation between 'wandering' and greater cognitive impairment. In a large recent study examining 638 community-based dementia sufferers, a prevalence of 17.4% (Klein *et al.* 1999) was reported. Wandering was significantly more frequent in patients with Alzheimer's disease, and in disease of longer duration and more severe cognitive impairment. Klien *et al.* also reported associations with other neuropsychiatric symptoms such as depression, delusions, hallucinations and sleep disorder.

Concepts and classification

The concept of 'wandering' is plagued with the same difficulties that beset 'agitation'. In a seminal paper on agitation, Cohen-Mansfield *et al.* (1992a) suggested three basic syndromes—aggressive behaviours, agitated behaviours and physically non-aggressive behaviours—within which they included increased motor activity. Other authors have separated the global term 'wandering' into three components: wandering outside at night, wandering outside the home during the day and getting lost throughout the home (Greene *et al.* 1982).

Stokes (1986) produced a classification of wandering based on his clinical experience of possible explanations for the behaviour. This classification system has the disadvantage of mixing descriptions of the behaviour with presumed causation. Stoke's list is as follows: separation anxiety; searching; boredom; loneliness; physical discomfort; coping with stress; apparent aimless wandering; disorientation; night-time wandering; and attention seeking.

In recent years, Tony Hope's group in Oxford has led the field in proposing 'a typology of wandering'. In their initial community-based study, Hope and Fairburn (1990) outline a nine-item descriptive typology on wandering in dementia and propose five fundamental components underlying the various wandering types (Table 5.1). They suggest that these components are constructs, which may help bridge the gap between a descriptive typology and an underlying aetiology of the behavioural disturbance. They propose that the following have a particular importance in the understanding of wandering.

- the overall amount of walking activity;
- avoidance of being alone;
- diurnal rhythm disturbance;
- navigational ability;
- faulty goal-directive behaviour.

These will be discussed in greater depth later in the chapter.

Albert (1992) re-analysed Hope and Fairburn's data using the method of Guttman scaling. As a result of this analysis, he suggested that the types of wandering described formed the basis of a scale. He concluded that 'the distribution of the types of wandering behaviour in the sample points to a single latent variable, with a hierarchical structure but demonstrates the centrality of purposeless behaviour in the class of wandering behaviours.' Hope and Fairburn disagree, believing that the underlying structure of wandering behaviour was more complex than the scale or model proposed by Albert. Hope *et al.* (1994) collected data on 83 elderly subjects suffering from either Alzheimer's disease or vascular dementia. This more recent study suggested that there were three main categories of wandering behaviour, one

Table 5.1 A descriptive typology of wandering in dementia (from Hope and Fairburn *et al.* 1990)

Checking/trailing	In checking, the subject repeatedly seeks the whereabouts of the carer (or occasionally another person). Trailing appears to be an extreme form of checking in which the subject tends to follow the carer (or another person) around excessively, walking closely behind as he or she walks around.
Pottering	The subject walks around the house and/or garden, apparently trying to carry out tasks (e.g. washing or drying up, cleaning, weeding) of own accord, but ineffectively.
Aimless walking	The subject walks around (either within the house or outside) without there being any evidence of a purpose. This category is not used if there appears to be a purpose, however bizarre, or if the walking meets the criteria for either checking/trailing or pottering.
Walking with inappropriate purpose	The subject's walking appears to be directed towards a purpose, but that purpose is inappropriate (e.g. the subject is searching for a deceased relative). Some definitive evidence for the purpose must be available (e.g. from what the subject says or does). If the purpose is inappropriate only because of excessive repetition of an appropriate purpose (e.g. subject goes shopping many times a day), then it is rated in the next category below.
Walking with appropriate purpose but inappropriate frequency	The subject's walking is directed towards an appropriate purpose (e.g. shopping) but is repeated with inappropriate frequency (e.g. goes to the greengrocer's six times a day).
Excessive activity	The subject is on the move for an abnormally large proportion of the time whilst awake. In the extreme form, the subject does not sit for more than a few minutes at a time. Subjects who are placed in this category will normally also fit into one of the preceding categories.
Night-time walking	The subject walks around inappropriately at night. This category is not used if the subject gets up only to go to the toilet.
Needs to be brought back home	The subject has been brought back to his or her place of residence on at least one occasion. This may be because the subject has been unable to get home without help, but not necessarily so. Others may be concerned and have brought the subject home even though the subjects could have got home by themselves. Often it is not possible to know whether or not the subject could have returned home unaided.
Attempts to leave home	The subject makes attempts to leave his or her place of residence, but carers prevent these attempts. The purpose of this category is to include those whose behaviour might fall into one of the other categories, were it not that their movements were restricted. In most cases the carers restrict the subject's movements because of previous problems associated with one of the other types of wandering.

of which is usefully divided into four subcategories. These authors proposed the following empirically determined structure of abnormal walking (activity disturbance) in dementia:

(1) reduced walking

(2) 'wandering'

    (a) trying to leave home;

    (b) being brought back home;

   (c) 'abnormal walking around'
      (i)   checking/trailing: frequent checking on whereabouts of carer or inappropriate following of carer;
      (ii) increased (hyperactive) aimless walking: walking around distinctly more than normal or without an obvious reason;
      (iii) pottering: ineffectively trying to do household or garden chores;
      (iv) inappropriate or 'over-appropriate' walking: walking around for a reason, but one that is inappropriate.

It is suggested that the latter four groupings are interrelated but that there was no worthwhile distinction between daytime and night-time wandering.

© John Wiley & Sons Limited. Reproduced with permission.

Aetiological basis for wandering-like behaviours

Biological factors

Clinicians have often seen a significant number of patients with motor over-activity which seems to have an underlying neurobiological basis. Some clinicians have termed this 'organic restlessness'. Animal studies have recorded specific brain lesions causing continuous pacing in their subjects (Skinner and Lindsley 1967, Lanier et al. 1975).

There may be some similarities with drug-induced akathisia, although in this clinical situation a subjective feeling of restlessness is crucial for the diagnosis. This often cannot be confirmed in a patient with cognitive impairment. There have been isolated cases of akathisia secondary to stroke disease in the basal ganglia. One author (Henderson et al. 1989) sees the typical cognitive deficits in Alzheimer's disease as responsible for wandering. Henderson describes 'spatial disorientation' as the parietal lobe dysfunction underpinning this behavioural change.

However, in the study of Hope and Fairburns (1990), the subjects who were repeatedly brought back home were not lost but were apparently trying to return to a former home. Therefore, the navigational ability appeared relatively intact, but the subjects suffered from a misidentification syndrome where they believed their real home was not their true home. It is not uncommon in clinical practice for wandering behaviours to be precipitated by the patient experiencing paranoid delusions or visual hallucinosis. The abnormal beliefs of being persecuted or seeing strangers in one's house causes the patient to leave home in terror or in search of safety.

Disturbances in the sleep–wake cycle and circadian rhythm have been suggested as a contributing factor to nocturnal wandering. A Japanese group has shown an absence of normal melatonin rhythm in approximately one-third of a small group of dementia patients when correlated with disturbed sleep–wake cycle and nocturnal wandering (Uchida et al. 1996). It is well known that the suprachiasmatic nucleus (SCN), also known as the 'biological clock', is involved in regulating circadian rhythms (Hoffman and Swaab 1994). The number of vasopressin-producing neurons in the human SCN decreases with normal ageing and is dramatically reduced in Alzheimer's disease. Circadian rhythms are adversely affected by poor light conditions. It has been suggested that institutionalized patients with Alzheimer's disease are generally exposed to less environmental light during the day than aged-matched controls, because they participate in few outdoor activities and watch too much television in dimly lit rooms. Some workers have found that 'bright light treatment' can prevent age-related loss of such neurons in an animal model. (Lucasson et al. 1995). This has been used clinically with some promising initial results (Satlin et al. 1992).

An interesting study in 1996 (Kamei et al. 1996) used a novel intracellular calcium antagonist, Fasudil, for wandering symptoms in patients with vascular dementia. Treatment effects were observed using ^{31}P-magnetic resonance spectroscopy and Xe-computed tomography (CT). Wandering symptoms disappeared in both patients during the treatment and reappeared a few days after discontinuation of the treatment. The magnetic resonance spectroscopy suggested that the wandering symptoms might have been related to a direct effect on intracellular energy metabolism.

A decrease in cell numbers in the SCN in Alzheimer's disease has been reported (Swaab et al.1985). They suggest that disturbance of diurnal rhythms could take one of two forms: either total disruption of rhythms or phase changes. Relatively few subjects in this study showed evidence of a phase shift and the authors remarked that, even in cases of extreme over-activity during the day, half of the subjects were inactive at night.

Psychological factors

It has been suggested that there is a relationship between wandering and premorbid lifestyle, work and ways of handling stress. Premorbid lifestyles were assessed by questionnaires sent to family members and calculation of energy expended on the Metabolic Cost of Activities (MET) scale. The analysis showed no significant correlations between premorbid lifestyle and the amount of wandering behaviour (Linton et al. 1997). Another study looked at premorbid personality and found that, for many people, wandering is an expression of a person's personality ingrained over a lifetime of development, rather than solely an expression of dementia (Thomas 1997). Wandering appeared significantly higher in patients categorized as extroverts with agreeable personality.

Separation anxiety has been identified as a significant component (Stokes 1986). This leads to the patient avoiding being alone and is likely to underlie the categories of checking and trailing described by Hope et al. (1990). The concept of separation anxiety is taken from attachment theory in child development. Hope et al. reported that, in their six subjects with checking and trailing behaviours, over-activity persisted even in the company of the carer, which implies that other factors were at work.

Environmental factors

Wandering commonly occurs with the person living at home and in a 24 h care setting. With regard to the former, being isolated, which can lead boredom and loneliness, can be an important factor. When a person is living alone, there are also, arguably, fewer ties with reality. This can lead to more marked temporal disorientation given the absence of external structure to cue a person's temporal orientation. Similar factors can operate in a 24 h care setting.

The loss of one's personal possessions and mementoes can exacerbate the problem. The practice of converting large Victorian houses into residential or nursing home accommodation, frequently on multiple levels and with labyrinthine corridors, further compounds the person with dementia's impaired spatial orientation. There is a growing consensus on the optimal design of buildings for people with dementia (Marshall 1997). People with dementia rely on visual cues in finding their way around. In a well-designed living space, the use of light, and the lack of complex and intricate wallpaper or carpet design greatly aid a demented person's ability to navigate their way through the home. In an interesting study within a dementia unit of a nursing home (Holmberg 1997), the value of adding a walking programme for physically active persons with severe dementia was assessed. *t*-Test analysis revealed a statistically significant reduction in the frequency of aggression in the 24 h period after the walkers' group. On average there was a reduction in aggressive events by approximately 30%. Other simple environmental manipulations have been suggested to avoid people walking into potentially dangerous areas. One such study (Hussian and Brown 1987) made use of the observation that many demented people perceive two-dimensional patterns as barriers. Grid patterns were made with masking tape over exit doors and there was a significant reduction in patients attempting to leave via these doors.

'Sundowning'

This term is widely used to describe patients who become more confused, agitated and prone to wandering at night. Some authors have quoted sources as far back as Hippocrates in noting this fact (Lipowski 1980, 1989). It is of interest that this phenomenon is not unique to patients with dementia. It has been documented that Parkinson's disease patients may show a greater tendency for 'sundowning' than patients with Alzheimer's disease (Bliwise 1994).

The first anecdotal work in this area was by Cameron (1941), who noted that 'sundowning' could be induced by bringing people with dementia into a dark room during the daytime. The first systematic study (Evans 1987) looked at 89 nursing home patients and found that 12% could be classified as 'sundowners'; this was associated with a more severe level of dementia, recent change of room and a greater number of medical diagnoses. In another study (Cohen-Mansfield *et al.*, 1992b). ratings were made every 3 min over a 24 h period with the Agitated Behavioural Mapping Instrument (ABMI). Vocalizations and physically aggressive behaviours were much more likely to occur between 4.30 p.m. and 11.00 p.m. Another study using systematic observations in nursing homes rated behaviours four times an hour, 24 hours a day over a 10 day period (Bliwise *et al.* 1990). These authors reported evidence to support the concept that sunset may be a vulnerable period for agitation. A contrasting view is held by Exum *et al.* (1993), who looked at the rate of prescribing *'as required'* medication over a 24 h period. These authors suggest that 'sundowning' is a factitious concept, merely reflecting a change of nursing shift at this time and as a result of over-reliance on psychotropic medication. A number of underlying mechanisms have been postulated to explain 'sundowning', including dysfunction of circadian rhythmicity (as described above) together with spontaneous and induced awakenings from sleep (Bliwise 1994).

Clinical assessment

When assessing wandering in a person with dementia, it is important to consider the environment in which the wandering behaviour takes place. This is discussed in full in Chapter 8. It is also helpful to describe the wandering behaviour in terms of the typology outlined above and devised by Hope and Fairburn (1990). The clinician needs to be aware of a number of conditions, which may present to the unwary as a primary problem with 'wandering'. These are outlined below and need to be considered during clinical assessment.

Agitated depression—this is usually obvious in clinical examination of the patient. Diurnal variation, neurovegetative upset and loss of pleasure in usual activities are helpful pointers in this diagnosis. Depressive illness in the elderly may present with marked panic and anxiety symptoms. These can leave to a patient feeling compelled to leave their own house and seek help, often with the fear that they are about to die.

Akathisia—this syndrome of motor restlessness and subjective sense of inner restlessness is commonly seen with neuroleptic medication. It is an extrapyramidal syndrome and is therefore particularly common when conventional neuroleptics are used. Useful clinical pointers are the lack of diurnal variation, inability to sit still even at rest and a likely temporal relationship with commencement or increase in neuroleptic medication. Treatment is to reduce and possibly stop the offending medication.

Psychosis—it is not uncommon for patients to wish to leave their own homes, often at inappropriate times, as a result of psychotic experiences. This often takes the form of visual hallucinations of strangers in their home who are perceived as a threat. Treatment of the primary psychosis is the best initial management.

REFERENCES

Albert, S. M. (1992). The nature of wandering in dementia: a Guttman scaling analysis of an empirical classification scheme. *International Journal of Geriatric Psychiatry*, **7**, 783–7.

Allan, K. (1994). Dementia in acute units: wandering. *Nursing Standard*, **9**(8), 32–4.

Ballard, C. G., Mohen, R. N. C., Bannister, C., Handy, S. and Patel, A. (1991). Wandering in dementia sufferers. *International Journal of Geriatric Psychiatry*, **6**, 611–14.

Bliwise, D. L. (1994). What is sundowning? *Journal of the American Geriatrics Society*, **44**, 1009–11.

Bliwise, D. L., Bevier, W. C., Bliwise, N. G., Edgar, D. M. and Dement, W. C. (1990). Systematic 24-hour behavioural observations of sleep wakefulness in a skilled care nursing facility. *Psychological Aging*, **5**, 16–24.

Bliwise, D. L., Watts, R. L., Watts, N., Rye, D. B., Irbe, D. and Hughes, M. (1994). Caregiver reports of disruptive nocturnal behaviour in Alzheimer's disease and Parkinson's disease. *Sleep Research*, **23**, 352–355.

Burns, A., Jacob, R. and Levy, R. (1990). Psychiatric phenomena in Alzheimer's disease. (IV): Disorders of behaviour. *British Journal of Psychiatry*, **175**, 86–94.

Cameron, D. E. (1941). Studies in senile nocturnal delirium. *Psychiatric Quarterly*, **5**, 47–53.

Cohen-Mansfield, J., Marx, M. S., Werner, P. and Freedman, L. (1992b). Temporal patterns of agitated nursing home residents. *International Psychogeriatrics*, **4**, 197–206.

Cohen-Mansfield, J., Marx, M. S. and Werner, P. (1992a). Agitation in elderly persons: an integrative report of findings in a nursing home. *International Psychogeriatrics*, **4** (Suppl. 4), 221–40.

De Leon, M. J., Potegal, M. and Gurland, B. (1984). Wandering and parietal signs in senile dementia of Alzheimer's type. *Neuropsychobiology*, **11**, 155–7.

Evans, L. K. (1987). Sundown syndrome in institutionalized elderly. *Journal of the American Geriatrics Society*, **35**, 101–8.

Exum, M. E., Phelps, B. J., Nabers, K. E. and Osbourne, J. G. Sundown syndrome: Is it reflected in the use of PRN medications for nursing home residents? *Gerontologist*, 1993, **33**, 756–61.

Greene, J. G., Smith, R., Gardiner, M. and Timbury, G. G. (1982) Measuring behavioural disturbance of elderly demented patients in the community and its effects on relatives: a factor analysis study. *Age and Aging*, **11**, 121–6.

Henderson, V. W., Mack, W. and White-Williams, B. (1989). Spatial disorientation in Alzheimer's disease. *Archives of Neurology*, **46**, 391–4.

Hoffman, M. A. and Swab, D. F. (1994). Alterations in circadian rhythmicity of vasopressin–producing neurones of the human suprachiasmatic nucleus (SCM) with aging. *Brain Research*, **651**, 134–42.

Holmberg, S. K. (1997). Evaluation of a clinical intervention for wanderers on a nursing unit. *Archives of Psychiatric Nursing*, **11**, 21–8.

Hope, R. A. and Fairburn, C. G. (1990). The nature of wandering in dementia: a community based study. *International Journal of Geriatric Psychiatry*, **5**, 239–45.

Hope, A., Tilling, K .M., Gedling, K., Keen, J. M. and Cooper, S. D. (1994). The structure of wandering in dementia. *International Journal of Geriatric Psychiatry*, **9**, 149–55.

Hussian, R. A. and Brown, D. C. (1987). Use of two dimensional grid patterns to limit hazardous ambulation in dementia patients. *Journal of Gerontology*, **42**, 558–60.

Kamei, S., Oishi, M. and Takasu, T. (1996) Evaluation of fasudil hydrochloride treatment for wandering symptoms in cerebrovascular dementia with ^{31}P-magnetic resonance spectroscopy and Xe-computed tomography. *Clinical Neuropharmacology*, **19**, 428–38.

Klein, D. A., Steinberg, M., Galik, E., Steele, C., Sheppard, J. M., Warren, A., Rosenblatt, A. and Lyketsos, C. E. (1999). Wandering behaviour in community-residing persons with dementia. *International Journal of Geriatric Psychiatry*, **14**, 272–9.

Lanier, I. P., Petit, T. L. and Zornetzer, S. F. (1975). Discrete anterior medial thalamic lesions in the mouse: the production of acute post-operative hyperactivity and death. *Brain Research*, **91**, 133–9.

Lipowski, Z. J. (1980). *Delirium. Acute Brain Failure in Man*. Charles C. Thomas, Springfield, Illinois.

Lipowski, Z. J. (1989). Delirium in the elderly patient. *New England Journal of Medicine*, **320**, 578–82.

Linton, A. D., Matteson, M. A. and Byers, D. (1997). The relationship between premorbid lifestyle and wandering behaviour in institutionalised people with dementia. *Aging (Milan)*, **9**, 415–18.

Lucasson, P. J., Hoffman, M. A. and Swaab, D. F. (1995). Increased light intensity prevents the age related loss of vasopressin-expressing neurones in the rat suprachiasmatic nucleus (SCN). *Brain Research*, **693**, 261–6.

Margo, J. L., Robinson, J. R. and Corea, S. (1980). Referrals to a psychiatric service from old people's homes. *British Journal of Psychiatry*, **136**, 396–401.

Manser, M. and Marshall, M. (1997). Better quality environments for people with dementia. In *Psychiatry in the Elderly*, 2nd edn (Jacoby, R. and Oppenheimer, C., eds), pp. 411–435. Oxford University Press, Oxford.

Rabins, P., Mace, M. and Lucas, M. (1982). The impact of dementia on the family. *Journal of the American Medical Association*, **248**, 333–5.

Sanford, J. (1975). Tolerance of disability in elderly dependants by supporters at home: its significance for hospital practice. *British Medical Journal*, **iii**, 471–4.

Satlin, A., Valicer, L., Ross, V., Herz, L. and Campbell, S. (1992). Bright light treatment of behavioural and sleep disturbances in patients with Alzheimer's disease. *American Journal of Psychiatry*, **149**, 1028–32.

Skinner, J. E. and Lindsley, D. B. (1967). Electrophysiological and behavioural effects of blockade of the non-specific thalamo-cortical system. *Brain Research*, **6**, 95–118.

Snyder, L. H., Ruppriecht, P., Pyrek, J., Brekhus, S. and Moss, T. (1978). Wandering. *Gerontologist*, **18**, 272–80.

Stokes, G. (1986). *Common Problems with the Elderly Confused. Wandering*. Winslow Press, London.

Swaab, D. F., Fliers, F. E. and Partiman, T. S (1985). The suprachiasmatic nucleus of the human brain in relation to sex, age, and senile dementia. *Brain Research*, **342**, 37–44.

Teri, L., Larson, F. B. and Reifler, B. V. (1988). Behavioural disturbance in dementia of the Alzheimer type. *Journal of the American Geriatrics Society*, **36**, 1–6.

Thomas, D. W. (1997). Understanding the wandering patient. A continuity of personality perspective. *Journal of Gerontological Nursing*, **23**, 16–24.

Uchida, K., Okamoto, N., Ohara, K. and Morita, Y. (1996). Daily rhythm of serum melatonin in patients with dementia of the degenerative type. *Brain Research*, **717**, 154–9.

6 Aggression

Introduction

Aggression is common amongst people with dementia. Aggressive behavioural problems are the single most common cause of referral into psychiatric services in old people's homes (Margo *et al.* 1980, Clarke *et al.* 1981) and it is the commonest cause for institutionalization (Reisberg *et al.* 1986). Up to 20% of the families of people with dementia report physical violence as a 'serious' care problems (Rabins *et al.* 1982, Argyle *et al.* 1985, Colerick and George 1986, O'Connor 1990, MacPherson *et al.* 1994, Coen *et al.* 1997). In addition, aggressive behaviour is a significant source of distress for formal carers within a nursing home setting (Everitt *et al.* 1991, MacPherson *et al.* 1994). It also is an important factor in the use of physical restraint (Werner *et al.* 1989) and over-medication (Cohen-Mansfield 1986, Billing *et al.* 1991, Martin *et al.* 1994).

The extent and importance of the problem

Despite the obvious importance of this behaviour, relatively little is known about its causes and treatment. Some authors speculate that there may have been a view that changes in behaviour are secondary to cognitive impairment and are therefore of relatively little interest (Fairburn and Hope 1998). Other authors see aggressive behaviour as an expression of personality change (Dian *et al.* 1990, Rubins *et al.* 1987a,b). A further problem has been that of syndrome definition. Aggressive behaviour has been mainly studied under the broad description of behavioural disturbance or 'agitated behaviour'. Recent research suggests that robust behavioural syndromes can be identified from among the widely heterogeneous behavioural changes, which occur in dementia (Hope *et al.* 1997). Aggressive behaviour forms one of these three distinct syndromes together with over-activity and psychosis.

Definitions and concepts

Aggression

There is no generally agreed definition of aggressive behaviour, particularly in patients with dementia. Most definitions of aggression include within them the notion of intention. For example, Moyer (1976) defined aggressive behaviour as 'overt behaviour involving intent to inflict noxious stimulation or to behave destructively towards another organism'. Possibly the most useful definition of aggression in the elderly with dementia is that 'aggressive behaviour is an overt act, involving the delivery of noxious stimuli to (but not necessarily aimed at) another organism, object or self, which is clearly not accidental' (Patel and Hope 1992a). These authors point out that the concept of intention is both difficult to identify and may be inappropriate to use with people who are cognitively impaired.

The definition of aggressive behaviours is compounded further by staff minimizing behavioural problems with the assumption that they are to be expected in people with dementia. Clear descriptions of the behaviours are encouraged. These should be observable manifestations with as few assumptions as possible. Whether an act is classified as aggressive or not, should not be dependent on the consequence of the behaviour, e.g. someone being hurt. Therefore, precise descriptions of behavioural manifestations within the dementias are the starting point for theories of aetiology, the existence of discernible behavioural syndromes (Hope *et. al.* 1997) and whether these correlate with particular dementia types or change as the dementia syndrome progresses.

Personality change

In clinical practice it is not uncommon to hear a problematic behaviour being attributed to a 'change in personality'. The concept of personality refers to a person's enduring and persistence responses across a variety of situations. When a person's automatic behaviours occur in a pervasive manner in a wide range of settings, there may be some justification for this view. However, there are difficulties when these concepts are applied to people with dementia or other brain damage:

(1) There is insufficient knowledge at present to be clear on the relationship between behaviour change and brain damage in dementia.

(2) The term 'personality' infrequently implies the core of a persons being, and therefore, any label such as 'an aggressive personality' is both judgmental and pejorative.

(3) It may also instil a false sense of therapeutic nihilism (Hope 1992, Hope and Patel 1993).

Agitation

This term is used frequently to describe disturbed behaviours in people with dementia. It is unsatisfactory on a number of levels:

(1) It is imprecise and can cover a range of conditions including delirium and depressive illness as well as behavioural problems associated with dementia.

(2) It implies a subjective experience of inner restlessness, which is often not possible to validate.

(3) The lack of precision in the term can also lead to a lack of sophistication in approach to managing the problem, which may result in the unthinking prescription of a sedative drug.

An operational definition of agitation has been developed by Cohen-Mansfield and Billing (1986) on the basis of studies done within a nursing home environment. These authors defined agitation as 'inappropriate verbal, vocal or motor activity that is not explained by needs or confusion *per se*'. They went on to describe it as always being inappropriate and that this was manifest in three categories of inappropriateness:

(1) the person may be abusive towards self and others;

(2) appropriate behaviour may be performed but with inappropriate frequency, such as constantly asking questions;

(3) behaviour may be inappropriate according to social standards for a specific situation.

Prevalence and incidence

Physical aggression occurs in 18–65% of patients with dementia (Rabins *et al.* 1982, Reisberg *et al.* 1987, Ryden 1988, Swearer *et al.* 1988, Burns *et al.* 1990, Hamel *et al.* 1990). More precise figures of incidence are difficult to define as patients with aggression are found within studies looking at imprecisely defined agitation.

Most studies report no firm association with age (Patel and Hope 1992, Shah 1993, Gibbons *et al.* 1997). There are some conflicting reports suggesting an association with physically violent behaviour in men (Eastley and Wilcock 1987). In terms of the relationship of aggresive behaviour with the natural history of their illness, Reisberg *et al.* (1989) found it to peak in patients with moderate to severe dementia. However, Mega *et al.* (1996) found that agitation increased from 47% in Alzheimer's disease patients with mild dementia (Mini Mental State Examinations (MMSE) score 21–30) to 85% in patients with severe dementia (MMSE score 0–10). These authors also reported a correlation between agitation and irritability. However, in patients with mild dementia it correlated with anxiety, whereas in patients with moderate dementia it correlated with only delusions and hallucinations. Mega *et al.* pointed out that these different associations might reflect changing determinants of agitation across the spectrum of severity of Alzheimer's disease.

A recent, prospective, 10 year longitudinal study of aggressive behaviour in dementia with autopsy follow-up (Keene *et al.* 1999) identified verbal aggression as the commonest and longest-lasting form of aggressive behaviour. Aggressive resistance and physical aggression are most likely to persist until death. Intimate care is the main factor precipitating aggressive behaviour. Keene *et al.* found no correlations between any type of aggressive behaviour and age, gender or duration of dementia. In another longitudinal study, Cohen-Mansfield and Werner (1998) described a follow-up study of 104 community-dwelling residents who attended daycare centres. People with increased verbal and physical aggressive behaviours had significantly greater decline in cognitive functioning and increased depression at baseline. Increases in physical aggression also correlated with greater cognitive impairment at baseline.

Other factors relating to aggression in patients with Alzheimer's disease are an inability to perform activities in daily living, such as dressing and bathing (Deutsch and Rovner 1991, Cohen-Mansfield *et al.* 1992, Dougherty *et al.* 1992), and a poor relationship between patient and carer (Hamel *et al.* 1990). A strong association exists between physical aggression and the presence of depressive and psychotic symptoms. It has been shown that these associations are robust, remaining significant over 4 years of follow up, and that they are independent of cognitive function, age, sex and duration of illness (Deutsch *et al.* 1991, Lopez *et al.* 1991, Aarsland *et al.* 1996 and Lyketos *et al.* 1999). McShane *et al.* (1998) in an important longitudinal study found that physical aggression was predicted by depressed mood whilst motor hyperactivity was predicted by persecutory ideas.

Neurobiological basis for aggressive behaviour

There is an increasing acceptance that behavioural disorder forms part of the fundamental core of the dementia syndrome. Taking this hypothesis further suggests there is a likely underlying pathological and neurochemical substrate for such behavioural abnormalities. It also provides a rationale for the treatment of behavioural disorder by psychotropic medication. The norepinephrine and serotonin (5-HT) neurotransmitter systems project from subcortical nuclei to the cortex and both are affected by Alzheimer's disease. This is supported by animal studies in which these pathways are lesioned (Foote *et al.* 1983). It is given further support by the knowledge that drugs acting on these systems are known to influence behaviour in both animals and humans (Glennon 1990).

Norepinephrine

There have been no studies directly linking norepinephrine with behavioural disturbance in Alzheimer's disease. However, there is some indirect evidence. Raskind *et al.* (1993) reported an exaggerated increase in cerebrospinal fluid (CSF) epinephrine secondary to α_2 receptor blockade in patients with Alzheimer's disease. This led to the development of agitation and psychotic symptoms. Other compensatory mechanisms include an increase in cortical β_2-adrenergic receptors (Kalaria *et al.* 1989). This may explain the therapeutic effects of propanolol, a β-adrenergic receptor antagonist which, in some open studies, reduces aggressive behaviour in Alzheimer's disease and other dementias (Yudofsky 1981, Petrie and Ban 1987, Weiler *et al.* 1988). Thus impaired noradrenergic production may be associated with depression (see Chapter 4) and over-compensation may induce psychosis or aggressive behaviour.

Serotonin

There is a reasonable body of evidence linking reduced serotonergic levels to aggressive behaviour in patients with schizophrenia and depression (Brown *et al.* 1982). The serotonergic system is affected by Alzheimer's disease pathology. This is confirmed by a number of strands of evidence ranging from autopsy studies (Cross *et al.* 1984) to reduced 5-hydroxyindoleacetic acid (5-HIAA), the 5-HT metabolite in CSF of patients with Alzheimer's disease (Soininen *et al.* 1981). This evidence is further supported by receptor-binding studies showing marked reductions in pre- and post-synaptic 5-HT receptor binding (Bowen *et al.* 1983, Cross *et al.* 1986, Palmer *et al.* 1987). These studies have found complex alterations in 5-HT in Alzheimer's disease. A detailed overview of the complex changes in neurochemistry in Alzheimer's disease is contained in a useful editorial (Esiri 1996).

There is evidence to suggest that the increased turnover of 5-HT in patients with Alzheimer's disease (as reflected by low CSF 5-HIAA) is normally compensated for in unmedicated Alzheimer's disease patients. However, in the presence of neuroleptic drugs, no such compensation takes place (Chen 1996). This adds further caution to the use of neuroleptics in patients with Alzheimer's disease (see Chapter 14).

Initial studies in humans appear consistent with the extensive animal studies showing a strong correlation between low 5-HT levels and aggression (Van Pragg 1991). The postulated mechanisms of reduced 5-HT and clinical depression and psychosis in Alzheimer's disease was reviewed in Chapters 3 and 4. There is some evidence linking these changes in 5-HT metabolism in Alzheimer's disease with aggressive behaviour. A prospective behavioural study found no correlation between neuronal loss in the raphe nucleus and behavioural disturbances (Chen 1994). There is a post-mortem study which found a significant link between cortical 5-HT and agitated behaviour (Palmer *et al.* 1988). A 'hyper-responsive' 5-HT system in Alzheimer's disease was suggested using the sereotonergic agonist *meta*-chlorophenylpiperazine (m-CPP) (Lawlor *et al.* 1989).

Acetylcholine

The central importance of reduced acetylcholine in Alzheimer's disease is widely accepted, as is the correlation between reduction in cholinergic transmission and the severity of cognitive impairment (Davies and Maloney 1976, Perry *et al.* 1978, Wilcock *et al.* 1982). There is a suggestion that aggressive behaviour may be mediated via cholinergic pathways (Smith *et al.* 1978). Similar changes have been shown in patients with dementia with Lewy bodies in whom they have been linked with psychosis (Perry *et al.* 1993).

Neuropathology

The most helpful study has been that of Förstl *et al.* (1993), based upon the Camberwell case register cohort. Key elements of Kluver–Bucy syndrome (hyperorality, rage reactions, hypermetamorphosis and visual agnosia) were associated with lower cell counts in the parietal cortex and parahippocampal gyrus. Interestingly, there was no association with the severity of pathology in subcortical nuclei. It is suggested, therefore, that decreased cortical inhibition in the presence of preserved subcortical structures may cause this neuropsychiatric syndrome. Relative preservation of subcortical structures is supported by a further study (Victoroff *et al.* 1996) who found that aggressive patients have better preservation of the substantia nigra than non-aggressive Alzheimer's disease patients.

Neuroimaging

Structural neuroimaging has shown that temporal lobe atrophy (Burns *et al.* 1990) and inferior parietal lobe atrophy (Swigar *et al.* 1995) show associations with aggressive behaviour. Functional neuroimaging using Positron Emission Tomography (PET) scanning shows that agitation is correlated with decreased frontal and temporal cortical metabolic rate (Sultzer *et al.* 1995, Sultzer 1996).

Classification of aggressive behaviours

The difficulties in constructing a satisfactory system for classifying these behaviours are manifold. These behaviours rarely occur as single isolated events but more often cluster with other psychiatric and behavioural symptoms (Baker *et al.* 1991). Baker's group reported that 57% of their Alzheimer's disease group had such a mixture of symptoms. Studies have frequently been anecdotal or, at best, a range of different behaviours have been subsumed under generalized terms such as 'agitation'. The semantic difficulties encountered with commonly used descriptive terms have been outlined above. A further confounding factor is that studies are often of different patient groups and of a variety of different settings ranging from in-patient psychogeriatric wards to community settings. Furthermore, classification of abnormal behaviour in dementia could take the form of an operational description of the behaviour or could be by the setting in which the behaviour occurred (for example, during intimate care). Despite these difficulties, some progress has been made in the use of multivariate statistics examining the relationship between different types of behavioural change.

Cohen-Mansfield *et al.* (1992) studied residents within nursing-home settings using the Cohen-Mansfield Agitation Inventory (CMAI) (see Table 6.1). Their results suggest a three-factor model of agitation (see Table 6.2):

Table 6.1 Behaviours rated on the Cohen-Mansfield Agitation Inventory

Pacing/aimless wandering	Scratching
Inappropriate dressing or undressing	Trying to get to a different place
Spitting	Intentional falling
Cursing or verbal aggression	Complaining
Constant unwarranted requests for attention or help	Negativism
	Eating inappropriate substances
Repetitive sentences or questions	Hurting self or others
Hitting	Handling things inappropriately
Kicking	Hiding things
Grabbing	Hoarding things
Pushing	Tearing things
Throwing things	Repetitious mannerisms
Making strange noises	Verbal sexual advances
Screaming	Physical sexual advances
Biting	General restlessness

Table 6.2 Subtypes of agitation (from Cohen-Mansfield *et al.* 1992)

Physically non-aggressive behaviours
- general restlessness
- repetitious mannerisms
- pacing
- trying to get to a different place
- handling things inappropriately
- hiding things
- inappropriate dressing or undressing
- repetitive sentences

Verbally non-aggressive behaviours
- negativism
- does not like anything
- constant requests for attention
- verbal bossiness
- complaining or whining
- relevant interruptions
- irrelevant interruptions

Physically aggressive behaviours
- hitting
- pushing
- scratching
- grabbing things
- grabbing people
- kicking and biting

Verbally aggressive behaviours
- screaming
- cursing
- temper outbursts
- making strange noises

(By Permission Cohen-Mansfield J., Marx M.S., Werner P. Agitation in elderly persons: an integrative report of findings in a nursing home. In International Psychogeriatrics, 4 Suppl. 4 221–40)

(1) aggressive behaviour, including physical and verbal aggression;

(2) physically non-aggressive behaviour, such as pacing, restlessness and wandering;

(3) verbally non-aggressive behaviour, such as repeated requests for attention.

It is of note, however, that not all the patients studied suffered from dementia.

Using the Behavioural Symptom Scale for Dementia (BSSD), Devanand *et al.* (1992) showed two main symptom groupings—the syndromes of disinhibition and apathy/indifference.

A more recent study (Hope *et al.* 1997) looked at patients in community settings using the Present Behavioural Examination (PBE). From this work emerged three robust syndromes (see Table 6.3):

Table 6.3 Brief definitions of the behavioural items in the three behavioural 'syndromes' (from Hope *et al.* 1997)

Over-activity	
• walking more	walking distinctly more than is normal
• aimless walking	walking aimlessly without an obvious reason
• trailing and checking	needing frequent reassurance of presence of carer either by following or by frequent checking location of carer
Aggressive behaviour	
• aggressive resistance	resisting attempt to help, or being uncooperative, usually in the context of intimate care
• physical aggression	e.g. hitting, kicking, scratching, pushing or spitting in an aggressive manner
• verbal aggression and hostility	speaking in an aggressive or cross tone or with voice raised in anger
Psychosis	
• hallucinations	hears or sees things that are not really there
• persecutory ideas	says something that suggests s/he thought people were trying to harm or plot against him/her or trying to steal property
• anxiety	very anxious or frightened (out of all proportion to stimulus)

(1) over-activity (walking more, walking aimlessly, 'trailing' their carer or checking where the carer was);

(2) aggressive behaviour (physical aggression, excessive resistance, verbal aggression);

(3) psychosis (anxiety, persecutory ideas and hallucinations).

These results confirm previous findings of a strong association between verbal and physical aggression (Cohen-Mansfield *et al.* 1992). It was, however, at odds with the proposed concept of 'agitated behaviour' by the same authors. Cohen-Mansfield *et al.* suggested that hyperactivity, aggressive behaviour and anxiety are closely linked justifying this concept of 'agitated behaviour'. However, the study of Hope *et al.* suggests that each of these types of behaviour is a distinct separate syndrome.

It has also been hypothesized that the setting in which aggressive behaviour occurs may relate to aetiology and optimal management (Ware *et al.* 1990). For example, whether a patient is physically or verbally aggressive may be of less aetiological significance than if the behaviour occurs during intimate care. Aggressive responses can commonly occur following having been told what to do, in response to having been prevented from undertaking an inappropriate task, at night, in response to aggressive behaviour in others, etc. This concept of the importance of the environment and social cues is developed further in Chapter 8.

Rating scales

Until relatively recently, the study of behavioural problems in the dementias has been handicapped by the lack of valid and reliable assessment instruments. As discussed earlier, early studies involved anecdotal unstructured descriptions of behaviour or a small series of cases. It is worth noting that unstructured reporting records five times fewer episodes of aggressive behaviour than structured daily ward reports (Lian *et al.* 1981). However, in the last decade a plethora of new scales has been published for assessing aggressive behaviour in demented elderly patients. These scales differ according to:

- the source of information (formal or informal caregiver);
- type of behaviour (mood or agitation);
- origin of the scale (imported from psychiatry or neurology or specifically designed for the demented elderly population);
- the proposed application of the rating scale (use in community or institutional settings);
- the availability of supportive psychometric data;
- the practicality of the test in terms of the training needs of the staff, the time interval of the assessment and the costs of the assessment in the widest sense.

Brief outline of rating scales in common use

Behavioural Pathology in Alzheimer's Disease (BEHAVE-AD) (Reisberg et al. *1987)*

This is a semi-structured interview that measures behavioural disturbance and psychotic symptoms by interviewing carers. The seven items address behaviour covering activity disturbances, aggressiveness and diurnal variation. There is good evidence of inter-rater reliability in Alzheimer's disease (Patterson *et al.* 1990, Sclan *et al.* 1996). The scale is discussed in more detail in Chapter 2.

The Present Behavioural Examination (PBE) (Hope and Fairburn 1992)

This is a semi-structured interview that was developed to be given by a trained interviewer and takes between 1 and 1.5 h to administer. The interview is with the main carer and a wide range of behaviour is covered. The PBE has been designed to be sensitive to change. There is evidence of good reproducibility and inter-rater reliability. There is also a section on mental and physical health. Subsections of the interview can be used separately, for example the aggressive behaviour subsection (Ware *et al.* 1990).

The Behaviour of Severity Rating Scale (BSRS) (Swearer et al. *1988)*

This looks at the relationship between disease severity and behavioural disturbance. It has nine behavioural items and two mood items. In the initial study the scale was rated on the basis of a telephone interview with the carer.

The Nurses Observation Scale for Geriatric Patients (NOSGER) (Spiegel et al. *1991)*

This has been developed for use by untrained nurses or caregivers for patients in care or at home. It is a 30-item scale measuring the frequency of different types of behaviour. Only 10 items measure behaviour (five social behaviour and five disturbed behaviour). The other items are concerned with memory, mood and activities of daily living. There was evidence of good reproducibility upon retesting and of concurrent validity.

The Caretaker Obstreperous Behaviour Rating Assessment (COBRA) (Drachman et al. 1992)

This measures the frequency and severity of 30 behavioural items including aggressive behaviour. Each item is operationally defined. Caregivers have been given formal training to use the instrument via videos. It has good reproducibility and inter-rater reliability.

The Nursing Home Behaviour Problem Scale (Ray et al. 1992)

This is a 29-item inventory designed to be used by nursing staff in care homes. It rates behavioural problems occurring over the preceding 3 days on a five-point scale. It has good inter-rater reliability, convergent validity and criterion validity.

The Disruptive Behaviour Rating Scale (DBRS) (Mungas et al. 1984)

This has been designed for use in nursing homes and measures behavioural disturbance over the previous 7 days. It utilizes behaviour checklists and interviews with nursing staff. It has good inter-rater reliability, concurrent and convergent validity though it can be time-consuming to administer.

Behavioural Syndrome Scale for Dementia (BSSD) (Devenand et al. 1992)

Twenty-four behavioural items are assessed using a semi-structured interview of caregivers over the preceding week on a seven-point rating scale. It shows good validity and reliability and is sensitive to change.

Behavioural Disturbance Scale (BDS) (Baumgarten et al. 1990)

This is a 28-item semi-structured interview by trained clinicians to community-dwelling caregivers of dementia sufferers. A range of behaviours are assessed, which may have occurred in the preceding week. There is good evidence of validity and reliability.

Memory and Behaviour Problem Checklist (Zarit et al. 1980)

This is a semi-structured interview administered by trained clinicians to caregivers of dementia suffers living at home. It provides three scores: a summed reaction to the presence of problems, a summed frequency of problem behaviour and a score relating to the product of the frequency and reaction scores. It measures 29 specific items and has an open-ended 'other problem item'. The scale includes items on aggressive behaviour, activities of daily living, apraxias and four items on 'spatial disorientation'. These four items are: wandering, getting lost indoors, getting lost in familiar streets, and inability to recognize familiar surroundings. These latter four items have been used in a study the relationship between visual spatial dysfunction and wandering (Henderson *et al.* 1989).

Cohen-Mansfield Agitation Inventory (CMAI) (Cohen-Mansfield 1986)

This is rated by nurses at the end of each 8 h shift over a 24 h period, therefore providing three sets of ratings. There are 29 behaviour items organized around four components of 'agitation', namely agitation, aggression, physical non-aggressive behaviour and hiding/hoarding. There are also items on abnormal eating behaviour. The CMAI has good inter-rater reliability and concurrent validity and has been used by a variety of different research groups in different settings.

Ryden Aggression Scale (RAS) (Ryden 1988)

This is a 25-item scale with three subscales: physical aggressive behaviour, verbal aggressive behaviour and sexual behaviour. It measures aggressive behaviour for up to 1 year previously. There is information on test–retest reproducibility but not on validity. The RAS is considered quick, user-friendly and cheap (Shah 1999).

Overt Aggression Scale (OAS) (Yudofsky et al. 1986)

This was originally developed for psychiatric in-patients and not specifically for the elderly. It has operationally defined components and is completed by nursing staff. There are 69 items, which measure verbal aggression, physical aggression against objects, physical aggression against self and others, and severity. There are inter-rater reliability data but this has not been studied in an in-patient psychogeriatric setting.

Staff Observation Aggression Scale (SOAS) (Palmsteirna and Wistedt 1987)

This scale analyses individual episodes of aggressive behaviour. It also measures potential precipitants of the behaviour. Data shows good reliability and construct validity. The SOAS uses the nature of staff intervention as an indicator of severity of behaviour.

Rating of Aggressive Behaviour in the Elderly (RAGE) (Patel and Hope 1992a)

This consists of 23 items, the majority of which are rated on a four-point scale of frequency. A global aggression score is obtained by adding all the ratings. It is used by nursing staff at the end of a 3 day period of observation. Psychometric studies show good reliability and validity, and sensitivity to change. Inter-rater reliability is significantly improved with the use of a ward checklist. RAGE has therefore been recommended for the longitudinal assessment of the natural history of aggressive behaviour and for treatment trials.

Brief Agitation Rating Scale (BARS) (Finkel et al. 1993)

This 10-item scale has been developed from the CMAI and is designed to be used by nursing assistants to measure agitation in nursing-home residents. It has been shown to have good inter-rater reliability and validity.

Despite the growing range of available scales to measure behavioural disturbance in the elderly with dementia, no single scale is deemed superiorto another. The majority have mixed components, often including neuropsychiatric symptoms and cognitive dysfunction in addition to behavioural problems. Other scales are focused on specific behavioural difficulties such as agressive behaviour. As research in this area continues, the relative usefulness of these various scales will become more apparent. The CMAI has good construct validity and has been the most widely used.

Clinical assessment of aggression

Information gathering and history taking

There are a number of broad-based principles underpinning clinical assessment of elderly people.

(1) Always take a collateral history, ideally from a relative or someone who has known the patient for a significant period of time. If a patient is in a residential/nursing home, the carer who knows most about the patient should be seen. It is most helpful to get the collateral history *before* interviewing and examining the patient. A good collateral history is worth more than multiple brain scans and blood tests!

(2) Get a clear description of the problematic behaviours together with the antecedents and consequences of these behaviours. Seek clarification if terms such as 'agitation' or 'resistive' are used.

(3) Find out the frequency and duration of the behaviour. Is there an emerging pattern? What was the event that precipitated this referral? Are there any warning signs that staff believe may herald the beginning of an episode of challenging behaviour?

(4) Premorbid personality is important, particularly previous aggressive behaviours, temper outbursts, etc.

Making a diagnostic formulation

It is useful to think of the behavioural presentation as a potential epiphenomenon of other primary physical and psychiatric disorders.

Physical problems—a wide range of conditions can present with a delirium (most commonly drug reactions, infections and organ failures). Useful clinical clues include fluctuating drowsiness, worsening at night, fleeting visual hallucinosis and failure to recognize the familiar (e.g. thinking a hospital ward is home or a relative is a stranger.)

Pain—a person with cognitive impairment may not find it easy to express that they are experiencing pain.

Constipation—a causal association between behavioural problems and bowel habit can be highlighted by observant nursing staff. Faecal incontinence in the absence of urinary incontinence suggests faecal impaction with overflow.

Depression—this may not present with symptoms of sadness of mood. Useful clues are a diurnal variation (worse in the morning), a past history of depression, loss of appetite, sleep disturbance and a loss of enjoyment of previously valued activities (e.g. visits from grandchildren). See Chapter 4 for further discussion.

Paranoid psychosis—due to its fleeting nature, this may be difficult to detect. Direct closed questions of carers are often required to elicit symptoms, e.g. 'Does your relative ever say or imply that people are trying to harm them or cause them trouble?' See Chapter 3.

Seizure disorder—in the absence of a generalized convulsion, this is often missed. Any episodes of *petit mal* occurring *de novo* in the elderly are, by definition, complex partial seizures, which can present with aggression. Other helpful clues are the sudden episodic unprovoked nature of the aggression, associated urinary incontinence, the presence of motor automatisms (e.g. lip smacking) and a tendency to go into a deep unrousable sleep after the episode. It is not uncommon for complex partial seizures to be misdiagnosed as transient ischaemic attacks.

In the absence of evidence of other primary physical or psychiatric conditions, it is reasonable to assume that the aggressive behaviour is a result either of primary brain changes from the dementia or of the interaction of these brain changes and the person's care environment. The assessment of the person in their environment is described in detail in Chapter 8.

REFERENCES

Aarsland, D., Cummings, J. L., Yenner, G. and Miller, B. (1996). Relationship of aggressive behaviour to other neuropsychiatric symptoms in patients with Alzheimer's disease. *American Journal of Psychiatry*, **153**, 243–7.

Argyle, N., Jestice, S. and Brook, C. P. B. (1985). Psychogeriatric patients: their supporters' problems. *Age and Aging*, **14**, 355–60.

Baker, F. M., Kokmen, E., Chandra, V. (1991). Psychomatic symptoms in cases of clinically diagnosed Alzheimer's disease. *Journal of Geriatric Psychology and Neurology*, **4**, 71–8.

Baumgarten, M., Becker, R. and Gauthier, S. (1990). Validity and reliability of the dementia behaviour disturbance scale. *Journal of the American Geriatrics Society*, **38**, 221–6.

Billing, N., Cohen-Mansfield, J. and Lipson, S. (1991). Pharmacological treatment of agitation in a nursing home. *Journal of the American Geriatrics Society*, **39**, 1002–5.

Bowen, D. N., Allen, S. J. and Benton, J. S. (1983). Biochemical assessment of serotonergic and cholinergic dysfunction and cerebral atrophy in Alzheimer's disease. *Journal of Neurochemistry*, **41**, 266–72.

Brown, G. L., Ebert, M. H., Goyer, P. F., Jimerson, D. C., Klein, W. J., Bunney, W. E. and Goodwin, F. K. (1982). Aggression, suicide and serotonin: relationship to CSF amine metabolites. *American Journal of Psychiatry*, **139**, 741–6.

Burns, A., Jacoby, R. and Levy, R. (1990). Psychiatric phenomena in Alzheimer's disease. IV: Disorders of behaviour. *British Journal of Psychiatry*, **157**, 86–94.

Chen, C. P., Eastwood, S. L. and MacDonald, B. (1994). Patterns and markers of cell loss in dorsal raphe nucleus in Alzheimer's disease. *Neuropathology and Applied Neurobiology*, **20**, 503.

Chen, C. P., Alder, J. T., Bowen, D. M., Esiri, M. M., McDonald, B., Tope, T., Jobst, K. A. and Francis, P. T. (1996). Presynaptic serotonergic markers in community-acquired cases of Alzheimer's disease: correlations with depression and neuroleptic medications. *Journal of Neurochemistry*, **66**, 1592–8.

Clarke, M. G., Williams, A. J. and Jones, P. A. (1981). A psychogeriatric survey of old people's homes. *British Medical Journal*, **283**, 1307–9.

Coen, R. F., Swanwick, G. R., Boyle, C. A. and Coakley, D. (1997). Behaviour disturbance and other predictors of carer burden in Alzheimer's disease. *International Journal of Geriatric Psychiatry*, **12**, 331–6.

Cohen-Mansfield, J. (1986). Agitated behaviour in the elderly. II: Preliminary results in the cognitively deteriorated. *Journal of the American Geriatrics Society*, **34**, 722–7.

Cohen-Mansfield, J. and Billing, N. (1986) Agitated behaviours in the elderly. 1: A conceptual review. *Journal of the American Geriatrics Society*, **34**, 711–21.

Cohen-Mansfield, J. and Werner, P. (1998). Longitudinal changes in behavioural problems in old age: a study in an adult day care population. *Journal of Gerontology Biological Sciences and Medical Sciences*, **53**, 765–71.

Cohen-Mansfield, J., Marx, M. S. and Werner, P. (1992). Agitation in elderly persons: an integrative report of findings in a nursing home. *International Psychogeriatrics*, **4** (Suppl. 4), 221–40.

Colerick, E. J. and George, L. K. (1986). Predictors of institutionalization among care givers of patients with Alzheimer's disease. *Journal of the American Geriatrics Society*, **34**, 493–8.

Cross, A. J., Crowe, T. J. and Ferrer, I. N. (1984). Serotonin receptor changes in dementia of Alzheimer type. *Journal of Neurochemistry*, **53**, 1574–81.

Cross, A. J., Crowe, T. J., Ferrer, I. N., Johnson, J. A., Peters, T. J. and Reynolds, G. P. (1986). The selectivity of a reduction of 5HT2 receptors in Alzheimer-type dementia. *Neurobiological Aging*, **7**, 3–7.

Cummings, J. L., Mega, M., Gray, K., Rosenberg, B., Thompson, S., Corusi, D. A. and Gornbein, J. (1994). The Neuropsychiatric Inventory: comprehensive assessment of psycho-pathology in dementia, *Neurology*, **44**, 2308–14.

Davies, P. and Maloney, A. R. J. (1976). Selective loss of central cholinergic neurones in Alzheimer's disease. *Lancet*, **ii**, 1403.

Deutsch, L. H. and Rovner, B. W. (1991). Agitation and other non-cognitive abnormalities in Alzheimer's disease. *Psychiatric Clinics of North America*, **14**, 341–51.

Deutsch, L. H., Bylsma, F. W. and Rovner, B. W. (1991). Psychosis and physical aggression in probable Alzheimer's disease. *American Journal of Psychiatry*, **148**, 159–63.

Devanand, D. P., Brockingham, C. D., Moody, B. J., Brown, R. R. P., Mayeux, R., Eendicott, J. and Sacheim, H. A. (1992). Behavioural syndromes in Alzheimer's disease. *International Psychogeriatrics*, **4** (Suppl. 2), 161–89.

Dian, L., Cummings, J. L., Petry, S. and Hill, M. A. (1990). Personality alterations in multi-infarct dementia. *Psychosomatics*, **4**, 415–19.

Dougherty, L. M., Bolger, J. P. and Preston, D. G. (1992). Effects of exposure to aggressive behaviour on job satisfaction of health care staff. *Journal of Applied Gerontology*, **11**, 160–72.

Drachman, D. A., Swearer, J. M., O'Donnell, B. F., Mitchell, A. L. and Maloon, A. (1992). The Caretaker Obstreperous-Behaviour Rating Assessment (COBRA) scale. *Journal of the American Geriatrics Society*, **40**, 463–80.

Eastley, R. J. and Wilcock, G. (1997). Prevalence and correlates of aggressive behaviours occurring in patients with Alzheimer's disease. *International Journal of Geriatric Psychiatry*, **12**, 484–7.

Esiri, M. M. (1996). The basis for behavioural disturbances in dementia (Editorial). *Journal of Neurology, Neurosurgery and Psychiatry*, **61**, 127–30.

Everitt, D. E., Fields, D. R., Soumerai, S. S. and Avorn, J. (1991). Resident behaviour and staff distress in the nursing home. *Journal of the American Geriatrics Society*, **39**, 792–8.

Fairburn, C. G. and Hope, R. A. (1988). Changes in behaviour in dementia: a neglected research area. *British Journal of Psychiatry*, **152**, 406–7.

Finkel, S. I., Lyons, J. S. and Anderson, R. L. (1993). A Brief Agitation Rating Scale (BARS) for nursing home elderly. *Journal for the American Geriatrics Society*, **41**, 50–52.

Foote, S. L., Bloom, F. E. and Aston-Jones, G. (1983). Nucleus locus ceruleus: new evidence of anatomical and physiological specificity. *Physiological Review*, **63**, 844–914.

Förstl, H., Burns, A., Levy, R. and Cairns, N. (1993). Neuropathological correlates of behaviour disturbance in confirmed Alzheimer's disease. *British Journal of Psychiatry*, **163**, 364–8.

Gibbons, P., Gannon, M. and Wrigley, M. (1997). A study of aggression among referrals to a community-based psychiatry of old age service. *International Journal of Geriatric Psychiatry*, **12**, 384–8.

Glennon, R. A. (1990) Serotonergic receptors: clinical implications, *Neuroscience and Biobehavioural Review*, **14**, 35–47.

Hamel, M., Gold, D. P. and Andres, D. (1990). Predictors and consequences of aggressive behaviour by community-based dementia patients. *Gerontologist*, **30**, 206–11.

Henderson, V. W., Mack, W. and White-Williams, B. (1989). Spatial disorientation in Alzheimer's disease. *Archives of Neurology*, **46**, 391–4.

Hope, R. A. (1992). Personality and behaviour in dementia and normal aging. In *Dementia and Normal Aging* (Huppert, F. A., Brayne, C. and O'Connor, D. W., eds), pp. 272–89. Cambridge University Press, Cambridge.

Hope, R. A. and Fairburn, C. G. (1992). The Present Behavioural Examination (PBE): the development of an interview to measure current behavioural abnormalities. *Psychological Medicine*, **22**, 223–30.

Hope, R. A. and Patel, V. (1993). Assessment of behavioural phenomena in dementia. In *Aging and Dementia—a Methodological Approach* (ed. A. Burns), pp. 221–6. Edward Arnold, London.

Hope, R. A., Keene, J., Fairburn, C., McShane, R. and Jacoby, R. (1997). Behavioural changes in dementia: are there behavioural syndromes? *International Journal of Geriatric Psychiatry*, **12**, 1074–8.

Kalaria, R. N., Andorn, A. C., Tabaton, M., Whitehouse, P. J., Harik, S. I. and Unnerstall, J. R. (1989). Adrenergic receptors in aging and Alzheimers disease: increased β_2-receptors in prefrontal cortex and hippocampus. *Journal of Neurochemistry*, **53**, 1772–81.

Keene, J., Hope, R. A., Fairburn, C. G., Jacoby, R., Gedling, K. and Ware, C. J. (1999). Natural history of aggressive behaviour in dementia. *International Journal of Geriatric Psychiatry*, **14**, 541–8.

Lawlor, B. A., Sunderland, T., Mellow, A. M., Hill, J. L., Molchan, S. E. and Murphy, D. L.

(1989). Hyper-responsively to the serotonergic agonist meta-chlorophenylpiperazine (m-CPP) in Alzheimer's disease: a controlled study. *Archives of General Psychiatry*, **46**, 542–9.

Lian, J. R., Snyder, W. and Merrill, J. L. (1981). Under-reporting of assaults on staff in a state hospital. *Hospital and Community Psychiatry*, **32**, 497–8.

Lopez, O. L., Becker, J. T. and Brenner, R. P. (1991). Alzheimer's disease with delusions and hallucinations: neuropsychological and electroencephalic correlates. *Neurology*, **41**, 906–12.

Lyketos, C. G., Steele, C., Galik, E., Rosenblatt, A., Steinberg, M., Warren, A. and Sheppherd, J. M. (1999). Physical aggression in dementia patients and its relationship to depression. *American Journal of Psychiatry*, **156**, 66–71.

MacPherson, R., Eastly, R., Richards, S. and Mian, A. (1994). Psychological distress among workers caring for the elderly. *International Journal of Geriatric Psychiatry*, **9**, 381–6.

Margo, J. L., Robinson, J. R. and Corea, S. (1980). Referrals to a psychiatric service from old people's homes. *British Journal of Psychiatry*, **136**, 396–401.

Martin, C., McKenzie, S. and Ames, D. (1994). Disturbed behaviour in dementia sufferers: a comparison of three nursing home settings. *International Journal of Geriatric Psychiatry*, **9**, 293–8.

McShane, R., Keene, J., Fairburn, C., Jacoby, R. and Hope, T. (1998). Psychiatric symptoms in patients with dementia predict the later development of behavioural abnormalities. *Psychological Medicine*, **28**, 1119–27.

Mega, M. S., Cummings, J. L., Fiorello, T. and Gornbein, J. (1996). The spectrum of behavioural changes in Alzheimer's disease. *Neurology*, **46**, 130–5.

Moyer, K. E. (1976). *The Psychobiology of Aggression*. Harper and Row, New York.

Mungas, D., Weiler, P., Franzi, C. and Henry, R. (1984). Assessment of disruptive behaviour associated with dementia: the Disruptive Behaviour Rating Scale. *Journal of Geriatric Psychiatry and Neurology*, **2**, 196–202.

O'Connor, D. W., Pollit, P. A., Roth, M., Brook, C. P. and Reiss, B. B. (1990). Problems reported by relatives in a community study of dementia. *British Journal of Psychiatry*, **156**, 835–41.

Palmer, A. M., Francis, P. T., Benton, J. S., Sims, N. R., Mann, D. M., Neary, D., Snowden, J. S. and Bowen, D. M. (1987). Presynaptic serotonergic dysfunction in patients with Alzheimer's disease. *Journal of Neurochemistry*, **48**, 8–15.

Palmer, A. M., Stratmann, G. C., Procter, A. W. and Bowen, D. M. (1988). Possible neuro-transmitter basis of behavioural changes in Alzheimer's disease. *Annals of Neurology*, **34**, 616–20.

Palmsteirna, B. and Wistedt, B. (1987). Staff observation aggression scale: presentation and evaluation. *Acta Psychiatrica Scandinavia*, **76**, 657–63.

Patel, V. and Hope, R. A. (1992a). A rating scale for aggressive behaviour in the elderly—the RAGE. *Psychological Medicine*, **22**, 211–21.

Patel, V. and Hope, R. A. (1992b). Aggressive behaviour in elderly psychiatric inpatients. *Acta Psychiatria Scandinavica*, **85**, 131–5.

Patterson, M. B., Schnell, A. H., Martin, R. J., Mendez, M. F., Smyth, K. A. and Whitehouse, P. J. (1990). Assessment of the behavioural and affective symptoms in Alzheimer's disease. *Journal of Geriatric Psychiatry and Neurology*, **3**, 21–30.

Perry, E. K., Tomlinson, B. E., Blessed, G., Bergmann, K., Gibson, P. H. and Perry, R. H. (1978). Correlation of cholinergic abnormalities with senile plaques and mental test scores in dementia. *British Medical Journal*, **ii**, 1457–9.

Perry, E. K., Marshall, E., Thompson, P., McKeith, I. G., Collerton, D., Fairbairn, A. F., Ferrier, I. N., Irving, D. and Perry, R. H. (1993). Monoaminergic activity in Lewy body dementia: relationship to hallucinosis and extrapyramidal features. *Journal of Neural Transmission, Parkinson's Disease Dementia Section*, **6**, 167–71.

Petrie, W. M. and Ban, T. A. (1987). Propanolol in organic agitation. *Lancet*, **324**, 327.

Rabins, P. V., Mace, N. L. and Lucas, M. J. (1982). The impact of dementia on the family. *Journal of the American Medical Association*, **248**, 333–5.

Raskind, M. A., Perskind, E. R., Wingerson, D., Pascualy, M., Dobie, D. J. and Veith, R. C. (1993) Enhanced cerebrospinal fluid norepinephrine response to yohimbine in aging and Alzheimer's disease. *Society of Neuroscience Abstracts*, **19**, 400.

Ray, W. A., Taylor, J. A., Lichtenstein, M. J. and Meador, K. G. (1992). The nursing home behaviour problem scale. *Journal of Gerontology*, **47**, 9–16.

Reisberg, B., Borenstein, J., Franssen, E., Shulman, E., Steinberg, G. and Ferris, S. H. (1986). Remedial behavioural symptomatology in Alzheimer's disease. *Hospital and Community Psychiatry*, **37**, 1199–201.

Reisberg, B., Borenstein, J., Salob, S. P., Ferris, S. H., Franssen, E. and Georgeotas, A. (1987). Behavioural symptoms in Alzheimer's disease: phenomenology and treatment. *Journal of Clinical Psychiatry*, **48** (Suppl. 5), 9–15.

Reisberg, B., Franssen, E. and Sclan, S. G. (1989). Stage specific incidence of potentially remediable behavioural symptoms in ageing and Alzheimer's disease. *Bulletin of Clinical Neuroscience*, **54**, 85–112.

Rubins, E. H., Morris, J. C., Storandt, M. and Berg, L. (1987a). Behavioural changes in patients with mild senile dementia of Alzheimer's type. *Psychiatric Research*, **21**, 55–62.

Rubins, E. H., Morris, J. C. and Berg, L. (1987b). The progression of personality change in senile dementia of Alzheimer's type. *Journal of the American Geriatrics Society*, **35**, 721–5.

Ryden, M. (1988). Aggressive behaviour in patients with dementia who live in the community. *Alzheimer's Disease and Associated Disorders*, **2**, 342–55.

Sclan, S. G., Saillon, A., Franssen, E., Hugonot-Diener, L. and Saillon, A. (1996). The Behavioural Pathology in Alzheimer's Disease Rating Scale (BEHAVE-AD): reliability and analysis of symptom category scores. *International Journal of Geriatric Psychiatry*, **11**, 819–30.

Shah, A. K. (1993). Aggressive behaviour among patients referred to a psychogeriatric service. *Medical Science Law*, **2**, 144–150.

Shah, A. K. (1999). Aggressive behaviour in the elderly. *International Journal of Psychiatry in Clinical Practice*, **3**, 85–103.

Smith, D., King, M. and Hocbelb, G. (1978). Lateral hypothalamic controls of killing: evidence of cholinergic mechanisms. *Science*, **167**, 900–901.

Soininen, H., MacDonald, E., Rekonen, M. and Rickkinen, P. J. (1981). Homovanillic acid and 5HIAA levels in CSF of patients with senile dementia of Alzheimer type. *Acta Neurologica Scandinavica*, **64**, 101–7.

Spiegel, R., Brunner, C., Erimini-Fundshilling, D., Monsch, A., Wotter, M., Puxty, J. and Tremmel, L. (1991). A new behavioural assessment scale for geriatric outpatients and inpatients—NOSGER (Nursing Observation Scale for Geriatric Patients). *Journal of the American Geriatrics Society*, **39**, 339–47.

Sultzer, D. L. (1996). Neuroimaging and the origin of psychiatric symptoms in dementia. *International Psychogeriatrics*, **8** (Suppl. 3), 239–43.

Sultzer, D. L., Mahler, M. E. and Mandelkern, M. A. (1995). The relationship between psychiatric symptoms and regional cortical metabolism in Alzheimer's disease. *Journal of Neuropsychiatry and Clinical Neuroscience*, **7**, 476–84.

Swearer, J. M., Drackman, D. A., O'Donnell, B. F. and Mitchell, A. L. (1988). Troublesome and disruptive behaviours in dementia: relationships to diagnosis and disease severity. *Journal of the American Geriatrics Society*, **36**, 784–90.

Swigar, M., Benes, F. and Rothman, S. (1985). Behavioural correlates of CT scan changes in older psychiatric patients. *Journal of the American Geriatrics Society*, **33**, 96–103.

Teri, L., Borson, S., Kiyak, H. A. and Yamagishi, M. (1989). Behavioural disturbances, cognitive dysfunction and functional skill. Prevalence and relationships in Alzheimer's disease. *Journal of the American Geriatrics Society*, **37**, 109–16.

Van Pragg, H. (1991). Serotonergic dysfunction and aggression control (Editorial). *Psychological Medicine*, **21**, 15–19.

Victoroff, J., Zarow, C., Mack, W. J., Hsu, C. and Chui, H. C. (1996). Physical aggression is associated with preservation of substantia nigra pars compacta in Alzheimer's disease. *Archives of Neurology*, **53**, 423–34.

Ware, C. J. C., Fairburn, C. and Hope, R. A. (1990). A community-based study of aggressive behaviour in dementia. *International Journal of Geriatric Psychiatry*, **5**, 337–42.

Weiler, P. G., Mungas, D. and Bernick, C. (1988). Propanolol for the control of disruptive behaviour in senile dementia. *Journal of Geriatric Psychiatry and Neurology*, **1**, 226–30.

Werner, P., Cohen-Mansfield, J., Braun, J. and Marx, S. (1989). Physical restraint and agitation in nursing home residents. *Journal of the American Geriatrics Society*, **37**, 1122–6.

Wilcock, G. K., Esiri, M. M., Bowen, D. M. and Smith, C. C. T. (1982). Alzheimer's disease: correlations of cortical choline acetyl transferase activity with severity of dementia and histological abnormalities. *Journal of Neurological Science*, **57**, 407–17.

Yudofsky, S. (1981). Propanolol in the treatment of rage and violent behaviour in patients with chronic brain syndrome. *American Journal of Psychiatry*, **138**, 218–30.

Yudofsky, S. C., Silver, J. M., Jackson, W., Endicott, J. and Williams, D. (1986). The overt aggression scale for the objective rating of verbal and physical aggression. *American Journal of Psychiatry*, **143**, 35–9.

Zarit, S. H., Reever, K. E. and Bach-Peterson, J. (1980). Relatives of the impaired elderly: correlations of feelings of burden. *Gerontologist*, **20**, 649–55.

7 Other behavioural and psychological symptoms in dementia

Introduction

There are almost as many types of behavioural and psychological symptoms in dementia (BPSD) as there are people with dementia. Although, for convenience and to facilitate treatment, they are usually grouped into clusters, some defy classification. For every problem, a better understanding is facilitated by a detailed description and evaluation; an approach which is far more helpful than trying to label a unique symptom 'artificially'. In addition, because BPSD have been classified in so many different ways, there are a number of partially overlapping terms in the literature, which frequently cause confusion; and a number of other features which are rarely manifest as clinically significant problems. There are, however, several additional BPSD which can be clinically important, and which merit separate discussion, but have not been covered in previous chapters.

Abnormal vocalizations

In clinical practice, abnormal vocalizations are usually seen in people with dementia who are residing in care facilities. The problem is usually referred to by care staff as 'shouting', 'screaming' or constant demands for 'attention'. Although the term 'abnormal vocalization' sounds a little over-elaborate, it does have the advantage of encompassing the broad range of manifestations, which include, for example, yelling/shouting, loud talking, mumbling, singing, chattering, sighing, howling, groaning and shrieking. The different characteristics of the sound production may be important in identifying the cause of the problem and hence have implications for treatment.

Evaluation and typology

The first study to characterize abnormal vocalizations (Ryan *et al.* 1988), based upon an evaluation of 400 residents of care facilities using staff informants, suggested six different forms:

(1) noise making that appears purposeless and perseverative;

(2) noise making in response to the environment;

(3) noise making that elicits a response from the environment;

(4) 'chatterbox' noise making;

(5) noise-making due to deafness;

(6) other noise making.

This system represented a major advance, in particular by highlighting the diversity of the problems categorized as abnormal vocalizations, and has been validated in a second independent cohort of more than 600 residents. It has, however, been criticized for omitting data regarding the type of sound produced, and for not identifying possible triggers for the behaviour (Cohen-Mansfield and Werner 1997). Cohen-Mansfield and Werner (1997) have subsequently published a more exhaustive dimensional system referred to as the 'typology of vocalizations'. Five dimensions are incorporated within the scale:

(1) type of sound;

(2) purpose of sound—e.g. requests for attention; pain; emotional distress; self-stimulation;

(3) response to the environment—including features of the physical environment (e.g. temperature, lighting, noise level or degree of isolation/crowdedness) and social environment (e.g. presence of other people, talking to other people and interactions related to specific activities such as washing or toileting);

(4) timing—how frequent is the behaviour and what is the pattern of occurrence?

(5) level of disruptiveness.

This system has the advantage of facilitating a very detailed assessment of a particular individual, and provides information that is very relevant to the planning of treatment interventions. The length of the evaluation may be prohibitive in some settings, although there is a shortened version tailored to the needs of routine clinical practice. Within each dimension, the various categories are not operationally defined, and many of the judgements depend upon clinical knowledge. Hence, although this is an excellent instrument, and although it acts to guide clinical evaluation, the quality of the data will be very dependent upon the skill and experience of the rater. Many different permutations of the dimensions are possible, although a correlation grid indicated three main patterns of vocalization:

(1) verbal behaviours associated with specific requests or needs, or with pain;

(2) verbal behaviours not associated with specific requests, but with general, undefined needs, e.g. calling for attention;

(3) verbal behaviours associated with self-stimulation.

The profile of the vocalization did predict response to different modes of treatment intervention, an important finding which is discussed further in Chapter 19.

Frequency and impact of abnormal vocalizations

All the available studies have focused upon abnormal vocalizations within care facilities. Whilst clinical experience certainly suggests that vocalizations are particularly common in residential care, nursing home and hospital environments; there is a considerable gap in our knowledge regarding the frequency of these behaviours amongst people with dementia living in the community. Within care facilities, a prevalence of 11–30% has been reported (Zimmer et al. 1984, Ryan et al. 1988, Cohen-Mansfield et al. 1990, Cariaga et al. 1991). The severity of the vocalizations is not clear in the majority of these reports, although Cohen-Mansfield and Werner (1997) reported that 87% of people reported as having abnormal vocalizations by care staff experienced the problem at a clinically significant level that was disruptive to staff and other residents, of whom 75% experienced the behaviour constantly. There are no data pertaining to the natural course of abnormal vocalizations.

Everitt et al. (1991) reported an association between abnormal vocalizations and caregiver distress. Abnormal vocalizations also frequently disturb other residents and their families (Meares and Draper 1999). This mirrors anecdotal clinical experience, where complaints by the relatives of other residents, or even people living in properties adjoining the care facility, are often the trigger for a clinical referral.

Associations of abnormal vocalizations

The most consistently reported associations of abnormal vocalizations are more severe cognitive impairment (Jackson et al. 1989, Cohen-Mansfield et al. 1990, Cariaga et al. 1991) and greater impairment of activities of daily living (Jackson et al. 1989, Cohen-Mansfield et al. 1990, Hallberg et al. 1990, Cariaga et al. 1991). Other associations related to illness characteristics include pain (Cohen-Mansfield et al. 1990, 1992, Cohen-Mansfield and Werner 1997), communication difficulties (Nasman et al. 1983, Cohen-Mansfield et al. 1992, Hallberg et al. 1993), deafness (Cohen-Mansfield and Werner 1997), depression (Greenwald et al. 1986, Cohen-Mansfield et al. 1990, 1992, Carlyle et al. 1991, Cohen-Mansfield and Werner 1997), psychosis (Hallberg et al. 1990), sleep disturbance (Cohen-Mansfield et al. 1990, Cariaga et al. 1991) and agitation (Cohen-Mansfield et al. 1990, Hallberg et al. 1990, Cariaga et al. 1991). Probably the most important associations from a management perspective are pain, deafness and depression, which should always be considered as possible triggers. Depression is particularly likely in people who are shrieking or sighing. Communication difficulties are also important, particularly receptive dysphasia, the severity and importance of which are not always appreciated by care staff. Often a detailed assessment may facilitate better resident–staff interaction and communication by highlighting simple single words, written material or pictures that a resident may be able to comprehend. The apparent associations with some of the other BPSD are more difficult to interpret. For example, both agitation and abnormal vocalizations are common in care facilities, and will therefore co-occur by chance in a moderate number of individuals; also, as a large proportion of residents with abnormal vocalizations experience them continuously whilst awake, they will be expressed during wakeful periods of the night. Apart from the association with the severity of the dementia and the related impairments, the other factors are potentially important for some people experiencing abnormal vocalizations, but will not apply to every or even the majority of individuals. This is largely a reflection of the diversity of the problem, and further emphasizes the importance of a detailed assessment. Possible associations with dementia type have not been evaluated, although anecdotal clinical experience suggests that vocalizations are particularly common in people experiencing communication difficulties in the context of a vascular dementia.

Various facets of the physical and social environment have also been highlighted as associations of abnormal vocalizations. Potentially important factors include social isolation (Cohen-Mansfield *et al.* 1990, Cohen-Mansfield and Werner 1995,1997), lack of involvement in activities (Hallberg *et al.* 1990, Cohen-Mansfield and Werner 1995), over-crowding (Cohen-Mansfield and Werner 1997), the quality of staff to resident interactions (Cohen-Mansfield *et al.* 1990, Hallberg *et al.* 1990, 1993, Cohen-Mansfield and Werner 1995, Edberg *et al.* 1995) and inadvertent re-inforcement of the behaviour (Ryan *et al.* 1988, Cariaga *et al.* 1991). Again, each of these possible associations may be important for some people with abnormal vocalizations. The importance of a detailed individual assessment is emphasized by the reported correlations between both under and over social stimulation respectively, and abnormal vocalizations. This highlights that triggers may be very diverse, reflecting differing patterns of likes and dislikes, and social preferences. The inadvertent re-inforcement of abnormal vocalizations is a frequent problem, which merits particular consideration. Some of these issues are explored in the case example at the end of this section.

Very little work has considered any potential biological correlates of abnormal vocalizations. This is probably not a significant omission, as it is unlikely—given the diversity of the behaviours encompassed within this category, and their relationship with environmental characteristics—that alterations in any specific cortical centre or neurotransmitter system will be responsible for this range of problems. It does, however, appear that vocalizations that serve to self-stimulate are not associated with environmental characteristics, and it is possible that biological factors may be more important in this group. Superficially, some of the vocalizations seen in this context bear some resemblance to the vocal tics seen in Gilles de la Tourette syndrome, which may offer some clues as to which neurotransmitter systems could be most profitably investigated.

Case example

Mr X, an 86 year old man with cognitive impairment, was admitted to a stroke unit following a second cerebrovascular accident, which resulted in receptive dysphasia. After Mr X's physical condition had stabilized, he was transferred to a rehabilitation ward. After he had been on the ward for several days, the nursing staff noticed that he was occasionally shouting 'help' or grunting loudly. Over a few days these vocalizations became louder and more frequent, and began to disturb other patients. Mr X was therefore moved to a side room at the end of the ward. Initially, this improved the situation for the other patients, although Mr X began shouting more loudly, until he was audible from the main ward. At this point it was decided that Mr X was not a good candidate for rehabilitation and that he should be discharged to a nursing home. The severity of his vocalizations was immediately apparent to the care staff, who felt that it would be best to nurse Mr X in his own room to minimize the impact on other residents, and to prevent relatives from complaining. As the problem continued to worsen, a 'behaviour training programme' was instigated. Mr X was informed that staff would ignore him if he was shouting. After 2 weeks the problem had not improved. One of the staff members decided to ask Mr X why he was shouting; he either continued to shout 'help' through the conversation, or gave lengthier replies which were not comprehensible. A different approach was then tried, of taking Mr X into the lounge for his meals, where he became particularly distressed and shouted even more loudly.

Although this case example has been exaggerated to make a series of points, elements of this history will be familiar to most people working in this field. At the time Mr X first began to shout, no attempt was made to make a detailed individualized appraisal of his problem. He may have had specific care needs, he may have been suffering from depression, or he may have been seeking reassurance. Perhaps he was finding the busy and crowded ward environment difficult to tolerate. Whatever the trigger for his shouting, it is likely to have been amplified by his inability to comprehend staff or express his own needs clearly. A formal evaluation of his receptive and expressive language skills at this stage may have facilitated better communication, perhaps by using short single words with picture prompts. In this way it might have been possible to make Mr X feel less isolated and possibly to identify specific care needs. By isolating Mr X in a side room, the only strategy available to Mr X was to shout more loudly to try and communicate his needs. Following his transfer to a nursing home, the badly thought-out behaviour-training programme would have had the same effect. In this particular situation, Mr X was probably unable to understand the boundaries of the programme. In general, trying to ignore any BPSD is usually ineffective, as the problem almost always escalates to the level where it can no longer be ignored. Although social isolation may have been an important factor, Mr X was probably not able to understand where he was being taken, and after a protracted period of isolation, a crowded dining room was probably a very frightening environment. The first step to effective intervention would clearly be a detailed evaluation of the situation, but particularly when problems have escalated to this degree, interventions may take a considerable period of time to improve the problem significantly. Consistence and patience is often required.

Eating disorders in Alzheimer's disease

Several different eating disorders are recognized in the context of dementia, including a change in preference for sweet foods (10–33%), increased (20–35%) or

decreased (22–41%) consumption, and eating non-food substances (3%) (Burns
et al. 1990, Cullen et al. 1997, Hope et al. 1997). The majority of these problems
rarely arise as clinical referrals, although an understanding of changing food
preference may help in the planning of care. If severe, reduced appetite can be associated with marked weight loss and can become an important risk to health. Eating
non-food substances is much less common but has the potential to be dangerous.
Other problems which may be clinically important, but have not been systematically
researched, include difficulties with feeding (such as coordinating cutlery, messy eating or drooling), forgetting that meals have been consumed and forgetting to eat.

A number of rating scales to evaluate psychopathology in dementia now include
an eating disorder subcategory (e.g. the Neuropsychiatric Inventory (Chapter 2)),
whilst other scales have been developed specifically to assess eating disorders in
Alzheimer's disease (AD) (e.g. Tully et al. 1997).

Inappropriate menu planning, depression (Cullen et al. 1997), clinical (Horner
et al. 1994) and subclinical (Feinberg et al. 1992) swallowing problems, poor dental
health and oropharyngo-oesophageal function can all be important associations of
poor food intake or reduced appetite. Abnormal eating attitudes, akin to those seen
in anorexia nervosa, may be linked to low weight and reduced food intake in some
people with mild cognitive impairment, but are often not recognized (Bartlett et al.
2000). The basic necessity of eating to maintain health, the frustration that disordered eating causes to caregivers and the increased risk of institutionalization and
death all make this an important topic (Riviere et al. 1999). Eating of inedible substances and hyperorality appears to be associated with widening of the third ventricle,
bilateral temporal lobe atrophy and other clinical features of Kluver–Bucy
syndrome (Burns et al. 1990). Hyperphagia may be linked to increased calorific need
in patients with motor restlessness, whilst younger people with more severe dementia
who are not restless may over-eat because they respond to any food stimulus, possibly
as a manifestation of frontal lobe pathology (Smith et al. 1998).

Abnormalities of eating appear to be more common in AD than in other dementias
(Cullen et al. 1997).

Several neurotransmitters have been putatatively linked to eating disorders in AD.
Reduced neuropetide Y and norepinephrine may be associated with anorexia, whilst
the action of galanin in the hypothalamus is thought to increase fat intake and affect
cholinergic hippocampal systems.

Sexual disinhibition

Although perceived sexual disinhibition is a common reason for clinical referrals,
but relatively little is known about its prevalence in people with AD. In a community-
dwelling cohort of 97 people with dementia, Hope et al. (1997) reported a prevalence of 5% for inappropriate sexual comments, but none of the people assessed
were displaying any inappropriate sexual behaviour or had exposed themselves.
Wright (1993) reported that 10% of a small sample of people with dementia living

with spouses in the community had experienced an increase in sexual desire. Clinical experience would suggest that the frequency of sexual problems is greater within care facilities, although the authors are unaware of any formal studies conducted within this setting. Clearly, sexual disinhibition is much more frequent in dementia of frontal lobe type (DFLT; Kertez *et al.* 1997) or other dementia conditions with prominent damage to frontal lobe areas.

Assessment

There are three main recurrent themes when assessing inappropriate sexual behaviour:

- distinguishing normal sexual expression from inappropriate sexual behaviour;
- identifying people who could, with simple guidance, normalise their sexual behaviour; and
- recognizing situations where a non-sexual behaviour may appear sexual.

There has been an increasing awareness of the need of elderly people, including those with dementia, to express their sexuality. This may vary from having one's hair styled, wearing perfume/aftershave or wearing nice clothes; to more overt sexual behaviours such as making sexual advances towards other people or masturbation. When two residents of a care facility both wish to engage in a mutual affectionate or sexual activity, this probably does not represent an inappropriate sexual behaviour, although it may raise other ethical issues depending upon the ability of the individuals concerned to give informed consent and the concerns of family members. Likewise, masturbation is not an inappropriate sexual behaviour if it is carried out discreetly in a private area. Difficulties may arise when people lose their social awareness and may need some guidance to help them maintain privacy. Similarly, if a female care assistant is aiding a male resident with an intimate personal care task, the potential for the resident to misinterpret the situation is understandable, given a certain level of impaired judgement. If such incidents are occasional, involve only mildly suggestive behaviour, are easily dissuaded by a clear verbal explanation and are non-recurrent, they too would probably fit into this second category of behaviour. A common example of a behaviour frequently interpreted as having a sexual motive, relates to males residing in care facilities who appear to expose themselves, but are actually trying to urinate. In such cases a toileting programme or a training programme to help the individual concerned to locate a toilet would be of greatest assistance.

Requests for affection or comfort can also be misunderstood. Many people with dementia, like many of the remainder of the population, find physical contact—such as holding a hand, or having a cuddle—very reassuring, as a normal means of emotional expression. In some circumstances it may be difficult to separate an attempt to elicit affection from a sexually motivated behaviour. If the contact has a possible sexual connotation that causes a degree of discomfort to the caregiver, a simple redirection as to a more appropriate means of expressing affection may be all that is required.

Although, in the absence of a well developed research literature, this section is mainly based upon clinical experience, the principles are very similar to the assessment of other BPSD problems, and depend upon a careful individualized evaluation. In addition to determining whether a behaviour is sexual, and, if so, whether it is inappropriate, an assessment following the principles of an Antecedent Behaviour Consequence (ABC) diary will clarify the frequency and severity of the problem, and will identify both potential triggers and possible reinforcers. The important themes are illustrated in the case examples at the end of Chapter 19.

Associations

There is a clear association between DFLT and frontal lobe damage and sexual disinhibition. Other associations are less well established, and probably vary between different individuals in different circumstances.

Sexual problems within a marital relationship

Within the context of a sexual relationship, additional problems arise, as individuals may lose the social skills that are important in setting the mood and scene for a fulfilling sexual encounter, or may experience physical difficulties in coordinating some aspects of a physical, sexual relationship. Many couples where one of the partners has dementia remain sexually active (Ballard *et al.* 1997), and a number of others would like to regain their sexual relationship. Because of the taboos surrounding sexual relationships in the elderly, particularly amongst people with dementia, these important issues are rarely addressed.

Anxiety

Whilst depression has been the focus of a number of studies in people with dementia, far less attention has been paid to anxiety. The sparse literature does suggest that anxiety symptoms are extremely common, with a prevalence in excess of 30% (Wands *et al.* 1990, Ballard *et al.* 1994, 1996, 1999, 2000, Hope *et al.* 1997). Of the specific symptoms, tension and subjective anxiety appear to be common, whilst panic attacks are unusual (Ballard *et al.* 1996). Diagnosis has been a problem as none of the anxiety scales have been specifically validated in people with dementia. There is really a need to design a specific scale, perhaps using principles similar to those utilized in the Cornell Depression Scale (Alexopoulos *et al.* 1988), where both patient and informant interviews are used to evaluate a checklist of key symptoms. Until this has been achieved it is suggested that a standard checklist of symptoms, such as that found within *DSM-IV* (APA 1994), is probably the best approach; although deciding at which point these symptoms become clinically significant is a problem. The Neuropsychiatric Inventory includes an anxiety subscale (Chapter 2), although the anxiety score quantifies the frequency, rather than the number or type, of anxiety features, most of the important information regarding individual symptoms is collected as part of the subscale. The BEHAV-AD (Chapter 2) collects standardized information regarding the severity of key anxiety symptoms, which can be very useful for symptom ascertainment; although it is unclear how it relates to a clinical diagnosis of an anxiety disorder.

Very little work has evaluated the potential associations of anxiety. Ballard *et al.* (1996) reported a possible association with milder cognitive impairment, and described several people with insight into some of their deficits who experienced related social anxieties. In an important study, Orrell and Bebbington (1996) indicated a possible association with life events. The loss of cognitive and problem-solving skills in people with dementia makes many situations anxiety provoking (Kitwood 1993), and anxiety is often one of the components within agitation or aggression. Developing a better understanding of how life events and day-to-day traumas within the environment precipitate and perpetuate anxiety is imperative.

Anxiety appears to be equally frequent in people with AD and dementia with Lewy bodies (Ballard *et al.* 1999); despite the high prevalence of anxiety after stroke (Schultz *et al.* 1997), it does not appear to be more frequent in vascular dementia (Ballard *et al.* 2000). There have been no studies examining the biological correlates of anxiety *per se*, although Chen *et al.* (1996) reported a relationship between loss of 5-hydroxytryptamine receptors in the frontal cortex and anxious depression. Given the link between white matter hyperintensities and late-life depression, this too merits examination as a potential association of anxiety arising in the context of dementia. Approximately half of people with anxiety disorders and dementia will have concurrent depression (Ballard *et al.* 1994).

REFERENCES

Alexopoulos, G. S., Abrams, R. C., Young, R. C. and Shamonian, C. A. (1988). Cornell Scale for Depression in Dementia. *Biological Psychiatry*, **23**, 271–84.

APA (1994). *Diagnostic and Statistical Manual of Mental Disorders*, 4th edn. American Psychiatric Association, Washington, DC.

Ballard, C. G., Mohan, R. N. C., Patel, A. and Graham, C. (1994). Anxiety disorder in dementia. *International Journal of Psychiatry*, **11**, 108–9.

Ballard, C., Boyle, A., Bower, C. and Lindesay, J. (1996). Anxiety disorders in dementia sufferers. *International Journal of Geriatric Psychiatry*, **11**, 987–90.

Ballard, C. G., Solis, M., Gahir, M., Cullen, P., George, S., Oyebode, F. and Wilcock, G. (1997). Sexual relationships in married dementia sufferers. *International Journal of Geriatric Psychiatry*, **12**, 447–51.

Ballard, C., Holmes, C., McKeith, I., Neill, D., Lantos, P., Cairns, N., Perry, E., Ince, P. and Perry, R. (1999). Psychiatric morbidity in dementia with Lewy bodies: a prospective clinical and neuropathological comparative study with Alzheimer's disease. *American Journal of Psychiatry*, **156**, 1039–45.

Ballard, C., Neill, D., O'Brien, J., McKeith, I., Ince, P. and Perry, R. (2000). Anxiety, depression and psychosis in vascular dementia: prevalence and associations. *Journal of Affective Disorders*. (In press.)

Bartlett, S., Shrimanker, J. and Ballard, C. (2000). Prevalence of abnormal eating amongst elderly people in residential care. *International Journal of Geriatric Psychiatry*. (In press.)

Burns, A., Jacoby, R. and Levy, R. (1990). Psychiatric phenomena in Alzheimer's disease. *British Journal of Psychiatry*, **157**, 86–94.

Cariaga, J., Burgio, L., Flynn, W. and Martin, D. (1991). A controlled study of disruptive vocalizations among geriatric residents in nursing homes. *Journal of the American Geriatrics Society*, **39**, 501–7.

Carlyle, W., Killick, L. and Ancill, R. (1991). ECT: an effective treatment in the screaming demented patient. *Journal of the American Geriatrics Society*, **39**, 637–9.

Chen, C. P. L.-H., Alder, J. T., Bowen, D. M., Eseri, M. M., McDonald, B., Hope, T., Jobst, K. A. and Francis, P. T. (1996). Presynaptic serotonergic markers in community-acquired cases of Alzheimer's disease: correlations with depression and neuroleptic medication. *Journal of Neurochemistry*, **66**, 1592–8.

Cohen-Mansfield, J. and Werner, P. (1995). Environmental influences on agitation: an integrative summary of an observational study. *American Journal of Alzheimer's Care and Related Disorders and Research*, **32–35**.

Cohen-Mansfield, J. and Werner, P. (1997). Typology of disruptive vocalizations in older persons suffering from dementia. *International Journal of Geriatric Psychiatry*, **12**, 1079–91.

Cohen-Mansfield, J., Werner, P. and Marx, M. S. (1990). Screaming in nursing home residents. *Journal of the American Geriatrics Society*, **38**, 785–92.

Cohen-Mansfield, J., Marx, M. S. and Werner, P. (1992). Agitation in elderly persons: an integrative report of findings in a nursing home. *International Psychogeriatrics*, **4**, 221–40.

Cullen, P., Abid, F., Patel, A., Coope, B. and Ballard, C. G. (1997). Eating disorders in dementia. *International Journal of Geriatric Psychiatry*, **12**, 559–62.

Edberg, A. K., Sandgren, A. N. and Hallberg, I.R. (1995). Initiating and terminating verbal interaction between nurses and severely demented patients regarded as vocally disruptive. *Journal of Psychiatric Mental Health Nursing*, **2**, 159–67.

Everitt, D. E., Fields, D. R., Soumerai, S. S. and Avorn. J. (1991). Resident behaviour and staff distress in the nursing home. *Journal of the American Geriatrics Society*, **39**, 792–8.

Feinberg, M. J., Ekberg, O., Segall, L. and Tully, J. (1992). Deglutition in elderly patients with dementia: findings of videofluorographic evaluation and impact on staging and management. *Radiology*, **183**, 811–14.

Greenwald, B. S., Marin, D. B. and Silverman, S. M. (1986). Serotonergic treatment of screaming and banging in dementia. *Lancet*, **ii**, 1464–5.

Hallberg, I. R., Norberg, A. and Eriksson, S. (1990a). Functional impairment and behavioural disturbances in vocally disruptive patients in psychogeriatric wards compared with controls. *International Journal of Geriatric Psychiatry*, **5**, 53–61.

Hallberg, I. R., Norberg, A. and Eriksson, S. (1990b). A comparison between the care of vocally disruptive patients and that of other residents at psychogeriatric wards. *International Journal of Geriatric Psychiatry*, **15**, 410–16.

Hallberg, I. R., Edberg, A. K., Nordmark, A., Johnsson, K. and Norberg, A. (1993). Daytime vocal activity in institutionalized severely demented patients identified as vocally disruptive by nurses. *International Journal of Geriatric Psychiatry*, **8**, 155–64.

Hope, T., Keene, J., Gedling, K., Cooper, S., Fairburn, C. and Jacoby, R. (1997). Behaviour changes in dementia. 1: Point of entry data of a prospective study. *International Journal of Geriatric Psychiatry*, **12**, 1062–73.

Horner, J., Alberts, M. J., Dawson, D. V. and Cook, G. M. (1994). Swallowing in Alzheimer's disease. *Alzheimer Disease and Associated Disorders*, **8**, 177–89.

Jackson, M. E., Drugovich, M. L., Fretwell, M. E., Spector, W. D., Sternberg, J. and Rosentein, R. B. (1989). Prevalence and correlates of disruptive behaviour in the nursing home. *Journal of Ageing Health*, **1**, 349–69.

Kertez, A., Davidson, W. and Fox, H. (1997). Frontal behavioural inventory: diagnostic criteria for frontal lobe dementia. *Canadian Journal of Neurological Sciences*, **24**, 29–36.

Kitwood, T. (1993). Person and process in dementia. *International Journal of Geriatric Psychiatry*, **8**, 541–6.

Meares, S. and Draper, B. (1999). Treatment of vocally disruptive behaviour of multifactorial aetiology. *International Journal of Geriatric Psychiatry*, **14**, 285–90.

Nasman, B., Bucht, G. and Eriksson, S. (1983). Behavioural symptoms in the institutionalised elderly—relationship to dementia. *International Journal of Geriatric Psychiatry*, **1**, 843–9.

Orrell, M. and Bebbington, P. (1996). Psychosocial stress and anxiety in senile dementia. *Journal of Affective Disorders*, **39**, 65–73.

Riviere, S., Lauque, S., Micas, M., Albarede, J. L. and Vellas, B. (1999). European programme: nutrition, Alzheimer's disease and health promotion. *La Revue de Geriatrie*, **24**, 121–6.

Ryan, D. P., Tainsh, S. M., Kolodny, V., Landrum, B. L. and Fisher, R. W. (1988). Noise amongst the elderly in long term care. *Gecrontologist*, **28**, 369–371.

Schultz, S. K., Castillo, C. S., Kosier, J. T. and Robinson, R. G. (1997). Generalized anxiety and depression. Assessment over 2 years after stroke. *American Journal of Geriatric Psychiatry*, **5**, 229–37.

Smith, G., Vigen, V., Evans, J., Fleming, K. and Bohac, D. (1998). Patterns and associates of hyperphagia in patients with dementia. *Neuropsychiatry, Neuropsychology and Behavioural Neurology*, **11**, 97–102.

Tully, M. W., Matrakas, K. L., Muir, J. and Musallam, K. (1997). The Eating Behaviour Scale. A simple method of assessing functional ability in patients with Alzheimer's disease. *Journal of Gerontological Nursing*, **23**, 9–15.

Wands, K., Merskey, H., Hachinski, V. C., Fishman, M., Fox, F. and Boniferro, M. (1990). A questionnaire investigation of anxiety and depression in early dementia. *Journal of the American Geriatrics Society*, **36**, 535–8.

Wright, L. (1993). *Alzheimer's Disease and Marriage*. Sage, CA.

Zimmer, J. G., Watson, N. and Treat, A. (1984). Behavioural problems among patients in skilled nursing facilities. *American Journal of Public Health*, **74**, 1118–21.

8 The person and the environment

Introduction

This chapter focuses mainly on the care of the person with dementia within institutional environments. While these settings are equipped to deal with problem behaviours, the environments are often associated with high levels of ill-being (Kitwood 1997). For example, Novaco (1993) claims that institutional settings are often conducive to the displaying of challenging behaviour. He argues that these environments tend to limit satisfaction and are intrinsically constraining, leading to frequent incidences of aggression and distress. Clegg (1993), describing parallel settings with people with learning difficulties, suggests that institutional environments foster lives of 'social emptiness'. Considering these difficulties, the main thrust of this chapter highlights the need to create environments that promote the health of all those living and working within them. To achieve this, people's environments are first examined from various perspectives: political, cultural, organizational, physical and social care. The work then goes on to examine the person's experience of having dementia within a particular setting. A framework is provided to help formulate the experience of the person with dementia. A case example is used to show how the framework can be put into practice in a care environment.

Impact of dementia

Dementia affects people on a number of levels and within a range of domains (physical, cognitive, emotional and social); the multidimensional nature of the impact is well represented in Table 8.1. Despite this wide range of impact, it is suggested that professionals working with people with dementia sometimes focus too much on the levels of pathology and impairment, being overly concerned with diagnosis and failing to take adequate account of the emotional, physical and social features of the person (Bender 1998). The importance of the wider picture is acknowledged within the World Health Organization's definition (WHO 1986), which describes dementia as the acquired global impairment of higher cortical functions, including memory, the capacity to solve problems of day-to-day living, performance of learned perceptuomotor skills, the correct use of social skills, all

Table 8.1   Level of impact of dementia

Dimensions	Nature of change
Pathology	changes in structure of the brain, e.g. brain atrophy, plaques and tangles
Impairment	changes at level of information processing, e.g. deficits in retrieval and storage abilities
Disability	impact on functional levels (cognitive and behavioural), e.g. inability to learn new information
Handicap	effects on integrated activities, e.g. inability to deal with novel situations
Quality of life	effects on social functioning, e.g. loss of confidence and greater social avoidance

aspects of language and communication and the control of emotional reactions in the absence of gross clouding of consciousness.

As the above definition highlights, dementia affects the person's emotional state, problem-solving capacity, temperament and interpersonal abilities and, in turn, his[1] ability to function in his environment. This emphasis on the psychosociological features of dementia is consistent with many of the current models of care, whereby support and treatment are delivered in ways that value the person's life experiences, personality and network of relationships. Using this approach, it is suggested that one can help the person with dementia to maintain his sense of dignity and even improve his state of well-being within his environment. To this end, it is important to assess both the environmental and intra-psychic (cognitive, emotional) influences on the person's well-being. Each of these features is discussed below, and a case example provides a practical illustration of how theory is used to guide practice.

The environment

Environmental influences are key features for people with dementia, and for older people in general, owing to the high level of dependency occurring within this group. The various spheres of environmental influence are highlighted in Fig. 8.1.

The interlocking representation suggests that each of the environmental spheres is influenced by the others. For example, the organizational structure will be influenced by political features, and the combined interaction of these two will affect the carers' social interface with the person with dementia.

The political environment

The role of government is clearly important in the allocation of health and welfare resources for people with dementia. The situation of people with dementia has undergone radical changes as a result of implementations of government policies

---

[1] In this chapter the person with dementia is discussed as a man. This has been done solely to improve the flow of the text.

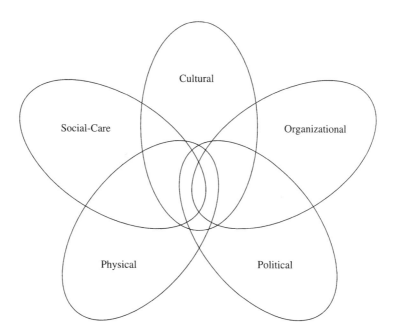

Fig. 8.1   The interlocking environmental spheres.

over the last 40 years. More recently, there have been a number of important publications highlighting the inadequacies of public-sector provision of welfare (Hadley and Hatch 1981, Barclay Report 1982, Audit Commission 1986, King's Fund 1987, Griffiths, 1988). In addition to this, there have also been concerns about the problems arising from public support of private residential care (Wagner Report 1988). Over the last three decades, successive Labour and Conservative governments in the UK have been worried about the growth in the number of economically dependent people in relation to those who are economically productive (see Parker and Penhale 1998). These concerns have resulted in a number of reformulations of the health and social care provision. Over this time, greater emphasis has been put on promoting private and voluntary provision of care. The current restructuring in the UK's National Health Service (NHS) will see further reorganization, with fund-holding systems being replaced by Primary Care Groups (PCGs). Such groups, which may evolve into Trusts, will cover populations of approximately 100,000 people. The changes are likely to see general practitioners (GPs), nurses and social service personnel taking responsibility for advising health authorities about commissioning services. In a recent article, Iliffe (1999) claims that the PCGs will potentially provide opportunities for a more coherent dementia service in which local strengths and needs would be better monitored. However, he points out that, unless the needs of people with dementia are well articulated, there is a risk that dementia will remain a low priority for primary care.

The cultural environment

Cultures have popular beliefs and myths associated with dementia, which serve to shape people's thoughts and fears about the condition. As professionals and members of this society, it is important for us to acknowledge the presence of such myths and fears because they often drive the values and rights we attribute to people with dementia. Thus our cultural background can influence treatment and funding strategies, and also determine the dysfunctional network of beliefs people take with them into later life.

It is worth noting that the term 'challenging behaviour' itself is a culturally bound label. Indeed, Emerson (1998) refers to challenging behaviour as 'culturally abnormal behaviour of such an intensity, frequency or duration that the physical safety of the person or others is likely to be placed in serious jeopardy, or behaviour which seriously limits use of, or results in the person being denied access to, ordinary community facilities' (Emerson 1998, p.127). This definition suggests that challenging behaviours are social constructions. Thus, in order to determine whether a behaviour meets the necessary criteria to qualify as a challenging behaviour, one must take account of the behaviour, the setting within which it occurs and the manner in which it is interpreted. For example, if a disruptive act is perceived as intentional and premeditated, it is far more likely to be seen as challenging. As Emerson (1998) states, the way in which the behaviour is perceived will determine how staff react to it. This may inform one whether to target change at the person with dementia, the environment or the staff's perceptions.

It is worth remembering also that people in the UK generally exist in multicultural and multiethnic environments, and thus there is a need to be aware of the heterogeneity of belief systems and expectations. Indeed, some of the behaviours that one might label as 'odd' might be perfectly explicable in a different culture (Patel *et al.* 1998; Patel and Mirza 2000). Jenkins (1998) has recently produced an article promoting the use of good communications skills with people with dementia from different cultures. The work stresses the importance of being aware of the significance of non-verbal nuances of language. For example, while Western cultures tend to promote 'good eye contact', this can be perceived as disrespectful, defiant and aggressive in other cultures.

The organizational environment

The management of dementia requires the provision of a great deal of resources and skills from many different organisations (NHS Trusts, Social Services, voluntary and private agencies), professional teams (GPs, old age psychiatrists, geriatricians, nurses, psychologists, occupational therapists, etc.) and non-professional groups (carers, members of voluntary groups). It has been suggested that the new PCGs and Trusts could play an important role in coordinating the activities of these disparate parties (Iliffe 1999). Under the PCGs' guidance, it is hoped that sensitive, evidence-based care can be provided within the local communities. However, in order for such a potentially unwieldy service to operate smoothly, service purchasers and providers must have a shared set of principles. Indeed, when groups within an organization are able to operate through shared principles, care can be delivered in a far more integrated way. The King's Fund have proposed the following set of guiding principles (King's Fund 1986):

- People with dementia, no matter the degree of severity, should be valued.
- They should be seen as individuals with varied needs and the same rights as other citizens.
- They have the right to forms of treatment and help that do not exploit family and friends.
- The value base for standard setting and service development should be adopted by all agencies (purchasers and providers).
- The framework should be regarded as non-negotiable because it applies to the values and rights of people with dementia as people first and sufferers of dementia second.

The Social Service Inspectorate (1990) claims that in those few situations where shared principles have actually been established between organizations, they have often been too 'fuzzy' and ambiguous, resulting in inconsistent service delivery. Thus, in order for principles, such as those suggested by the King's Fund, to have the necessary positive impact on the life of a person with dementia, they need to be operationalized in terms of appropriate care plans. These care plans should examine people's needs rather than problems, and be monitored closely to ensure that the principles are being adhered to adequately.

The physical environment

The importance of dementia-friendly design is well recognized (Sixsmith *et al.* 1993, Cohen-Mansfield and Werner 1998, Marshall *et al.* 1998). A number of features are known to reduce levels of well-being and functioning in institutional settings. For example, it is recognized that large, high-ceilinged rooms tend to distort speech and distance perception; small rooms often lead to a sense of enclosure and anxiety; uniformity of appearance sometimes promotes aimless wandering and disorientation; difficulty in finding the toilet can result in incontinence. Some of these features can be remedied by good designs through the use of signposts, symbols and colour coding. Thus, with a bit of thought, rooms can be made more accessible, attractive and appropriate for the needs of the person with dementia. The following principles represent key features which help improve quality of life and reduce disorientation:

- providing space for both privacy and social interaction;
- promoting people's ability to make safe decisions and choices within the environment;
- using clear cueing and way-finding features;

- providing stimulation within the environment;
- promoting a sense of security by employing familiar and age-appropriate objects (piano, wireless, etc.);
- allowing the person to personalize his environment.

Good quality research regarding the physical environment is sadly lacking. However, there is evidence that room designs can promote social interaction (Annerstedt *et al.* 1993) and that floor design can reduce unsafe attempts to use exit doors (Hussian and Brown 1987, Hewawasam 1996). The findings of a unique cross-agency project on design conducted in Glasgow are currently proving extremely helpful (Dick 1999). In this project, a team of politicians, architects, academics, people with dementia and their families and carers worked together to create a comprehensive design guide (Rogan 1998). The team are presently producing a blueprint of good practice for architects and designers creating new and refurbished environments for people with dementia.

While such projects give valuable insight on how to design the environment, it is still essential that one continues to conduct appropriate assessments at the level of the individual. Sometimes, even the most careful and well-meaning planning can result in difficulties, as in the case of Mr J. Mr J was a 78 year old man relocated from his home into a residential setting. In order to personalize his new bedroom, his 'favourite' armchair was taken from his home and placed in his new room. However, in this particular case it was inappropriate to attempt to produce an analogue environment because Mr J had associated this particular chair with a traumatic burglary he had experienced prior to moving into a residential home. It was later determined that he had been tied to this chair during the attack, and thus when the chair was brought into the new home he experienced high levels of arousal and agitation. This example illustrates that it is important to consult with the person with dementia, his relatives and carers when creating a suitable physical environment.

The social care environment

Whether the individual is at home or in residential placement, his interpersonal surroundings will influence his presentation. Indeed, it is important to recognize that humans are sociotropic beings, who value strong and validating interpersonal relationships. Kitwood (1997) was a champion of such perspectives. Together with his colleagues in Bradford, he suggested that people's levels of well-being were related to the opportunities provided for them to engage in fulfilling relationships and activities. Kitwood placed particular emphasis on the social setting within which the person with dementia lived, claiming that states of ill-being often occurred when the person's social environment was negative. Indeed, he stated that, in situations where the person's well-being was continually undermined, the person with dementia would experience the processes associated with a 'malignant social psychology'. It was suggested that malignant social environments would be characterized by poor

Table 8.2 Examples of personal detractors

Type of detractor	
Treachery	using some form of deception in order to distract or manipulate a person, or force them into compliance
Disempowerment	not allowing a person to use the abilities that he still has; failing to help him to complete action that he has initiated
Infantilization	treating a person very patronizingly, as an insensitive parent might treat a young child
Intimidation	inducing fear in a person, through the use of threats of physical power

quality of life and high levels of negative social interaction. Kitwood and his colleagues termed these negative interactions 'personal detractions' (Table 8.2). Seventeen detractors have been described, and four of them are presented below.

It is important to note that the impact of the carers' interaction may sometimes be so extreme that it constitutes abuse—physical, sexual or psychological—and may even involve inappropriate physical restraint.

As one can see, Kitwood (Bradford Dementia Group 1997) places a great deal of emphasis on the type of care and support provided to the person with dementia. One of Bradford's main achievements in this area has been the development of the Dementia Care Mapping (DCM) system, an observational tool designed to assess the quality of life of people with dementia (Kitwood and Bredin 1992). The DCM process involves raters (mappers) observing about half the individuals in a residential or specialist care setting over a period of 5–6 h. The behavioural data obtained in such a map are coded and assessed in terms of the relative degree of well-being of a person with dementia. Information is also collected about negative and positive examples of staff engagement. Following the observational phase, the data are collated and fed back to the care team, and work is then done with the team to promote improvements.

The DCM procedure is currently being adapted as a staff-training tool by researchers in Newcastle (James and Reichelt 2000). While the core of the observational procedure has been left unchanged, greater emphasis is being placed on monitoring and quantifying positive examples of staff members' social interactions. As such, this work recognizes staff training as a crucial element in the delivery of good care. Unfortunately, to date, much of the training into care settings has been badly organized and shown to be ineffective in the long term (Moniz-Cook *et al.* 1998). Moniz-Cook *et al.* suggest that the plight of staff in homes could be greatly improved by delivering training programmes that provided them with the opportunity to discuss their own ideas and initiatives. It is proposed that this would foster a culture of collaboration and reciprocity, and reduce the level of staff burnout. Thus, such 'staff-centred' approaches complement Kitwood's (1997) notion of 'person-centred' work with people with dementia.

Having discussed environmental influences, it is important to examine the person's inner experience of his condition. In order to do this, one is required to produce a comprehensive formulation for the person. The formulation will help to determine both the person's needs and elucidate the mechanisms underpinning any problematic behaviours.

Formulating the person's inner experience

Until relatively recently, formulations were not widely used with people with dementia (Bender 1998). However, researchers are finally beginning to value formulations for this group. Kitwood (1997) used a conceptual model to help develop appropriate formulations designed to access the person's experience of dementia. This model has been adapted by one of the present authors (I. J.), and now includes a mental health component in order to provide a more comprehensive framework (Fig. 8.2). By exploring every element of this equation, one can arrive at a comprehensive formulation of the individual's problems. The components within Figure 8.2 are described below:

(1) *Cognitive status.* The way in which a person with dementia experiences an event will be affected by his ability to process information in a coherent way. For example, deficits in memory and/or problem-solving may lead to distress, particularly when the person has insight into his difficulties. In addition, some of the features displayed by the person with dementia (behaviour, emotions) may reflect changes in brain pathology. Clearly, this must be taken into account when attempting to understand the individual. Because each form of dementia is associated with changes in different cortical and subcortical areas, each one tends to have its characteristic profile. The progressive dementias also have varying temporal and developmental profiles.

(2) *Personality.* Despite dementia being described as a process in which a person 'loses his personality', it is important to appreciate that a person's premorbid personality will be apparent throughout many aspects and phases of the condition. Indeed, it is common for an individual with even severe dementia to want to express lifestyle preferences (e.g. about accommodation, religious practices, food, sexual orientation). While some of the personality changes will be related to changes in brain pathology, others will be associated with psychological sequelae. For example, owing to an emerging sense of vulnerability, a

Cognitive   +   Personality   +   History   +   Physical   +   Environmental   +   Mental health
status   status   status   status

= Person's experience of dementia

Fig. 8.2   An adapted version of Kitwood's (1997) model.

person with dementia may become more emotional and seek more physical attention.

(3) *History.* Aspects of long-term and procedural memory remain relatively preserved in many of the dementias, so the knowledge of the person's history is helpful in understanding the person's behaviour and communications. Information about the individual's life, relationships and roles will also be important. Indeed, it is common to observe historical themes (losses, traumas) re-emerging during the development of the dementing illness.

(4) *Physical health status.* Apart from cognitive impairment associated with head injury, dementia tends to be an illness of old age, and hence it often occurs in a context of declining physical health (e.g. visual and auditory problems) and age-related illness (e.g. arthritis, backache, cancer, toothache, constipation and chiropody ailments). These health-related issues will be important to include within the formulation.

(5) *Mental health status.* The prevalence of mental health problems, particularly within older populations in general, is such that it is important to acknowledge their potential influence. Premorbid difficulties may well interact with current problems to produce affective disorders. A high level of psychiatric morbidity is common following the onset of dementia. For example, Burns *et al.* (1990) showed that 16% of their patients with Alzheimer's disease had delusions, usually concerning theft; a further 20% were experiencing persecutory ideations. Relatively high incidences of psychotic and perceptual disorders have also been found in both multi-infarct (Berrios and Brook 1985, Rubin *et al.* 1988) and subcortical dementia (Cummings 1985).

(6) *Environmental status.* Environmental features have been considered above, but in addition to these it is worth checking whether a person's problematic behaviour is due to him being too hot, too cold or hungry. It is also appropriate to check that the person with dementia is not suffering from excessive unwanted stimulation (e.g. a loud television or radio) and not experiencing any situation that could be defined as abusive.

The development of a formulation, comprised of the above components, helps one to obtain insight into the experience of the whole person, including his past and current perception of the illness. Once the latter has been constructed, one is in a better position to both help and intervene in appropriate ways (James 1999a,b), that is, to act in a manner that resolves any acute difficulties (depression, anxiety, challenging behaviour), while simultaneously promoting the person's dignity and well-being.

A case study is presented in the following section which illustrates the development of the formulation described in Fig. 8.2. The case reveals a typical assessment process, relying on the gathering of data from a variety of key sources using both the person with dementia and people within his environment. Once the information has been developed into a coherent formulation, a set of appropriate and realistic intervention strategies can be produced.

Case study

Background

Mr T is a 79 year old widower. He used to work as a bank manager in the locality and has been living in a residential home for 4 months. The staff at the residential home asked for assistance when they became very concerned about his excessive wandering and aggression.

Mr T was diagnosed 4 years ago with Alzheimer's disease, with particular memory and orientation problems. He suffered a left hemisphere stroke last year, resulting in mild/moderate mobility problems and mild expressive aphasia.

He was recently moved into a residential home because he was assessed to be a risk to himself and his neighbours. For example, he was forgetting to switch off domestic appliances, failing to lock the front door and refusing help from Social Services. For the last 3 years he has been living with his son and daughter-in-law in an annexe of their house. His daughter-in-law has health problems and is no longer able to care for him. Another reason for Mr T's move was the difficulties his daughter-in-law and her husband were having in coping with his constant false accusations of her infidelity.

Initially, Mr T appeared to be settling well in his new home, but after a number of weeks he became increasingly agitated. He was often found wandering the corridors asking to go home. During one recent incident, he hit a fellow resident with his walking stick. He was considered to be depressed and agitated and was prescribed a course of neuroleptics.

The assessment process, and its development into a formulation, will be discussed below:

The initial assessment interview was conducted with Mr T by himself, and then with his son. A second assessment interview was carried out with the staff, and a third involved a period of behavioural observations.

Assessment

Summary of the initial assessment

(i) *History.* Mr T is the eldest of two sons. He was brought up in an upper-working class home in Newcastle. His mother was forced to leave the family home when Mr T was 15 years of age when it was discovered that she was having an affair. He attended grammar school, before entering a bank as a clerk. After 30 years of service, he became manager of his local bank. He married his childhood sweetheart at 21, and after two miscarriages they had one son. His wife died 5 years ago following a stroke. It was around this time that people first noticed

Mr T's cognitive difficulties. His dementia was initially misdiagnosed as depression.

Prior to moving into the residential home. Mr T lived in a terraced house with his son and daughter-in-law. He had lived there for 3 years. He used to get daily support from his family and received regular visits from his vicar. Until 6 months ago, he did some of his own shopping at the corner shop. This stopped when he became increasingly disorientated outside of his home. Prior to his stroke (13 months ago), he cleaned the house himself and kept his room meticulously clean.

(ii) *Personality*. Mr T's son described him as an intelligent, articulate man who was also rather private. Apart from his relationship with his wife, he has had few intimate friends and was commonly described by others as quiet and aloof. His son remarked that his father liked order and discipline, and abhorred over-familiarity. His family described him as frugal and 'a little obsessive' regarding his finances. Over recent years he had become increasingly worried about his finances, and repeatedly sought reassurances regarding his fiscal status.

(iii) *Physical health*. Mr T is generally a healthy individual, although he has prostrate problems and has recently experienced a period of confusion and incontinence resulting from a urinary tract infection. A year ago, a stroke (left partial anterior cerebral infarct) left him weak on his right-hand side. He has mild semantic anomia (naming difficulties), which he is very embarrassed about.

(iv) *Cognitive*. A global screening assessment of his cognitive status using the Middlesex Elderly Assessment of Mental Status (MEAMS) (Golding 1989) and subtests of the WAIS-R (Wechsler Adult Intelligence Scale 1981), revealed memory problems, visuospatial and problem-solving difficulties. These results are consistent with the fact that Mr T finds it difficult to function outside of his normal, routinized environment.

(v) *Environment*. Mr T currently lives in a downstairs room (3.5 m $\times$ 6 m) in a residential home. He dislikes the communal nature of the home and spends a lot of time by himself in his room. When asked about this, he said that he finds the common room intimidating, being dominated by 'aggressive' women and the noisy television. Despite his liking of structure, he finds the 'inflexibility' of the home's regime upsetting, particularly with respect to the rigid meal and bed times. He also fails to see why he cannot go for a walk in the garden before breakfast, although he is aware that there might be some 'confounded' regulations against it. He thinks that staff regard him as an 'ungrateful trouble-maker'. He dislikes their over-familiarity when addressing him, and feels particularly embarrassed by the jocular manner of the young female care assistants when they are engaged in his personal care (toileting, bathing).

Over recent months, Mr T has begun to feel more and more lonely, and this is partly because his son is visiting him less regularly. His son claimed that he was finding it particularly difficult to deal with his father's accusations of his wife's infidelity.

The second stage of the assessment involved an interview with the home's warden and Mr T's key-worker; this was part of the environmental assessment.

Staff assessment

It became evident from the interview with staff that there had been some organizational changes over recent months. This had resulted in a number of staff leaving the home and the re-allocation of key-workers with respect to the residents. Therefore the current key-worker was not very familiar with Mr T's background and was even rather sketchy about his current level of well-being. When we examined Mr T's care plan, it was interesting to note that many of the issues were described in terms of problems rather than needs.

This conversation also revealed that staff viewed Mr T as a rather stubborn person, and some staff felt that he regarded himself as somewhat superior to them. It was accepted that these attitudes probably had a negative impact on staff members' interactions with him. Indeed, it seemed that often carers were quite happy for him to stay in his room as he was 'out of the way'.

Observational assessment

The third form of assessment looked at the problematic behaviours in more detail. These observational assessments of Mr T operating within his environment were key to the assessment process. A research assistant was used as an independent observer to provide accurate and unbiased data (i.e. the information was freer from institutional and cultural biases). It was also felt important to ask the staff to engage in observational work too, as it required them to examine Mr T's behaviour in more detail and also to identify some of the triggers which might be contributing to the behaviours.

The data from the staff were combined with information from the research assistant. The assistant was asked to monitor Mr T's behaviour over 3 days. A number of important observations were made with respect to both the wandering and the aggression.

Two forms of wandering were identified. In the morning Mr T's wandering seemed to have a purpose, and often involved him wandering around the corridors. He appeared to follow a routine, occasionally trying to access the garden through doors which looked out on to it. A more aimless form of walking was identified later in the day, which seemed to be associated with peak visiting hours. At such times he would frequently be agitated, asking for his coat. He often hovered around the front door, requesting to be taken either home or to his bank.

One of the staff observing this first form of walking felt that it had a 'social' quality about it. She suggested that the wandering provided Mr T with the opportunity for some social contact with other people in the home. She noted that it was common for him to nod and smile as he passed by other people in the corridor. Based on what was known about his background (i.e. his dislike of intimate contact with people), the member of staff's hypothesis seemed plausible. Indeed, Mr T's walking may well have provided him with a level of social contact that he found most acceptable.

The few episodes of aggression were all connected with perceived invasion of Mr T's privacy. For example, on one occasion another resident entered his room without knocking on the door, and in a different incident he became upset when a female resident tried to hug him.

The observations also revealed that Mr T was very embarrassed by the fact that he required help in the toilet. Indeed, it appeared that two episodes of incontinence were due to him failing to ask for the help he required to get to the toilet in time.

Formulation

The information gathered was used to develop a formulation, resulting in the generation of a hypothesis concerning the triggers and maintaining factors associated with Mr T's behaviour.

The formulation provided insight into Mr T's condition and, in conjunction with the organization's philosophy of care, realistic interventions were proposed which were appropriate and practical for his situation.

Interventions

A meeting was arranged at which the formulation was presented to Mr T, his family and representatives from the home. Owing to Mr T's deteriorating cognitive abilities, particularly his memory problems, it was decided that the most effective

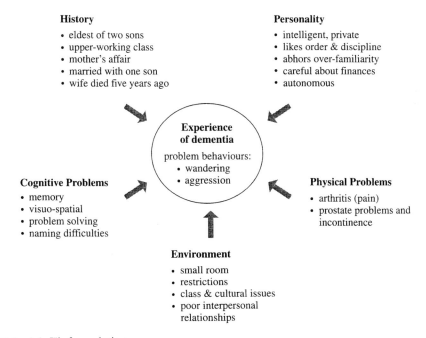

History
- eldest of two sons
- upper-working class
- mother's affair
- married with one son
- wife died five years ago

Personality
- intelligent, private
- likes order & discipline
- abhors over-familiarity
- careful about finances
- autonomous

Experience of dementia
problem behaviours:
- wandering
- aggression

Cognitive Problems
- memory
- visuo-spatial
- problem solving
- naming difficulties

Physical Problems
- arthritis (pain)
- prostate problems and incontinence

Environment
- small room
- restrictions
- class & cultural issues
- poor interpersonal relationships

Fig. 8.3 Mr T's formulation.

treatments would be behavioural and social modification strategies, as opposed to direct counselling techniques.

These strategies were to be directed at Mr T's perceived needs, which were derived from the formulation. Five major needs were identified.

(1) *to provide Mr T with the appropriate level of privacy*—Mr T was moved to the end room of the corridor, next door to a man with whom he had recently begun to strike up a relationship. He was given a key to the door, and a sign was placed on the door saying 'Please knock before entering'. A referral was sent to the continence service in order to provide advice for an appropriate toileting regime. A new seating arrangement was created in an area of the common room, furthest away from the television, which permitted a small group of people to sit and chat. Here residents were encouraged to be a part of the wider community, but at the same time enjoyed a greater degree of privacy.

(2) *to get the staff to address Mr T in a socially validating manner*—Mr T's formulation was presented at a staff meeting. The hypothesis regarding his disruptive behaviours was discussed together with the reasons why it was felt appropriate for him to be addressed in a more formal manner. The staff agreed that some of Mr T's current behaviours might be a reflection of his premorbid personality. Indeed, some of his actions previously seen as challenging could be interpreted as him striving to maintain formality, order and privacy. The observations made by the member of staff regarding the 'social' nature of the wandering helped the staff to reformulate Mr T's behaviour. As a result, the staff were better able to see the therapeutic aspect of this feature. It helped them to tolerate the activity better, making them less likely to perceive it as challenging behaviour.

(3) *to support his son in making regular visits in order to combat his father's loneliness*—this required a counselling session with the son, in order to help him deal with the tricky issue regarding the claims of infidelity against his wife. During the session, it was explained that it was common for people who are feeling vulnerable to reactivate themes that had previously caused trauma. In the case of his father, the plight of his own mother is likely to have left him feeling insecure, and thus he was now revisiting this theme at a time of great insecurity. It was also suggested that more regular visits might reduce his father's insecurity and in turn reduce the level of accusations. The son was also advised that, when he met his father, he should open the conversation by orientating Mr T to his wife and the marital status. For example, he might say 'Hi Dad. My wife Joan asked me to send her best wishes. She's keeping well. Obviously, being married to me for 25 years must be doing her some good.'

(4) *allowing Mr T to walk in the garden at times when he was feeling tense*—some of his wandering behaviour was thought to be his attempt to relieve tension. The staff did not think it was possible for him to be allowed into the garden before breakfast, owing to safety issues, but they suggested that he could walk in the

garden immediately after breakfast. However, before this could be tried out, it was necessary to put a more secure lock on the garden gate.

(5) *to go with him to the bank*—it was also suggested that Mr T should be taken to the bank once a month by his son to get a bank statement about his finances. His son brought in a ledger in which his father could record any financial transactions that he chose to. This latter feature needed to be monitored carefully to ensure that Mr T did not start accusing the staff of stealing any fictitious monies.

Outcome

Mr T's aggressive behaviours reduced markedly as a result of the interventions. It is interesting to note, however, that one of the nurses suggested that some of the improvement may have been due in part to the staff relabelling his actions. For example, acts that were previously labelled as challenging were now more likely to be recognized as communication strategies. Thus they were dealt with appropriately, usually before they became more extreme and dysfunctional.

Mr T's wandering behaviour remained fairly constant. It was evident, however, that he gained pleasure from his morning stroll in the garden.

General discussion

The approach described here puts the person with dementia at the centre of the formulation and thus can be described as person-centred. Over the last 20 years, there has been a great development in person-centred approaches. At the heart of the approach is the aim of working to reduce the distress of the person by identifying and treating the reversible causes of physical, behavioural, cognitive and mental difficulties in ways that preserve the person's dignity and promote his independence. In the described case, it was known that Mr T valued his privacy, particularly when engaging in self-care activities. It was deemed important to preserve his range of functioning, especially with respect to his mobility and attempts to control his own finances. However, it was necessary to recognize that these opportunities could only be given within realistic and safe boundaries.

The interventions employed in this case involved mainly modifications of Mr T's environment, but other therapeutic strategies could have been employed. Indeed, owing to his reaction caused by the loss of his mother early in his life, a course of resolution therapy might have been appropriate (see Chapter 10). In an ideal setting, one would implement an integrated care package that contained both environmental modification and psychological components (validation, reality orientation, and cognitive therapies). However, in reality, such interventions are rarely effective unless staff and managers are willing to commit resources, including a commitment to staff training (see Chapter 12).

The presented case also demonstrates the negative impact of an impoverished interpersonal environment, with Mr T experiencing problems in all of his proximal relationships. For example, he had difficulties with his son and daughter-in-law, with his fellow residents and with the staff. This sociotropic feature was felt to be a particularly important source of distress, because good quality relationships, which validate and individuate the person, are essential in maintaining self-esteem. This case describes a number of interventions to facilitate better social interactions between Mr T and his son and fellow residents, but the formulation suggested that the greatest amount of work needed to be done with the staff.

A feature that underlay many of the difficulties in Mr T's case was a cultural difference between Mr T and the staff. This upper working-class man found it difficult to settle in a community that he perceived as being brash and irreverent. On the other hand, the staff referred to him as 'snooty' and perceived him as someone who felt superior to them. Such perceptions are powerful, greatly influencing the nature of social interactions. As outlined earlier, they can occur with respect to both social class and ethnic differences and are often overlooked in conceptualizations.

This case study also highlights a rather reactive approach to the distress experienced by a person with dementia. For example, the above interventions were driven mainly by attempts to solve Mr T's challenging behaviours. A more holistic approach would have assessed all the important areas of his life, his strengths, weaknesses, likes and dislikes. Relevant quality-of-life questions would also have been asked, both problematic and non-problematic (is he sufficiently intellectually stimulated?; to what degree is he sexually/sensually satisfied?).

It is suggested that these holistic approaches are much better at promoting greater levels of well-being across the whole range of a person's biological, physical and psychological needs. In the above case, the role of medication was not outlined. It is important to note, however, that medication played a complementary role in the treatment of Mr T. In accordance with good practice, Mr T's tolerance of the neuroleptics was assessed carefully and his progress on them monitored over time.

Conclusion

Traditional psychotherapy has often been criticized for focusing too much on 'intrapsychic' phenomena, i.e. mental processes, thoughts and feelings (Milne *et al.* 1999). For obvious reasons this has not been the case in the field of dementia, owing to the conditions affecting the cognitive abilities of a person with dementia. Indeed, it may even be the case that, until recently, workers in this field have concentrated on environmental and behavioural issues and failed to pay sufficient attention to the inner experience of a person with dementia. The present chapter has attempted to readdress these features. It has examined the person's experience in terms of his environment and sense of personhood. The case study suggests that, in order to understand a person's behaviour, it is vital to produce a formulation that provides a window into his experience. Once having gained such access, it is then more likely that one can arrive at interventions that are both realistic and appropriate for the person.

Acknowledgements

Thank you to F. Katharina Reichelt for her intellectual contribution to this work, and to Tricia Roe for her help in the preparation of the chapter.

REFERENCES

Annerstedt, L., Gustafson, L. and Nilsson, K. (1993). Medical outcome of psychological intervention in demented patients: one year clinical follow-up after relocation into group living units. *International Journal of Geriatric Psychiatry*, **8**, 833–41.

Audit Commission (1986). *Making a Reality of Community Care.* HMSO, London.

Barclay Report (1982). *Social Workers: Their Role and Tasks*. Bedford Square Press, London.

Bender, M. (1998). Shifting our focus from brain to mind. *Journal of Dementia Care*, **6**, 20–22.

Berrios, G. and Brook, P. (1985). Delusions and the psychopathology of the elderly with dementia. *Acta Psychiatrica Scandinavia*, **68**, 263–70.

Bradford Dementia Group (1997). *Evaluating Demetia Care. The DCM Method: The Dementia Care Mapping Manual*, 7th edn. University of Bradford, Bradford.

Burns, A., Jacoby, R. and Levy, R. (1990). Psychiatric phenomena in Alzheimer's disease. 1: Disorders of thought content. *British Journal of Psychiatry*, **157**, 72–6.

Clegg, J. A. (1993). Putting people first: a social constructionalist approach to learning disability. *British Journal of Clinical Psychology*, **32**, 389–406.

Cohen-Mansfield, J. and Werner, P. (1998). The effects of an enhanced environment on nursing home residents who pace. *Gerontologist*, **38**, 199–208.

Cummings, J. (1985). Organic delusions: phenomenology, anatomical correlations and review. *British Journal of Psychiatry*, **146**, 184–97.

Dick, R. (1999). Just another disability: design on dementia. *Journal of Dementia Care*, **7**, 20–22.

Emerson, E. (1998). Working with people with challenging behaviour. In *Clinical Psychology and People with Intellectual Disabilities* (Emerson, E., Hatton, C., Bromley, J. and Caine, A., eds), pp. 127–153. John Wiley and Sons, Chichester.

Golding, E. (1989). *The Middlesex Elderly Assessment of Mental State*. Thames Valley Test Company, Bury St Edmunds.

Griffiths, R. (1988). *Community Care: Agenda for Action*. HMSO, London.

Hadley, R. and Hatch, S. (1981). *Social Welfare and the Failure of the State*. George Allen and Unwin, London.

Hewawasam, L. (1996). Floor patterns limit wandering of people with Alzheimer's. *Nursing Times*, **92**, 41–4.

Hussian, R. A. and Brown, D. C. (1987). Use of two-dimensional grid patterns to limit hazardous ambulation in demented patients. *Journal of Gerontology*, **45**, 558–60.

Iliffe, S. (1999). Commissioning dementia care—an emergency strategy. *Journal of Dementia Care*, **7**, 14–15.

James, I. A. (1999a). Using a cognitive rationale to conceptualize anxiety in people with dementia. *Behavioural and Cognitive Psychotherapy*, **27**, 345–51.

James, I. A. (1999b). Cognitive conceptualisations of distress in dementia. *Clinical Psychology Forum*, **134**, 21–5.

James, I. A. and Reichelt, F. K. (2000). Promoting dementia care mapping's role as a supervision tool. *PSIGE Newsletter*. British Psychological Society, **72**, 34–7.

Jenkins, C. (1998). Bridging the divide of culture and language. *Journal of Dementia Care*, **6**, 22–4.

King's Fund (1986) *Living Well Into Old Age.* King's Fund, London.

King's Fund (1987). *Facilitating Innovation in Community Care.* King's Fund, London.

Kitwood, T. (1997). *Dementia Reconsidered.* Open University Press, Buckingham.

Kitwood, T. and Bredin, K. (1992). A new approach to the evaluation of dementia care. *Journal of Advances in Health and Nursing Care*, **1**, 41–60.

Marshall, M., Judd, S. and Phippen, P. (1998). *Design for Dementia.* Hawker Publications, London.

Milne, D., Dickson, S., Blackburn, I.-M., and James, I. (1999). All in the head? A content analysis of cognitive therapy trainees and experts. *Journal of Cognitive Psychotherapy*, **13**, 203–13.

Moniz-Cook, E., Agar, S., Silver, M., Woods, R., Wang, M., Elston, C. and Win, T. (1998). Can staff training reduce behavioural problems in residential care for the elderly mentally ill? *International Journal of Geriatric Psychiatry*, **13**, 149–58.

Novaco, R. W. (1993). Clinicians ought to view anger contextually. *Behaviour Change*, **10**, 208–18.

Parker, J. and Penhale, B. (1998). *Forgotten People: Positive Approaches to Dementia Care.* Arena, Aldershot.

Patel, N. and Mirza, N. R. (2000) Care for ethnic minorities: the professional's view. *Journal of Dementia Care*, **8**, 26–8.

Patel, N., Mirza, N. R., Lindblad, P., Samaoli, O. and Marshall, M. (1998). *Dementia and Minority Ethnic Older People: Managing Care in the UK, Denmark and France.* Russell House, Lyme Regis.

Rogan, F. (1998). Dementia-friendly design guidelines. *Journal of Dementia Care*, **6**, 10–18.

Rubin, E., Drevets, W. and Burke, A. (1988). The nature of psychotic symptoms in senile dementia of the Alzheimer's type, *Journal of Geriatric Psychiatry and Neurology*, **1**, 16–20.

Sixsmith, A., Stilwell, J. and Copeland, J. (1993). 'Rementia': challenging the limits of dementia care. *International Journal of Geriatric Psychiatry*, **8**, 993–1000.

Social Service Inspectorate (1990). *All Change from Hospital to Community.* HMSO, London.

Wagner Report (1988). *Residential Care: a Positive Choice.* HMSO, London.

Wechsler, D. (1981). *WAIS-R Manual.* The Psychological Corporation. New York.

WHO (1986). Dementia in later life: research and action: report of a WHO scientific group on senile dementia. World Health Organization, Geneva.

9 Depression and burden in dementia carers: the role of behavioural and psychological symptoms

Introduction

The majority of people with dementia live in the community, usually supported by one main informal carergiver, on whom the greatest share of responsibility falls. Indeed, the day-to-day rigours of caregiving are extremely demanding, a point made very well in the publication *The 36 Hour Day* (Mace and Rabins 1981). Caregivers have important mental health needs in their own right, their well-being has a key impact upon the quality of life of the person that they are looking after and they represent the cornerstone of any community care package, without whom institutional care would become necessary for many more dementia sufferers. Supporting caregivers effectively is hence also important for economic reasons. Many aspects of the caregiving role are stressful, although the presence of behavioural and psychological symptoms in dementia (BPSD) appears to be one of the key factors, both as a precipitant of burden and depression, and as a factor that leads to the breakdown of community care packages. The relationship between psychiatric morbidity in caregivers, BPSD symptoms and some of the implications for care are the focus of this chapter.

The term BPSD covers a diverse cluster of behaviour disturbances, such as restlessness (Hope *et al.* 1994), aggression (Patel and Hope 1992), shouting (Cohen-Mansfield and Werner 1997) and a variety of psychiatric symptoms, including delusions (Burns *et al.* 1990), hallucinations (Holroyd and Sheldon-Keller 1995), depression (Greenwald *et al.* 1989) and anxiety (Ballard *et al.* 1996a). Such symptoms are extremely common in dementia sufferers. The current chapter will review the evidence that these symptoms are important associations of burden and depression in caregivers, and will make some preliminary suggestions regarding priorities for intervention studies.

The concepts of burden and depression

A number of different concepts have been used to try to capture the essence of the practical and emotional demands of caregiving. These include broadly defined terms such as burden (Montgomery *et al.* 1985), stress (Knight *et al.* 1993) and caregiver strain (Cantor 1983), as well as more tightly defined specific measures of psychiatric morbidity, particularly depression. The majority of reports focus upon burden, which is usually subdivided into the categories of objective and subjective burden (Grad and Sainsbury 1965). However, burden is relative, usually assessed by a score on a burden questionnaire; there is no such thing *per se* as excess burden. 'Objective burden' refers to the level of disability and problem behaviours with which the carer has to cope; 'subjective burden' focuses upon the emotional response of carers to the practical demands placed upon them. The latter incorporates a variety of items such as exhaustion, distress and overload. The constituents do vary slightly between the different burden scales, but there is good internal consistency between the component elements (Pearlin *et al.* 1990), and they are effective in capturing the essence of the emotional experience of caregiving.

Psychiatric morbidity has been measured in the majority of studies by scores on specific rating scales for depression (Fitting *et al.* 1986, Dura *et al.* 1990, Schulz *et al.* 1990) or by more general measures of psychiatric dysfunction (Brodaty and Hadzi-Pavlovic 1990, Draper *et al.* 1992), although some studies have used operationalized clinical diagnosis. Even though one would expect some overlap between subjective burden and psychiatric morbidity, the two concepts are essentially different and capture different aspects of the reaction to the caregiving process (see Fig. 9.1).

This framework highlights a number of important points. For example, it clearly distinguishes between objective features (BPSDs) and the resulting distress (burden and psychiatric morbidity). It also illustrates the important role that cognitions play both in the form and level of distress experienced (Lazarus 1993). Indeed, as illustrated, in situations where the carer appraises himself/herself as having appropriate coping resources, he/she may achieve a sense of mastery by dealing with the situation adequately.

The framework also presents a conceptual template on which to base both therapeutic assessment and intervention strategies. For example, it suggests the need to assess the nature of the BPSD, together with the carer's subjective appraisal of them. In addition, it implies the need to enhance the carer's coping strategies, and where appropriate get them to re-evaluate any dysfunctional appraisal biases (catastrophizing; minimizing the positive and maximizing the negatives, etc.).

The importance of BPSD

BPSD are associated with patient distress (Gilley *et al.* 1991, Ballard *et al.* 1995b) and are perceived to be the most difficult symptoms to cope with by carers (Rabins

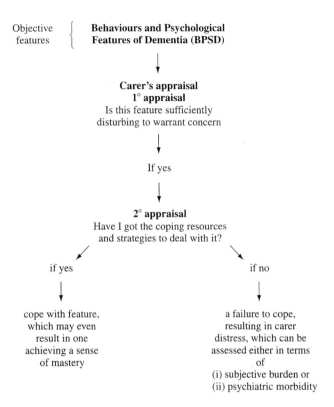

Fig. 9.1   A framework demonstrating the relationship between carer coping and the objective and subjective features of stress.
(By Permission Ballard C., Lower K., Powell I., O'Brien J. and James I. (2000) Impact of Behavioural and Psychological Symptoms of Dementia on Caregivers. In International Psychogeriatrics, **12** (supp. 1) 93–105)

et al. 1982). They are associated with an increased rate of cognitive decline (Rosen and Zubenko 1991, Förstl *et al.* 1993), increased rates of institutionalization (Steele *et al.* 1990) and have been associated with physical abuse in one recent study (Compton *et al.* 1997).

BPSD have also been shown to damage the patient–carer relationship (Greene *et al.* 1982, Deimling and Bass, 1986). Mood changes and withdrawal are particularly important, resulting in changes in the caregiver's feelings towards the patient, hence disrupting the bonds of affection that are vital in maintaining interpersonal relationships (Horowitz and Shindelman 1983). It is therefore not surprising that BPSD are a common precipitant of family discord (Rockwell *et al.* 1994).

Hence, one would expect that BPSD would be an important trigger for increased burden and depression amongst dementia carers. However, this cannot be assumed, and the evidence must be evaluated carefully.

BPSD as an association of caregiver burden

BPSD have been consistently associated with an increased level of carer burden. Apart from the report of Zarit *et al.* (1980), all studies focusing upon this area have identified a significant association between some aspect of BPSD and caregiver burden (Table 9.1), with many studies finding BPSD to be the strongest correlate. Many of these studies used an overall score of behavioural disturbance, which can in some cases be difficult to interpret. Thus comparisons, and overall conclusions, are difficult to make because some scales incorporate items pertaining to disabilities, such as incontinence, whilst others do not operationally define the BPSD symptoms in question. Nevertheless, a pattern does emerge, suggesting that withdrawal, apathy (Greene *et al.* 1982, Logiudice *et al.* 1995), mood disturbance (Donaldson *et al.* 1997), aggression (Gilleard *et al.* 1982) and restlessness (Gallagher-Thompson *et al.* 1992) may be the most important individual symptoms. The evidence is not as strong for an association between psychotic symptoms and caregiver burden, although a significant link was reported by Donaldson *et al.* (1997).

Hence, overall there is an overwhelming weight of evidence suggesting a significant relationship between BPSD and carer burden. Details of these studies are given in Table 9.1. Further work is still required to examine the relationship with specific BPSD, in studies which define the individual behavioural and psychiatric disturbances more stringently.

The issue of caregiver burden is an extremely important feature to address because the impact on the carer is so great. In addition to the distress and psychiatric morbidity experienced by caregivers, the subjective burden they experience also influences a number of other key parameters. For example, Brown *et al.* (1990) demonstrated a significant link between increased use of support and clinical services and the level of carer distress; whilst Katon *et al.* (1982) demonstrated that the level of stress in caregivers is associated with an increased number of visits to the general practitioner and a greater number of prescriptions. It is also clear that the level of carer burden is an extremely important predictor of subsequent institutionalization (Steele *et al.* 1990).

Therefore, in addition to the implicit distress experienced by the caregiver, it is likely that increased carer burden also affects the quality of life and symptoms experienced by the patient, as well as having major health and economic implications.

BPSD as an association of depression in dementia caregivers

The relationship between BPSD and caregiver depression is rather less clear-cut than the association between BPSD and burden. Although several studies have reported significant associations between 'demanding behaviour', or the overall level of behavioural disturbance in patients, and depression in their caregivers (Gilleard *et al.* 1982, Deimling and Bass, 1986, Pruchno and Resch, 1989, Baumgarten *et al.* 1992; Gallagher-Thompson *et al.* 1992, Ballard *et al.* 1996, Cullen *et al.* 1997, Lowery *et al.* 1999), a number of other studies (Hayley *et al.* 1987, Brodaty and Hadzi-Pavolic, 1990, Ballard *et al.* 1995) have failed to identify any significant relationship. On balance, the evidence does suggest a possible association between BPSD and caregiver depression, although the case is unproven.

Perhaps one of the explanations for disparity between studies lies in the nature of depression amongst dementia carers. Ballard *et al.* (1996) followed up a cohort of carers monthly for 1 year. Although cross-sectionally at the time of the baseline evaluation, <30% of the cohorts were depressed, the majority of the carers developed depression at some stage over the year of follow up. A large proportion of the carers experienced a month or two of minor depression, followed by recovery. Given the transient and recurring nature of depression, a cross-sectional model may therefore be inappropriate. Although Ballard *et al.* (1995a) were not able to demonstrate an association between BPSD and caregiver depression in a cross-sectional analysis, they demonstrated a strong association between the number of months of depression over the follow-up year and the total problem behaviour score (Ballard *et al.* 1996b). The only other longitudinal study (Gallagher-Thompson *et al.* 1992) also reported a significant association between BPSD and caregiver depression. Clearly there is a need for further longitudinal studies in this area. It is likely that BPSD is a much better predictor of depression longitudinally than in a cross-sectional evaluation. The studies discussed in this section are summarized in Table 9.1.

Despite the equivocal evidence regarding an association, there is ample evidence of high levels of depression in carers. For example, the reported prevalence of depression in the carers of dementia sufferers varies from 14% (Morris *et al.* 1988) to 78% (Harper *et al.* 1993), with the main body of work reporting prevalences between 30% and 50% (Pagel *et al.* 1985, Williamson and Schultz, 1993). The majority of these studies used standardized cut-offs on depression rating scales, although Pagel *et al.* (1985) applied research diagnostic criteria (RDC; Spitzer *et al.* 1978) to the rating scale data. Coope *et al.* (1995) reported a prevalence of 29% for case-level depression using the AGECAT system, from a standardized psychiatric assessment; with a further 4% of carers experiencing case levels of anxiety and 12% experiencing subcase levels of depression. There was a high level of concordance between RDC and AGECAT diagnoses. It is hence clear that in cross-sectional studies, clinically significant depression is common amongst the carers of dementia sufferers. Only a quarter of these depressed carers, however, experienced a depressive illness categotized as major by RDC (Coope *et al.* 1995).

Coping strategies

Using a stress/coping conceptual model of caregiving (Fig. 9.1), it has been postulated that coping strategies may be an intermediate variable, predicting the development of increased subjective burden and psychiatric morbidity (Williamson and Schulz 1993), in response to the rigours of caregiving. There is certainly anecdotal literature (Haley *et al.* 1987) suggesting that individuals who use more active coping

Table 9.1 Summary of methodology and design of the studies reviewed

Study	Patients		Caregivers		Source of patient/caregiver subject dyads	Design	Data analysis techniques	Main measure of outcome
	n	diagnosis	n	relationship[a]				
1	29	senile dementia	29	spouse and daughters	research and training centre; out-patients	C/S	correlations	burden
2	46	dementia	46		psychogeriatric day hospital patients	C/S	correlations and multiple regression analysis	burden and depression
3	38	senile dementia	38		geriatric day hospital attenders	C/S	correlations	
4	586	mentally impaired elderly	586	spouses and children	cross-sectional study of intra-household caregiving	C/S	path analysis	depression
5	40	dementia	40	children	screening survey investigating mental status in patients from a general practice register	C/S	correlations	burden
	39	controls	39					
6	54	dementia	54	relatives	dementia caregiver support group; social services and healthcare agencies; professional referrals; media advertisements	C/S	correlations	depression
7	262	Alzheimer's disease	262	spouses	public announcements; carer support groups; community and religious groups; hospitals	C/S	analysis of variance	burden and depression
8	53	dementia	53	relatives	dementia caregiver support groups	C/S	correlations	depression
9	120	dementia	120	relatives	general practice registers	C/S	correlations	burden
	107	controls	107	relatives				
10	409	dementia	409	spouses and children	dementia caregiver support groups	C/S	multiple regression analysis	burden
11	103	dementia	103	spouses and children	geriatric assessment unit; out-patients	C/S	analysis of variance and multiple regression analysis	depression
12	115	controls	115	relatives	patients undergoing cataract surgery senile dementia out-patients	L	correlations and multiple regression analysis	depression
	29	Alzheimer's	29	spouses				
13	51	dementia	51		referrals to a community rehabilitation and geriatric service	C/S	correlations	burden
	48	controls	48					

14	140	dementia	140		Alzheimer's diagnostic centre; out-patients	C/S	correlations	burden
15	213	dementia	213	relatives	hospitals; day-care centres; community health clinics; carer support groups	L	multiple regression analysis	burden
16	201	Alzheimer's	201	children	cross-sectional study of adult child caregivers of Alzheimer's patients	C/S	multiple regression analysis	burden and depression
17	42	cognitively impaired elderly	42		hospital aged care assessment centre	C/S	correlations and multiple regression analysis	burden
18	100	dementia	100	carers	patients known to old-age psychiatry services	C/S	correlations and analysis of variance	burden
19	109	dementia	109	relatives	consecutive referrals to clinical old-age psychiatry services	C/S	multiple regression	depression
20	100	dementia	100	relatives	referrals to old-age psychiatry services	C/S	Mann-Whitney U-test	depression
21	90	dementia	90	relatives	from Canberra longitudinal study of the elderly	C/S	multiple regression analysis	depression
22	50	dementia	50	primary carers	clinical convenience sample	C/S	multiple regression analysis	burden
23	85	dementia	85	relatives	patients followed up from 1995 study	L	correlations and multiple regression analysis	depression

1, Zarit et al. 1980; 2, Gilleard et al. 1982: 3, Greene et al. 1982; 4, Deimling and Bass 1986; 5, Eagles et al. 1987; 6, Haley et al. 1987; 7, Pruchno and Resch 1989; 8, Brodaty and Hadzi-Pavlovic 1990; 9, O'Connor et al. 1990; 10, Harper and Lund 1990; 11, Baumgarten et al. 1992; 12, Gallagher-Thompson et al. 1992; 13, Draper et al. 1992; 14, Farran et al. 1993; 15, Reis et al. 1994; 16, Weiler et al. 1994; 17, Logiudice et al. 1995; 18, Donaldson et al. 1998; 19, Ballard et al. 1995a; 20, Lowery et al. 2000; 21, Cullen et al. 1997; 22, Coen et al. 1997; 23, Ballard et al. 1996.
[a] Caregiver samples included relatives and non-relatives, except where specified.
C/S, cross-sectional; L, longitudinal.

strategies, such as problem solving, experience fewer symptoms of depression than carers who rely on more passive methods. Supporting this work, Saad *et al.* (1995) reported significant associations between positive strategies for managing disturbed behaviour and active strategies for managing the implications of the illness respectively, and reduced levels of caregiver depression. Nolan *et al.* (1997) suggest that an important role of professionals is in helping carers enhance their coping skills, supporting existing skills and helping to develop new ones.

Conclusion

Burden and psychiatric morbidity in caregivers are important predictors of patient and carer distress, as well as service utilization, and are therefore important targets for further research. BPSD are strong predictors of caregiver burden and also predict psychiatric morbidity amongst caregivers in longitudinal studies. The coping strategies adopted by caregivers may be important in determining whether they experience increased burden or psychiatric morbidity in response to BPSD symptoms.

REFERENCES

Ballard, C. G., Saad, K., Coope. B., Graham, C., Gahir, M., Wilcock, G. K. and Oyebode, F. (1995a). The aetiology of depression in the carers of dementia sufferers. *Journal of Affective Disorders*, **35**, 59–63.

Ballard, C. G., Saad, K., Patel, A., Gahir, M., Solis, M., Coope, B. and Wilcock, G. (1995b). The prevalence and phenomenology of psychotic symptoms in dementia sufferers. *International Journal of Geriatric Psychiatry*, **10**, 477–85.

Ballard, C., Boyle, A., Bowler, C. and Lindesay, J. (1996a). Anxiety disorders in dementia sufferers. *International Journal of Geriatric Psychiatry*, **11**, 987–90.

Ballard, C. G., Eastwood, C., Gahire, M. and Wilcock, G. (1996b). A follow up study of depression in the carers of dementia sufferers. *British Medical Journal*, **312**, 947–8.

Baumgarten, M., Battista, R. N., Infante-Rivard, C., Hanley, J. A., Becker, S. and Gauthier, S. (1992). The psychological and physical health of family members caring for an elderly person with dementia. *Journal of Clinical Epidemiology*, **45**, 61–70.

Brodaty, H. and Hadzi-Pavlovic, D. (1990). Psychosocial effects on carers living with persons with dementia. *Australian and New Zealand Journal of Psychiatry*, **24**, 351–61.

Brown, L. J., Potter, J. F. and Foster, B. G. (1990). Caregiver burden should be evaluated during geriatric assessment. *Journal of the American Geriatrics Society*, **38**, 455–60.

Burns, A., Jacoby, R. and Levy, R. (1990). Psychiatric phenomena in Alzheimer's. *British Journal of Psychiatry*, **157**, 72–96.

Cantor, M. H. (1983). Strain among caregivers: a study of experience in the United States. *Gerontologist*, **23**, 597–604.

Cohen-Mansfield, J. and Werner, P. (1997). Typology of disruptive vocalisations in older persons suffering from dementia. *International Journal of Geriatric Psychiatry*, **12**, 1079–91.

Coen, R. F., Swanwick, G. R. J., O'Boyle, C. A. and Coakley, D. (1997). Behaviour disturbance and other predictors of carer burden in Alzheimer's disease. *International Journal of Geriatric Psychiatry*, **12**, 331–6.

Compton, S. A., Flanagan, P. and Gregg, W. (1997). Elder abuse in people with dementia in Northern Ireland: prevalence and predictors in cases referred to a psychiatry of old age service. *International Journal of Geriatric Psychiatry*, **12**, 632–5.

Coope, B., Ballard, C., Saad, K., Patel, A., Bentham, P., Bannister, C., Graham, C. and Wilcock, G. (1995). The prevalence of depression in the carers of dementia sufferers. *International Journal of Geriatric Psychiatry*, **10**, 237–42.

Cullen, J. S., Grayson, D. A. and Jorm, A. F. (1997). Clinical diagnoses and disability of cognitively impaired older persons as predictors of stress in their carers. *International Journal of Geriatric Psychiatry*, **12**, 1019–28.

Deimling, G. T. and Bass, D. M. (1986). Symptoms of mental impairment among elderly adults and their effects on family caregivers. *Journal of Gerontology*, **41**, 778–84.

Donaldson, C., Tarrier, N. and Burns, A. (1997). The impact of the symptoms of dementia on caregivers. *British Journal of Psychiatry*, **170**, 62–8.

Draper, B. M., Poulos, C. J., Cole, A. M., Ehrlich, F. and Poulos, R. G. (1992). A comparison of caregivers for stroke and dementia victims. *Journal of the American Geriatrics Society*, **40**, 896–901.

Dura, J. R., Haywood-Niltes, E. and Kiecolt-Glaser, J. K. (1990). Spousal caregivers of persons with Alzheimer's and Parkinson's disease dementias: a preliminary comparison. *Gerontologist*, **30**, 332–6.

Eagles, J. M., Craig, A., Rawlinson, F., Restall, D. B., Beattie, J. A. and Besson, J. A. (1987). The psychological well-being of supporters of the demented elderly. *British Journal of Psychiatry*, **150**, 293–8.

Farran, C. J., Keane-Hagerty, E., Tatarowicz, L. and Scorza, E. (1993). Dementia care-receiver needs and their impact on caregivers. *Clinical Nursing Research*, **2**, 86–97.

Fitting, M., Rabins, P., Lucas, J. M. and Eastham, J. (1986). Caregivers for dementia patients: a comparison of husbands and wives. *Gerontologist*, **26**, 248–52.

Förstl, H., Besthorn, C., Geiger-Kabisch, C., Sattel, H. and Schreiter-Gasser, U. (1993). Psychotic features and the course of Alzheimer's disease: relationship to cognitive electro-encephalographic and computerised tomography. *Acta Psychiatrica Scandinavica*, **87**, 395–9.

Gallagher-Thompson, D., Brooks, J. O., Bliwise, D., Leader, J. and Yesavage, J. A. (1992). The relations among caregiver stress, 'sundowning' symptoms, and cognitive decline in Alzheimer's disease. *Journal of the American Geriatrics Society*, **40**, 807–10.

Gilleard, C. J., Boyd, W. D. and Watt, G. (1982). Problems in caring for the elderly mentally infirm at home. *Archives of Gerontology and Geriatrics*, **1**, 151–8.

Gilley, D. W., Whalen, M. E., Wilson, R. S. and Bennett, D. A. (1991). Hallucinations and associated factors in Alzheimer's disease. *Journal of Neuropsychiatry*, **3**, 371–6.

Grad, J. and Sainsbury, P. (1965). An evaluation of the effects of caring for the aged at home. In *Psychiatric Disorders in the Aged*. WPA Symposium. Geigy, Manchester.

Greene, J. G., Smith, R., Gardiner, M. and Timbury, C. G. (1982). Measuring behavioural disturbance of elderly demented patients in the community and its effects on relatives: a factor analytic study. *Age and Ageing*, **11**, 121–6.

Greenwald, B. S., Kramer-Ginsberg, E., Marin, D. B., Laitman, L. B., Hermann, C. K. and Mohs, R. C. (1989). Dementia with co-existent major depression. *American Journal of Psychiatry*, **146**, 1472–8.

Haley, W. E., Levine, E. G., Brown, S. L. and Bartolucci, A. A. (1987). Stress, appraisal, coping and social support as predictors of adaptational outcome among dementia caregivers. *Psychology and Aging*, **2**, 323–30.

Harper, S. and Lund, D. A. (1990). Wives, husbands and daughters caring for institutionalized and non-institutionalized dementia patients: toward a model of caregiver burden. *International Journal of Aging and Human Development*, **30**, 241–62.

Harper, D. J., Manasse, P. R., James, O. and Newton, J. T. (1993). Intervening to reduce distress in caregivers of impaired elderly people: a preliminary evaluation. *International Journal of Geriatric Psychiatry*, **8**, 139–45.

Holroyd, S. and Sheldon-Keller, A. (1995). A study of visual hallucinations in Alzheimer's disease. *American Journal of Geriatric Psychiatry*, **3**, 198–205.

Hope, T., Tilling, K., Gedling, K., Keene, J. M., Cooper, S. D. and Fairburn, C. G. (1994). The structure of wandering in dementia. *International Journal of Geriatric Psychiatry*, **9**, 149–55.

Horowitz, A. and Shindelman, L. W. (1983). Reciprocity and affection: past influences on current caregiving. *Journal of Gerontological Social Work*, **5**, 5–20.

Katon, W., Kleinman, A. and Rosen, G. (1982). Depression and somatization: a review. *American Journal of Medicine*, **72**, 127–35.

Knight, B. G., Lutzky, S. M. and Macofsky-Urban, F. (1993). A meta-analytic review of interventions for caregiver distress: recommendations for future research. *Gerontology*, **33**, 240–48.

Lazarus, R. S. (1993). Coping theory and research: past, present, and future. *Psychosomatic Medicine*, **55**, 234–47.

Logiudice, D., Waltrowicz, W. and McKenzie, S. (1995). Prevalence of dementia among patients referred to an aged assessment team and associated stress in their carers. *Australian Journal of Public Health*, **19**, 275–9.

Lowery, K., Mynt, P., Aisbett, J., Dixon, T., O'Brien, J. and Ballard, C. (2000). Depression in the carers of dementia sufferers: a comparison of the carers of patients suffering from dementia with Lewy bodies and the carers of patients with Alzheimer's disease. *Journal of Affective Disorders*. **59**, 61–5.

Mace, N. L. and Rabins, P. V. (1981). *The 36 Hour Day.* Johns Hopkins University Press, Baltimore, MD.

Montgomery, R. J. N., Gonyea, J. G. and Hooyman, N. R. (1985). Caregiving and the experience of subjective and objective burden. *Family Relations*, **34**, 19–26.

Morris, R. S., Morris, L. W. and Britton, P. G. (1988). Factors affecting the emotional well-being of the caregivers of dementia sufferers. *British Journal of Psychiatry*, **153**, 147–56.

Nolan, M., Grant, G. and Keady, J. (1997). *Understanding Family Care.* Open University Press, Buckingham.

O'Connor, D. W., Pollitt, P. A., Roth, M., Brook, C. P. and Reiss, B. B. (1990). Problems reported by relatives in a community study of dementia. *British Journal of Psychiatry*, **156**, 835–41.

Pagel, M. D., Becker, J. and Coppel, D. B. (1985). Loss of control, self-blame and depression: an investigation of spouse caregivers of Alzheimer's disease patients. *Journal of Abnormal Psychology*, **94**, 169–82.

Patel, V. and Hope, R. A. (1992). Aggressive behaviour in elderly psychiatric in patients. *Acta Psychiatrica Scandinavica*, **85**, 131–5.

Pearlin, L. I., Mullen, J. T., Semple, S. J. and Skaff, M. M. (1990). Caregiving and the stress process: an overview of concepts and their measures. *Gerontology*, **30**, 583–94.

Pruchno, R. A. and Resch, N. L. (1989). Aberrant behaviours and Alzheimer's disease: mental health effects on spouse caregivers. *Journal of Gerontology*, **44**, S177–82.

Rabins, P. V., Mace, N. L. and Lucas, M. J. (1982). The impact of dementia on the family. *Journal of the American Medical Society*, **248**, 333–5.

Reis, M. F., Gold, D. P., Andres, D., Markiewiez, D. and Gauthier, S. (1994). Personality traits as determinants of burden and health complaints in caregiving. *International Journal of Aging and Human Development*, **39**, 257–71.

Rockwell, E., Jackson, E., Vilke, G. and Jeste, D. V. (1994). A study of delusions in a large cohort of Alzheimer's disease patients. *American Journal of Psychiatry*, **2**, 157–64.

Rosen, J. and Zubenko, G. S. (1991). Emergence of psychosis and depression in the longitudinal evaluation of Alzheimer's disease. *Biological Psychiatry*, **29**, 2224–32.

Saad, K., Hartman, J., Ballard, C., Kurian, M., Graham, C. and Wilcock, G. (1995). Coping by the carers of dementia sufferers. *Age and Ageing*, **24**, 495–8.

Schulz, R., Visintainer, P. and Williamson, G. (1990). Psychiatric and physical morbidity effects of caregiving. *Journal of Gerontology and Psychological Science*, **45**, 181–91.

Spitzer, R. L., Endicott, J. and Robins, E. (1978). Research diagnostic criteria: rationale and reliability. *Archives of General Psychiatry*, **35**, 773–82.

Steele, C., Rovner, B., Chase, G. A. and Folstein, M. (1990). Psychiatric symptoms and nursing home placement of patients with Alzheimer's disease. *American Journal of Psychiatry*, **147**, 1049–51.

Weiler, P. G., Chiriboga, D. A. and Black, S. A. (1994). Comparison of mental status tests: implications for Alzheimer's patients and their caregivers. *Journal of Gerontology*, **49**, S44–51.

Williamson, G. M. and Schulz, R. (1993). Coping with specific stressors in Alzheimer's disease caregiving. *Gerontologist*, **33**, 747–55.

Zarit, S. H., Reever, K. E. and Bach-Peterson, J. (1980). Relatives of the impaired elderly: correlates of feelings of burden. *Gerontologist*, **20**, 649–55.

10 Psychological therapies and approaches in dementia

Introduction

This chapter examines the most common and widely practised therapies for people with dementia: behaviour therapy, reality orientation, validation, reminiscence and life review. While behaviour therapy is a direct method of intervening with people displaying challenging behaviours, other approaches aim to reduce the incidence of challenging behaviours by promoting higher levels of contentment, orientation and social interaction. It is important to note that, when describing these various therapies, some of the distinctions being made will be rather artificial, and open to debate. This is because there is a lot of overlap between the approaches, and the therapies are rarely practised in their pure form. The therapies are often complementary, so it is necessary for a clinician to have knowledge of each of the approaches to be able to draw from a well-resourced database. The latter section of this chapter examines future directions and developments.

Rationale for people's behaviour

Before discussing strategies for managing challenging behaviours, it is worth examining their nature. The list given in Table 10.1 was developed for people with learning disabilities, yet is equally applicable for people with dementia. A person with dementia might display several of these behaviours.

When attempting to understand challenging behaviours, Emerson (1998) claims that there are three important aspects to take into account:

- *Challenging behaviour is a social construct*—challenging behaviours usually transgress some social rule within a particular context. The significance of the transgression will depend on the nature of the behaviour, the setting and how carers interpret it.

- *Challenging behaviours have wide-ranging personal and social consequences*—the behaviours tend to affect not only the quality of life of the person with dementia, but also that of the carers and others in close proximity (e.g. fellow residents).

Table 10.1   Forms of challenging behaviour (adapted from Emerson 1998)

• Biting others	• Pinching others
• Biting self	• Pinching self
• Destructive behaviours	• Pulling other's hair
• Eating inedible objects	• Pulling own hair
• Excessive drinking	• Regurgitating food
• Hitting others	• Repetitive 'persisting'
• Hitting others with objects	• Repetitive screaming
• Hitting own body with hand	• Running away
• Hitting own body with objects	• Scratching others
• Hitting own head against objects	• Scratching self
• Hitting own head with hand	• Smearing faeces
• Inappropriate sexual behaviour	• Stripping in public
• Meanness or cruelty	• Stuffing fingers in body openings
• Non-compliance	• Teeth grinding
• Outbursts of temper	• Theft
• Over-activity	• Verbal aggression

How these individuals respond to the person with dementia is likely to have a major impact on his/her behaviour. Some responses may include abuse, exclusion and deprivation, which clearly will adversely affect the well-being of the person with dementia. Thus when devising appropriate interventions, a therapist must both reduce the impact of the behaviour (frequency, duration) and attend to any negative reactions and consequences associated with the challenging behaviour.

• *Challenging behaviours are defined by their presentation and impact*—challenging behaviours vary greatly in their manifestation and aetiology (see Table 10.1). Thus no one management approach alone will be appropriate for dealing with all forms of challenging behaviour.

As the above definition highlights, an important issue concerning challenging behaviours is how they are interpreted. For example, aggression is usually seen as being more challenging if perceived as intentional. Indeed, the degree to which the person with dementia is perceived to have intended his/her disruptive behaviour is crucial in determining the carer's reaction to that behaviour. The notion of intentionality opens up a philosophical minefield (Searle 1980). For example, Nisbett and Wilson (1977) have debated whether people are consciously aware of why they make a decision to perform a particular action. They suggest that, in many situations, people do not have conscious access to the reasoning behind their mental processing and actions. This feature raises important issues regarding the mental processes underpinning the actions of a person with dementia and the staff's perceptions of those actions.

Adler (1927) provided a useful framework for analysing the mechanisms behind a person's actions at a more concrete level. He suggested looking for evidence for each of the elements listed in Table 10.2.

The above section has highlighted the fact that challenging behaviours come in

Table 10.2 Adler's explanation for behaviours

Does the person's dysfunctional behaviour help:
* to initiate an emotional state?
* to stop an emotional state?
* to avoid an emotional state?
* to reduce the intensity of an emotional state?
* to intensify an emotional state?
* to maintain an emotional state?
* to elicit a response from the physical environment?
* to elicit a response from the interpersonal environment?
* to act in a way that is consistent with personal values, standards and goals?

many forms and have a wide-ranging impact on people and the environment. It suggests that people's responses to the individual displaying the challenging behaviour are likely to have a significant effect on the person with dementia and the manifestation of the behaviour; in some cases exacerbating the disruptive behaviour. A crucial feature in determining carers' abilities to manage challenging behaviour is their interpretation of its causal roots. This section has also provided a useful checklist to help examine the underlying mechanisms behind challenging behaviours.

In the following, management strategies will be discussed in more detail with particular attention to functional and dysfunctional methods of responding to disruptive behaviours. In addition, approaches are outlined that indirectly affect challenging behaviours, reducing their likelihood of future occurrence by creating positive therapeutic milieus.

The therapies and approaches

Behaviour therapy

Behavioural approaches have made the greatest contribution to professionals' understanding and interventions in the area of challenging behaviour. Traditional behaviour therapy has been based on principles of conditioning (classical and operant) and learning theory. In recent years, positive programming methodologies (La Vigna and Donnellan 1986) have helped produce major advances. The latter techniques have moved away from strategies aimed at suppressing or eliminating challenging behaviours, employing non-aversive contingencies in helping to develop more functional behaviours. The following sections will first examine traditional behaviour therapy approaches, principally operant conditioning, and then move on to discuss positive programming.

Traditional behaviour therapy
Detailed descriptions of the fundamentals of classic and operant conditioning are widely available (Rimm and Masters 1974, Perrin 1996), and thus are not discussed

extensively here. Both approaches are based on the premises that challenging behaviours are often learned and therefore can be unlearned and that most challenging behaviours have recognizable patterns to their development and maintenance.

Classical conditioning theory states that a triggered automatic response (fear) can be elicited in the presence of a neutral stimulus (e.g. a chair), in situations where the neutral stimulus has previously been paired with the original trigger (a fear-inducing trigger). For example, a man who suffered an assault in his home, frequently became anxious whenever he sat in the chair in which he had been sitting when the attack took place. In this situation, the chair became a 'conditioned stimulus' and the fear elicited in its presence the 'conditioned response'. In order to deal with this problem, classical conditioning suggests a programme of response extinction. The man, having been taught relaxation skills, was repeatedly asked to sit in the chair over longer periods. Over time, he learned that sitting in the chair did not automatically lead to either an attack or to an overwhelming sense of dread and fear.

The operant techniques (sometimes termed instrumental techniques) have proved extremely useful in the area of challenging behaviour. The operant approach suggests that people learn to act in a particular way because environmental responses reinforce the behaviour, making the action either more or less likely to occur in the future. Table 10.3 summarizes the most common reinforcers that produce and maintain behaviours. Knowledge of the impact of different forms of reinforcement is vital with respect to a therapist's interventions, because the same mechanisms that maintain actions are used to eliminate and change them. There are many other forms of reinforcer. The interested reader is advised to consult Perrin (1996) and Rimm and Masters (1974).

Reinforcement patterns are often complicated and require detailed assessment to achieve an understanding of the links between the triggers, behaviours and reinforcers (i.e. the antecedents, behaviours and consequences (A-B-C)). However, it is not only the type of reinforcer which influences the expression of a behaviour, but also its timing and scheduling. The main types of scheduling are continuous, fixed

Table 10.3 Description of types of reinforcer

Positive reinforcement	occurs when a feature is added which increases the likelihood of a desired behaviour being performed again
Negative reinforcement	occurs when a feature is withdrawn (usually an unpleasant stimulus) which increases the likelihood of a desired behaviour
Extinction	occurs when a positive reinforcer is withheld following the occurrence of an unwanted behaviour; this may involve not responding to or ignoring the behaviour
Punishment	occurs when an aversive stimulus is applied following the occurrence of an unwanted behaviour; there are major ethical and practical problems regarding the use of punishment, as it may lead to escape behaviours, or the occurrence of further challenging behaviours (see Parker and Penhale 1998, p.80).

interval and variable interval. In continuous reinforcement a reinforcer is provided every time the target behaviour is expressed. In interval forms, the reinforcer occurs at specific time intervals (e.g. every 10 s or every 5 min) or after a specified number/ratio of the behaviours have been observed (e.g. every other time, or every 10th time). As the name suggests, the variable form (also known as either variable ratio or intermittent reinforcement) indicates that the reinforcer occurs inconsistently, sometimes randomly. This is one of the most powerful forms of scheduling. Behaviours generated using this form of reinforcement pattern are particularly difficult to extinguish. This is because the inherent unpredictability of the scheduling results in the classic 'gambler's' form of excitement (i.e. 'Will I be rewarded this time, or maybe the next?'). As an example of this, when staff are required to treat someone displaying chronic aggression, it is not uncommon for individual carers to use different approaches to deal with the challenging behaviour. Some staff will be confrontational, some will ignore it, while others will acquiesce to whatever demands are being made. This combination of reinforcement strategies, with different scheduling patterns, is likely to reinforce the aggressive behaviour strongly. In such situations an agreed response strategy is required. This should be consistent and provide supportive strategies to allow the person with dementia to communicate and obtain his/her needs in a more socially acceptable manner (see Meares and Draper, 1999 for an illustrative case example).

Assessment and intervention

Behaviour therapy requires a detailed assessment period in which the A-B-C relationships are unravelled. The interventions are based on this analysis. Emerson (1998) suggests that the aims of assessment are to:

- identify what it is that the person does which is challenging;
- describe the impact of the challenging behaviour upon the quality of life of a person with dementia; and
- attempt to understand the processes underlying the person's challenging behaviour.

In order to identify the challenging behaviour (i.e. the how, what, where and when), one must obtain a detailed and specific description of the behaviour. The use of terms such as 'shouting' or 'self-injurious behaviour' are far too general. Hope and Patel (1993) and Stokes (1996) are particularly critical of the unclear and unstructured descriptions of behaviours. As Stokes (1996, p.602) says, 'Before we are able to understand challenging and intervene to change that behaviour, we must employ a language that is meaningful and unambiguous.'

In order to get an adequate idea of the manifestation of the challenging behaviour and knowledge of the sequence of actions leading up to it, the therapist often needs to use some form of recording device like a diary or chart. Carr *et al.* (1994) propose a functional assessment procedure under the headings 'description', 'categorization' and 'verification' to identify the underlying processes of challenging behaviours. Thus, when describing the behaviour, Carr *et al.* use a semi-structured interview, asking specific questions about the immediate impact and contextual control of the challenging behaviour. Such an interview might include the following questions:

- What are the activities or settings in which the behaviour typically occurs?
- Does the behaviour appear to be influenced by environmental factors (noise, number of people, lighting, music, temperature)? Please describe in detail.

Within the categorization process, the therapist must determine the main function of the challenging behaviour, as well as any secondary functions. In addition, he/she should identify whether any features within the environment predict which of the various functions were being fulfilled at any one time (see Table 10.2).

The verification procedure involves checking out a conceptual hypothesis that may have been developed based on one's information from the assessment. This process is often done by performing a very detailed naturalistic observation of the challenging behaviour.

It is relevant to note that recording devices can be fraught with problems, and hence Emerson (1998) suggests that they are kept as simple and practical as possible. He also recommends that any recording system being used on a ward should be developed in partnership with the staff.

The detailed assessment procedures described above provide insight into the disposition of the person with dementia and his/her reasons for engaging in a challenging behaviour. They help to develop guidelines for managing the challenging behaviour and to identify possible alternatives which could replace the challenging behaviour; as such, they build the basis for the intervention phase.

In the intervention phase the therapist must design and implement an appropriate therapeutic strategy. Emerson (1998) suggests focusing on three key features: taking account of the person's preferences; changing the context in which the challenging behaviour takes place, and using reinforcement strategies and schedules that disrupt the challenging behaviour.

An awareness of the individual's preferences of, for example, diet, activities and music, is important when establishing rewards for positive reinforcement schedules. Where a challenging behaviour is associated with a particular activity or setting, the most straightforward intervention is often a contextual change, i.e. to eliminate the triggering scenarios. For example, if the person does not like eating at a communal table, it is appropriate to put him/her on a separate table in the dining room. Such direct procedures are often effective because they are usually easy to implement and produce quick results. However it may sometimes be impossible to manipulate the environment appropriately, e.g. when safety issues are involved.

In attempting to change the context of the challenging behaviour, the therapist's role is to intervene at the level of the setting (triggering events). For example, the therapist may be able to reduce the rates of disruptive behaviours by enriching the environment of the person with dementia, through either increasing incidences of positive interactions or introducing new materials (e.g. Favell *et al.* 1982, Mace *et al.* 1989). Changing the schedule is helpful where challenging behaviours occur in connection with routinized behaviour (dressing, toileting). In such circumstances, staff often try to rush through these procedures in order to minimize distress and to reduce the risk of personal harm. However, this approach can lead to an increase in agitation. By changing this schedule by merely slowing down one's level of activity, over-stimulation can be avoided and 'escape' reactions prevented.

The interventions discussed so far have not involved any direct work on the reinforcement schedules or the contingencies maintaining the challenging behaviour. However, as outlined earlier, a major part of the work of the therapist is to select the most appropriate regime and scheduling programme to tackle disruptive actions (see Table 10.3). For example, if a person learns that he/she can get carers' attention by shouting, he/she will be more likely to shout, whereas if the behaviour is ignored it may cease.

In order to carry out behavioural strategies successfully, one must obtain the support of staff and management. The strategies are often time-consuming and are sometimes tedious and slow. It is essential that staff are able to offer a consistent approach, otherwise the technique may serve to further reinforce the problem behaviour, as described above.

Positive programming

A different approach to treat challenging behaviours is positive programming, which is most commonly associated with the field of learning disabilities, and is illustrated in the work of La Vigna and Donnellan (1986). The researchers 'offer a constructional approach that celebrates, rewards and extends each person's existing current valuable repertoire' (Kushlik *et al.* 1997, p.142). The approach aims to maintain high quality of life in an ordinary environment. The methodology comprises of three overlapping components:

- *Assessment*—this involves a comprehensive assessment of both the person's strengths and needs and the functions of the challenging behaviour. A functional analysis is carried out to determine the factors associated with a behaviour. Particular attention is paid to whether the challenging behaviours are an attempt by the person to express his/her needs or feelings.

- *Use of proactive interventions*—based on the assessment, staff can be advised how to deal with the person in the 'hot' situation. Staff are specifically taught how to help the person with dementia communicate his feelings and needs using strategies and techniques that do not require him to resort to challenging behaviours. When devising alternative strategies to be used by the person with dementia, it is important that these have the same function as the challenging behaviour (e.g. providing the person with a more functional way to signal that he is hungry, bored or in pain).

- *Implementation of safety strategies*—as well as the proactive strategies used in the previous stage, additional strategies must be implemented to keep staff and residents safe. Steps also need to be taken to limit the negative effects of the challenging behaviours until the proactive strategies start working effectively.

Staff require training in order to implement the strategies over the long periods of time required to achieve success. It is specifically suggested that the people with dementia and the staff are trained in 'frustration tolerance' to enable them to cope with the transition phases of treatment.

Efficacy

Only a small number of studies have demonstrated the effectiveness of behavioural interventions in dementia. For example, there is evidence of successful reductions in wandering, incontinence and other forms of stereotypic behaviours (see Holden and Woods 1982, Bakke 1997, Woods 1999). Meares and Draper (1999), Bird *et al.* (1995) and Rapp *et al.* (1992) present case studies testifying to the efficacy of behaviour therapy. In their reports, all of the authors noted that the challenging behaviours had diverse causes and maintaining factors, and they proposed that interventions must be tailored to each individual case. For example, in Wisner and Green's (1986) case study of a man with vascular dementia, the significant reduction in aggression was attributed to the tailored addition of cognitive features to the behaviour strategies. In the study by Bird *et al.* (1995), the person with dementia was trained to respond to cues which were gradually faded once the associations had been established. Signs and symbols, together with portable alarm systems (set at predetermined intervals) were typically used to cue people. These strategies have also helped to reduce incidents of incontinence, the number of times people went into fellow residents' bedrooms, and wandering and inappropriate sexual conduct (Hussian 1981). Behaviour therapy was also used successfully by Rinke *et al.* (1978), who improved the degree of self-care in six people in residential homes. Pinkston and Linsk (1984) performed similar work in a family setting. Typically residents were asked on a regular basis whether they would like to go to the toilet and were assisted with their toileting when they responded in the affirmative.

It is important to note that behavioural programmes depend heavily on the co-operation of staff. Challenging behaviours are often very difficult to treat, so it is frequently impossible to return an individual to his/her premorbid level of functioning. The modest level of impact can reduce the morale and motivation of the staff asked to engage in behaviour therapy programmes. It is therefore important to involve staff in setting collaborative and realistic goals.

Reality orientation

Reality orientation was one of the most widely used management strategies for dealing with people with dementia (for a review see Holden and Woods 1995). It helps people deal with memory loss and disorientation by reminding them of facts about themselves and their environment. The aim is to reduce the anxiety caused by confusion, the frustration due to lack of stimulation, and the dependence caused by a sense of helplessness. There are two forms of reality orientation, formal and informal. Formal, or classroom, reality orientation is typically used for groups of well-matched residents and their staff. A wide range of activities and materials are used to orientate the individuals to features in their environment. The daily or weekly sessions usually involve providing the names of those in the group, and the date, time and place of the meeting. Current information and themes of interest are also discussed, and these features are supported through the use of diaries, clocks and information sheets.

Informal, or 24 h, reality orientation was originally developed as a way of reinforcing the formal approach. However, it is now perceived to be the more practical of the two methodologies. It involves a number of changes to the environment, with clear sign-posting being employed around the ward or home, extensive use of notices and other memory aids, and a consistent orientating approach by all staff. In later versions of the approach, staff are trained to take a more reactive stance, orientating only when specific questions about time, history and place have been requested (Reeve and Ivison 1985, William *et al.* 1987).

There is a wide range of opinions regarding the efficacy of reality orientation, but two findings emerge consistently. Firstly, reality orientation sessions can increase people's verbal orientation as compared with untreated control groups (Bleathman and Morton 1988; see Holden and Woods 1995). Secondly, 'real life' change is difficult to obtain using this form of therapy. Nevertheless, there is some evidence that behavioural changes can be achieved using reality orientation techniques (Hanley *et al.* 1981, Williams *et al.* 1987), but specific targeting seems to be required.

Reality orientation has been much criticized as being rather mechanical, inflexible, insensitive, adopting a confrontational style and having an over-emphasis on cognitive aspects. Furthermore, Goudie and Stokes (1989) claim that the approach can sometimes remind the person with dementia about their deterioration. Tentative evidence in support of this latter perspective comes from Baines *et al.* (1987), who found that there was an initial lowering of mood in those attending reality orientation sessions. Finally, it has also been suggested that reality orientation may increase carers' frustration 'when endlessly having to correct confused conversation with little noticeable effect' (Hitch 1994, p.51). Thus it is evident that other therapeutic and management strategies needed to be developed either to support or to replace reality orientation. One of the most promising methodologies has been validation therapy.

Validation therapy

Validation therapy was developed by Naomi Feil in the 1960s in the USA as 'fantasy therapy' (Feil 1967) and was renamed 'validation therapy' in 1978. Feil was disillusioned with the reality orientation approach and suggested that some of the features associated with dementia (repetition and retreating into the past) were active strategies on the part of the person with dementia to avoid stress, boredom and loneliness. She argued that the present reality is often too painful for the person with dementia, and therefore he retreats into an inner reality (fantasy), which is based on feelings rather than intellect.

Validation therapy attempts to help the person with dementia deal with his/her feelings by validating them, and subsequently helping him/her to move from his/her inner world to the shared reality of the present. In this form of therapy, one empathizes with the hidden meanings and feelings behind the confused speech and behaviour. It is claimed that validation therapy promotes communication with the severely confused older person on his own terms, on subjects that he chooses to discuss and issues that are important to him. In validation therapy it is assumed that all the words and actions of a person with dementia have a real sense of purpose and value. The rambling words and strange actions may seem nonsensical to an observer, but may be perceived as coherent and communicative to the person with dementia. Goudie and Stokes (1989) suggested that the confused messages may be attempts to make sense of the world, express needs or highlight distress.

Validation therapy can be initiated in groups or with individuals. According to Jones (1997), validation therapy can be used as a milieu approach (24 h a day) by all people coming into contact with the person with dementia. It uses a staged set of interventions aimed at targeting different features being displayed during the various phases of the dementing process (there are four overlapping stages identified, see Jones 1997). People coming into contact with the person with dementia are not expected to know all the facts about that person's history, but are encouraged to focus on the emotional content of what is being said and to attempt to understand the person in whatever reality he is experiencing. Topics of conversation may centre around past conflicts and problems; orientation to current here-and-now reality is irrelevant.

Feil's work (1989, 1993) provides some useful validation techniques that can be successfully applied to help restore a sense of emotional well-being to severely confused people. Her communication-orientated strategies are based on the counselling skills of reflective listening, exploration, warmth and acceptance (Rogers 1951). It is important to note, however, that carers must avoid making too complicated interpretations of behaviour when applying the validation approach. The danger is that obvious explanations for the confused actions might be missed and, more importantly, simple solutions to identify problems may be overlooked.

Validation therapy was originally developed for people with Alzheimer's disease and multi-infarct dementia. It is not known how useful the approach is for other forms of dementia, or for people with long histories of psychiatric difficulties (Jones 1997). In Hitch's (1994) review of working therapeutically with people with dementia, she notes that validation therapy promotes contentment, results in less negative affect and behavioural disturbance, produces positive effects (smiles, social interaction) and provides the individual with insight into external reality (Feil 1982). However, a number of cautionary notes were also sounded. Indeed, it was suggested that therapists could become too focused on confused communication and fail to identify basic uncomplicated details (e.g. pain or hunger). There is also a danger that staff and other professionals may succumb to the temptation of colluding with the delusion (Jones 1985, Goudie and Stokes 1989).

There have been few empirical studies testifying to the efficacy of validation therapy (Feil 1967, Mitchell 1987). Indeed, only a small number of 'quality' trials concerning validation therapy have been carried out (Peoples 1982, Pretczynski 1991; see Bleathman and Morton 1992), although several less robust case studies have been reported (Fritz 1986, Miesen and Jones 1997).

Reminiscence therapy

It was once thought harmful to encourage a person with dementia to relive their past and recall their childhood and adolescence. However, since the 1960s, reminiscence therapy has been recognized as an effective way of restoring high levels of well-being in people with dementia. Reminiscence therapy involves helping the person with dementia to think about and relive positive past experiences, especially those considered personally significant (e.g. family holidays or weddings). The aim is to provide pleasure and cognitive stimulation by focusing on happy memories. Reminiscence therapy can be carried out individually on an informal basis, or in group sessions. The group sessions may be structured or free-flowing, and they may include a variety of activities such as art, music, use of artefacts, outings, cooking, etc. Each group session is generally focused around a particular topic such as childhood or adolescence. The group may serve the purpose of creating historical records.

O'Donovan (1993) states that there is little evidence of cognitive improvements from using reminiscence work, but some evidence of improvements in behaviour, well-being, social and self-care and motivation (Baines *et al.* 1987, Gibson 1994; for a review see also Woods and McKiernan 1995). It is suggested that the approach is particularly good at enhancing self-esteem and life satisfaction, as it validates a person's treasured memories and interests (Haight 1988, Osborn 1990). It has also been claimed that aspects of the personality of people with dementia, thought to be lost, may remerge during reminiscence work (Woods 1999).

The advantage of this form of therapy is its great flexibility; it can be adapted to the ability of the individual person with dementia. Even the severely disabled individual can gain pleasure from listening to an old record or by engaging in a procedurally learned activity (e.g. knitting, or spinning a top). This approach also encourages staff to see the person behind the illness; during the reminiscence the patient is expert.

Life-review therapy

Life-review work is often confused with reminiscence therapy. However, careful examination of the literature suggests a clear distinction. Reminiscence focuses

mainly on happy memories (Oliveria 1977), while life review is concerned with negative memories (Haight 1988, Haight and Burnside 1993). Thus, while reminiscence
may be included in the life-review process, it is unlikely that reminiscence will
include life review. Buechel (1986) describes life review as a process of re-evaluation,
resolution and reintegration of past conflicts, perhaps giving new significance to
one's life. Therefore, it attempts to help the person achieve adaptation and is particularly appropriate for those with difficult pasts. It is thought to be most effective on
a one-to-one basis, but may also be carried out as group therapy. It is a natural
process whereby the elderly person takes stock of his/her life. For the therapist, this
involves taking a detailed history of the person's life to establish previous coping
mechanisms. These can be used to resolve past problems and thus come to terms
with the present and future more readily.

The benefits of life-review therapy are believed to be similar to those of reminiscence therapy. It is suggested that, by coming to terms with the past, the person can
approach the future more positively (Sullivan 1982, Osborn 1989). However, one
must take care when encouraging a person to talk about distressing issues from the
past because the person might no longer retain the coping mechanisms to deal with
the issues well. In addition, owing to the negative biases associated with low affect
(see Chapter 11), which is a common state within this group, the therapist must be
careful to distinguish between negative interpretations of events and the factual
details. For example, when talking about their past, a person's description of their
unhappy childhood might be a reflection of a negative selective memory bias. In
such circumstances the therapist must take care not to reinforce perceptions, while
empathizing with the patient's distress.

The future

As the field of dementia moves into the new millennium, there is a greater degree of
integration regarding therapeutic strategies, with a sharing of skills from different
orientations (behaviour therapy, humanistic, cognitive therapy and psychodynamic)
and specialties (learning disability, general psychiatry, health psychology, organizational psychology). The present section outlines some of the most promising
approaches currently being developed within behaviour therapy, psychotherapy and
information-processing theory.

Behaviour therapy

Over the last 20 years, behaviour therapy has produced a number of new and
interesting models of assessment and conceptualization (O'Donohue and Krasner
1995). Many of these models have been influenced by cognitive and problem-
solving therapies; nevertheless, at their heart they retain the familiar A-B-C chains
(or stimulus, organismic mediator, response and consequence (SORC)). For example,
the 'clinical pathogenesis map' framework (Nezu and Nezu 1989, 1993) and the

'functional analytic causal model (FACM; Haynes 1994, O'Brien and Haynes 1995) seem particularly useful in outlining causal relationships within affective and behavioural problems. Indeed, Nezu *et al.* (1997) have recently provided a case study describing how their frameworks can be used to conceptualize challenging behaviour (sexual aggression) displayed by an adult with cognitive impairment. As part of the framework, they assessed the person's intellectual capacity, cognitive biases and misinterpretations, problem-solving skills, self-control skills and social skills, and the impact of the environment on the behaviour. They produced an elegant conceptual model which examines the above features under four categories:

- current dysfunctional system;
- developmental history;
- recent stress; and
- relevant stimuli.

Such approaches appear extremely helpful in understanding the background and maintaining features of challenging behaviours. However, despite their apparent validity, the models have yet to receive empirical support.

Interpersonal psychotherapy

Another form of therapy that has proven to be as effective as cognitive therapy in a number of major trials for the treatment of depression within a general psychiatric setting is interpersonal psychotherapy (IPT; Elkin *et al.* 1989, Frank *et al.* 1990). In IPT the therapist tackles a person's problems in terms of four areas: interpersonal conflict, interpersonal deficits, grief, and role transitions (Miller and Silberman 1996; see Table 10.4).

IPT takes a problem-solving perspective and, being less structured than other forms of 'handbook-based' therapies, it is flexible and therefore particularly suited for use with older people (Sholomskas *et al.* 1983, Frank *et al.* 1993). The main value of this approach is that it focuses the treatment on fundamental areas that are commonly associated with human distress. Hence, it is a pantheoretical approach that can be used systematically with the person with dementia and his/her carers. Indeed, the simplicity and clarity of IPT make it easy to use in a collaborative fashion with staff and fellow professionals.

Information processing

One of the most helpful of the information-processing frameworks is the interactive cognitive subsystem (ICS) model (Barnard 1985, Teasdale and Barnard 1993). This approach provides comprehensive conceptual frameworks which are directing assessment and intervention strategies in clinical psychology and psychiatry (Teasdale 1996). In recent years the model has been applied to older people (Williams 1995, Woods 1999).

The model hypothesizes that conscious awareness, which is language-based, is

Table 10.4 The four treatment areas in interpersonal psychotherapy (IPT)

Interpersonal conflict	This feature may stem from changes in personality as a result of executive (i.e. 'frontal') problems. Many challenging behaviours bring the person into conflict with other people, including carers and fellow residents.
Interpersonal deficits	These may be associated with cognitive impairment and an inability to solve problems in current settings. Challenging behaviours may result from a loss of ability to inhibit inappropriate behaviour or emotion, or a loss of ability to communicate effectively. The deficits can also be connected to low mood, resulting in decreased energy and motivation to make good quality relationships. If the person displays challenging behaviour frequently, over a period of time he may begin to lose the ability to engage another person positively.
Grief	People with dementia may experience a sense of loss regarding their cognitive abilities and independence. They may also experience grief because of deaths among their family and peer group. Owing to memory difficulties, the sense of loss may be a recurrent theme for them.
Role transitions	Transitions can be related to deteriorating health, wealth and status. Relocation into a care setting can exacerbate the above difficulties; such moves may also lead to dropping of formerly satisfying activities (e.g. working in the garden).

only one form of awareness, and that most cognitive information is processed within non-language-based systems. ICS emphasizes the important role played by non-verbal processing mechanisms, and highlights their influence on a person's emotions. Hence, it is a useful framework to explain why sensory therapies (e.g. touch, music and aromatherapy) are able to alleviate distress in people with dementia. For example, it is recognized that during a conversation with someone it is often not the content of the speech that determines the listener's feeling about the conversation, but how the information is conveyed (speaker's tone, body posture, facial expression) as well as their own current state (tired, relaxed, low). In other words, the person receives all sorts of verbal, non-verbal, environmental and internal stimuli which influence mood during the conversation.

At a more mechanistic level, ICS suggests that the cognitive system is continuously processing and exchanging qualitatively different kinds of information (features of sound, touch, sight, smell, etc.). These details are registered and transformed between the various systems within the cognitive architecture, and then, at some stage, a degree of meaning is extracted from these interactions. It is hypothesized that two levels of meaning are being extracted, one specific and the other generic. The specific level is language-based and 'conveys information about specific states of the world that can be verified by reference to evidence' (Teasdale 1996, p.29). For example, a person opening a door to a room containing a toilet and hand basin can confirm that this is a WC. This fact-based information is then fed back into the system in order to provide data for the 'generic' level. At the generic meaning level (non-language-based), all of the various forms of information (smell, sound, specific meaning, etc.) are synthesized in order to produce a holistic or implicit meaning (i.e. a sense of state of being). In the above example, opening the door might have resulted in a state of relief, confusion or embarrassment, depending on the situation and contextual features.

The ICS model also emphasizes the important part played by pattern-recognition processes within people's brain. It suggests that people unconsciously recognize and store regular patterns of information (memory traces) at various levels, linking the 'raw input' levels to the 'meaning' levels. These pattern-recognition systems provide a mechanism by which distress can be triggered by a specific sensory cue and then generalized across a range of situations (see Fig. 10.1). Thus, once a memory trace is established, it can be elicited by cues which are in some way related to the initial distressing situation. These cues can also generate memories, bodily sensations and states of ill-being.

In terms of a clinical example, a memory trace leading to depression may be activated by the person smelling a fragrance that was previously experienced during a period of low mood. As this theory predicts, feedback occurs both latterly and vertically along the neural network, hence, the smell may trigger other depressive features in the memory trace. Thus the person may begin to adopt a wearisome body posture and/or selectively attend to negative features in his/her environment.

Having outlined the architecture and processes, one can now see how the ICS model is helpful when working with people with dementia. For example, it recognizes that the routines common in many care settings are ideal for establishing memory traces. It would predict that, once a negative trace has been established for a person with dementia in a home, then there would be sufficient similarities across situations for negative states of ill-being to be generalized widely. Therefore, a great deal of importance is placed on guarding against the establishment of negative traces and attempting to promote positive traces. The positive traces may be generated and established through traditional language-based therapy, but also through physical and sensuous means, exercise, massage and good interpersonal communication (Teasdale 1996). To quote from Teasdale (1996, p.44), 'We noted earlier the potential contribution of interventions directed at changing specific meanings and related negative automatic thoughts. The ICS analysis suggests that interventions targeted at creating changes at the bodily level (e.g. by physical exercise, changing posture, facial expression, etc.) also have a contribution to make.'

Woods' (1999) recent review of therapy for dementia also reflects on how the ICS model could help explain why people with dementia frequently seek security by requesting either people or things from their past (e.g. 'I want my mother'; 'I want to go home and make my husband's tea'). Extending the ideas of Williams (1995), Woods suggests that while the generic (emotional) meaning level remains intact in dementia, the specific level (associated with language and language-based learning) is frequently impaired. Owing to this deficit, when a person with dementia is feeling low, they may be unable to make sense of this feeling in the current context. Thus in an attempt to explain the emotion, the person with dementia may generate memories of occasions when he or she previously felt low, lonely or abandoned. In turn, this

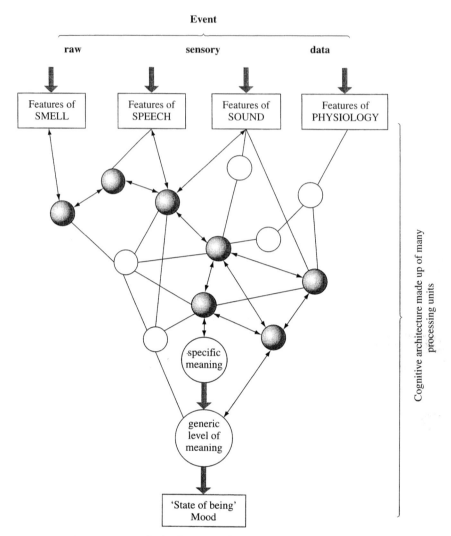

Fig. 10.1   An adapted (simplified) representation of the ICS model. An event is processed by a number of subsystems within the cognitive network/architecture (smell, touch, sound, etc). The resulting neural activation produces a pattern of response, leading to the two levels of meaning (specific and generic) being generated. Only the generic level is associated with feelings (depression, anxiety, anger—i.e. a state of being). If this network is repeatedly activated, a memory trace is formed, which links together all the units that have been activated during the processing of the event. It is suggested that any one unit within the memory trace has the capacity to trigger the other units into action at a future date.

may result in the person with dementia retrieving comforting memories (memories or themes that provide a sense of security) from the past by way of compensation.

ICS, would appear particularly relevant for treating people with dementia, especially in situations where the person with dementia has poor comprehension, receptive and memory abilities. The model supports the importance of validation approaches, and therapies that appropriately stimulate the senses of the person with dementia. Thus *snoezelen*, (a form of multisensory therapy) aromatherapy and music therapy are useful approaches when working with the ICS framework.

Conclusion

Clinicians have debated whether the notions of therapy and treatment are applicable in the field of dementia. Indeed, many would argue that the best one can ever hope for is the development of appropriate management techniques. However, this chapter has shown that a great deal of positive work can be done to improve the lot of people with dementia.

It is important to note that most approaches outlined in this chapter are complementary and should not be implemented in a purely prescriptive fashion. Each one initially requires a detailed assessment procedure, leading to a set of hypotheses regarding the establishment and maintenance of the challenging behaviour. As most challenging behaviours have a multifactorial aetiology, the assessment procedure will need to be comprehensive and the interventions wide ranging, often requiring the assistance of staff and management. The role of staff in the management of challenging behaviours is particularly important (see Chapter 12); because much of the work in homes is carried out by untrained staff, one must work closely with staff to ensure that they are not unintentionally reinforcing problematic behaviours. In addition, it is worth discussing the goals of the treatment programme with the carers at the outset (Meares and Draper 1999). If their expectation is that the challenging behaviour can be eliminated entirely, any partial success may not be sufficient to motivate them to maintain a particular regime. Thus clear goals, which are specific, observable, relevant, realistic and agreed, are vital.

There is relatively little quality research in this field. Most studies have tended to use small sample sizes and only a few have used controls (Hinchliffe *et al.* 1995). Despite these shortcomings, there now seems to be a renewed interest in the field. New treatment strategies, such as positive programming, IPT and ICS, are providing helpful conceptual models to enable professionals to work effectively with people with dementia.

Acknowledgements

Thank you to F. Katharina Reichelt for her intellectual contribution to this work, and to Tricia Roe for her help in the preparation of the chapter.

REFERENCES

Adler, A. (1927). *The Practice and Theory of Individual Psychology.* Harcourt Brace, New York, NY.

Baines, S., Saxby, P. and Ehlert, K. (1987). Reality orientation and reminiscence therapy: a controlled cross-over study of elderly confused people. *British Journal of Psychiatry*, **151**, 222–31.

Bakke, B. L. (1997). Applied behaviour analysis for behaviour problems in Alzheimer's disease. *Geriatrics,* **52** (Suppl. 12), 40–43.

Barnard, P. (1985). Integrating cognitive subsystems: a psycholinguistic approach to short-term memory. In *Progress in the Psychology of Language* (Ellis, A., ed.), Vol. 2, pp. 197–258. Erlbaum, London.

Bird, M., Alexopoulos, P. and Adamowicz, J. (1995). Success and failure in five case studies: use of cued recall to ameliorate behaviour problems in senile dementia. *International Journal of Geriatric Psychiatry*, **10**, 305–11.

Bleathman, C. and Morton, I. (1988). Validation therapy and the demented elderly. *Journal of Advanced Nursing*, **13**, 511–14.

Bleathman, C. and Morton, I. (1992). Validation therapy: extracts from 20 groups with dementia sufferers. *Journal of Advanced Nursing*, **17**, 658–66.

Buechel, H. (1986). Reminiscence: a review and prospectus. *Physical and Occupational Therapy in Geriatrics*, **5**, 25–37.

Carr, E. G., Levin, L., McConnachi, G., Carlson, J. I., Kemp, D. C. and Smith, C. E. (1994). *Communication-based Intervention for Problem Behaviour: a User's Guide for Producing Positive Change.* Brookes, Baltimore, MD.

Elkin, J., Shea, M., Watkins, J. T., Imber, S. D., Sotsky, S. M., Collins, J. F., Glass, D. R., Pilkonis, P. A., Leber, W. R., Docherty, J. P., Fiester, S. J. and Parloff, M. B. (1989). National Institute of Mental Health Treatment of Depression Collaborative Research Program: general effectiveness of treatment. *Archives of General Psychiatry*, **46**, 971–83.

Emerson, E. (1998). Working with people with challenging behaviour. In *Clinical Psychology and People with Intellectual Disabilities* (Emerson, E., Hatton, C., Bromley, J. and Caine, A., eds), pp. 127–153. John Wiley and Sons, Chichester.

Favell, J. E., McGirney, J. F. and Schell, R. M. (1982). Treatment of self-injury by providing alternate sensory activities. *Analysis and Intervention in Developmental Disabilities*, **2**, 83–104.

Feil, N. (1967). Group therapy in a home for the aged. *Gerontologist*, 7, Part 1.

Feil, N. (1982). *Validation: The Feil Method.* Edward Feil Productions, Cleveland, OH.

Feil, N. (1989) The validation: an empathic approach to the care of dementia. *Clinical Gerontology*, **8**, 89–92.

Feil, N. (1993). *The Validation Breakthrough: Simple Techniques for Communicating with People with 'Alzheimer's-type' Dementia.* Health Profession's Press, Baltimore, MD.

Frank, E., Kupfer, D. J., Perel, J. M., Cornes, C., Jarrett, D. B., Mallinger, A. G., Thase, M. E., McEachran, A. B. and Grochocinski, V. J. (1990). Three-year outcomes for maintenance therapies in recurrent depression. *Archives of General Psychiatry*, **47**, 1093–9.

Frank, E., Frank, N., Cornes, C., Imber, S. D., Miller, M. D., Morris, S. M. and Reynolds, C. F. (1993). Interpersonal psychotherapy. In *The Treatment of Late-life Depression in New Applications of Interpersonal Psychotherapy* (Klerman, G. L. and Weismann, M., eds), pp. 167–98. American Psychiatric Press, Washington, DC.

Fritz, P.A. (1986). The language of resolution among the old-old: the effect of validation therapy on two levels of cognitive confusion. Paper presented at the Speech Communication Association Convention. Chicago, IL, 12–16 November, 1986.

Gibson, F. (1994). What can reminiscence contribute to people with dementia? In *Reminiscence Reviewed: Evaluations, Achievements, Perspectives* (Bornat, J., ed.), pp. 46–60. Open University Press, Buckingham.

Goudie, F. and Stokes, G. (1989). Understanding confusion. *Nursing Times*, **85**, 35–7.

Haight, B. K. (1988). The therapeutic role of a structured life review process in homebound elderly subjects. *Journal of Gerontology*, **43**, 40–44.

Haight, B. K. and Burnside, I. (1993). Reminiscence and life review: explaining the differences. *Archives of Psychiatric Nursing*, **7**, 91–8.

Hanley, I. G., McGuire, R. J. and Boyd, W. D. (1981). Reality orientation and dementia: a controlled trial of two approaches. *British Journal of Psychiatry*, **138**, 10–14.

Haynes, S. N. (1994). Clinical judgement and the design of behavioural intervention programmes: estimating the magnitudes of intervention effects. *Psicologia Conductual*, **2**, 165–84.

Hinchliffe, A. C., Hyman, I. L., Blizard, B. and Livingston, G. (1995). Behavioural complications of dementia—can they be treated? *International Journal of Geriatric* Psychiatry, **10**, 839–847.

Hitch, S. (1994). Cognitive therapy as a tool for the caring elderly confused person. *Journal of Clinical Nursing*, **3**, 49–55.

Holden, U. P. and Woods, R. T. (1982). *Reality Orientation: Psychological Approaches to the Confused Elderly*. Churchill Livingstone, Edinburgh.

Holden, U. P. and Woods, R. T. (1995). *Positive Approaches to Dementia Care*, 3rd edn. Churchill Livingstone, Edinburgh.

Hope, R. A. and Patel, V. (1993). Assessment of behavioural phenomena in dementia. In *Ageing and Dementia: a Methodological Approach* (Burns, A., ed.), pp. 221–36. Edward Arnold, London.

Hussian, R. A. (1981). *Geriatric Psychology: a Behavioural Perspective*. Van Nostrand Reinhold, New York.

Jones, G. M. M. (1985). Validation therapy: a companion to reality orientation. *Canadian Nurse*, **81**, 20–23.

Jones, G. M. M. (1997). A review of Feil's validation method for communicating with and caring for dementia sufferers. *Current Opinion in Psychiatry*, **10**, 326–32.

Kushlik, A., Trower, P. and Dagnan, D. (1997). Applying cognitive-behavioural approaches to the carers of people with learning disabilities who display challenging behaviour. In *Cognitive-behaviour Therapy for Older People with Learning Disabilities* (Kroese, B. S., Dagnan, D. and Loumidis, K., eds), pp. 141–61. Routledge, London.

La Vigna, G. and Donnellan, A. (1986). *Alternative to Punishment: Solving Behaviour Problems with Non-aversive Strategies*. Irvington, New York, NY.

Mace, F. C., Yankanich, M. A. and West, B. (1989). Toward a methodology of experimental analysis and treatment of aberrant classroom behaviour. *Special Services in the School*, **4**, 71–88.

Meares, S. and Draper, B. (1999). Treatment of vocally disruptive behaviour of multifactorial aetiology. *International Journal of Geriatric Psychiatry*, **14**, 285–90.

Miesen, B. and Jones, G. (eds) (1997). *Care-giving in Dementia*. Tavistock Routledge, London

Miller, M. D. and Silberman, R. L (1996). Using interpersonal psychotherapy with depressed elders. In *A Guide to Psychotherapy and Aging: Effective Clinical Interventions in a Life Stage Context* (Zarit, S. and Knight, B. G.). APA, Washington, DC.

Mitchell, G. J. (1987). An analysis of the communication process and content with confused elderly clients during validation therapy. Master's thesis, University of Toronto, School of Nursing.

Nezu, A. M. and Nezu, C. M. (eds) (1989). *Clinical Decision Making in Behaviour Therapy: a Problem-solving Perspective.* Research Press, Champaign, IL.

Nezu, A. M. and Nezu, C. M. (1993). Identifying and selecting target problems for clinical interventions: a problem-solving model. *Psychological Assessment*, **5**, 254–63.

Nezu, A. M., Nezu, C. M., Friedman, S. H. and Haynes, S. N. (1997). Case formulation in behaviour therapy: problem-solving and functional analytic strategies. In *Handbook of Psychotherapy Case Formulation* (Eells, T. D., ed.), pp. 368–401. Guilford Press, New York, NY.

Nisbett, R. E. and Wilson, T. D. (1977). Telling more than we can know: verbal reports on mental processes. *Psychological Review*, **84**, 231–59.

O'Brien, W. H. and Haynes, S. N. (1995). A functional analytic approach to the conceptualisation, assessment and treatment of a child with frequent migraine headaches. *In Session*, **1**, 65–80.

O'Donohue, W. and Krasner, L. (1995). Theories in behaviour therapy. philosophical and historical context. In *Theories of Behaviour Therapy: Exploring Behaviour Change* (O'Donohue, W. and Krasner, L., eds), pp. 1–22. American Psychological Association, Washington, DC.

O'Donovan, S. (1993). The memory lingers on. *Elderly Care*, **5**, 27–31.

O'Donovan, S. (1996). A validation approach to severely demented clients. *Nursing Standard*, **11**, 48–52.

Olds, J. (1995). Strategies of care for patients with dementia. *Dementia*, **10**, 585–7.

Oliveria, O. H. (1977). Understanding old people: patterns of reminiscing in older people and their relationship to life satisfaction. Dissertation. University of Tennessee, Knoxville, TN.

Osborn, C. (1989). Reminiscence. When the past eases the present. *Journal of Gerontological Nursing*, **15**, 6–12.

Osborn, C. (1990). *A Practical Guide to Reminiscence Work.* Age Exchange, London.

Parker, J. and Penhale, B. (1998). *Forgotten People: Positive Approaches to Dementia Care.* Ashgate, Arena, Aldershot.

Peoples, M. (1982). Validation therapy versus reality orientation as treatment for disorientated institutionalised elderly. Master's thesis, College of Nursing, University of Akron, OH.

Perrin, T. (1996). *Problem Behaviour and the Care of the Elderly.* Winslow, Bicester.

Pinkston, E. M. and Linsk, N. L. (1984). *Care of the Elderly—a Family Approach.* Pergamon, New York, NY.

Pretczynski, J. (1991). Examining validation. Doctoral thesis, University of Reims, France.

Rapp, M. F., Flint, A. J., Hermann, N. and Roulx, G. B. (1992). Behavioural disturbances in the demented elderly phenomenology, pharmacotherapy and behavioural management. *Canadian Journal of Psychiatry*, **37**, 651–7.

Reeve, W. and Ivison, D. (1985). Use of environmental manipulation and classroom and modified informal reality orientation with institutionalised, confused elderly patients. *Age and Ageing*, **14**, 119–21.

Rimm, D. C. and Masters, J. C. (1974). *Behaviour Therapy: Techniques and Empirical Findings.* Academic Press, New York, NY.

Rinke, C. L., Williams, J. J., Lloyd, K. E. and Smith-Scott, W. (1978). The effects of prompting and reinforcement on self-bathing by elderly residents of a nursing home. *Behaviour Therapy*, **9**, 873–81.

Rogers, C. (1951). *Client-centred Therapy.* Houghton Miffin, Boston, MA.

Searle, J. R. (1980). The intentionality of intention and action. *Cognitive Science*, **4**, 47–70.

Sholomskas, A. J., Chevron, E. S., Prusoff, B. A. and Berry, C. (1983). Short-term interpersonal psychotherapy (IPT) with the depressed elderly: case reports and discussion. *American Journal of Psychotherapy*, **37**, 552–66.

Stokes, G. (1996). Challenging behaviour in dementia: a psychological approach. In *Handbook of the Clinical Psychology of Ageing* (Woods, R. T., ed.), pp. 601–28. John Wiley and Sons, Chichester.

Sullivan, C. A. (1982). Life review: a functional review of reminiscence. *Physical and Occupational Therapy in Geriatrics*, **2**, 39–52.

Teasdale, J. D (1996). Clinical relevant theory: integrating clinical insight with cognitive science. In *Frontiers of Cognitive Therapy* (Salkovskis, P. M., ed.), pp. 26–41. Guilford Press, New York, NY.

Teasdale, J. D. and Barnard, P. J. (1993). *Affect, Cognition and Change: Remodelling Depressive Thought*. Erlbaum, Hove.

Williams, J. M. G. (1995). Interacting cognitive subsystems and unvoiced murmurs: A review of 'Affect, Cognition, and Change' by John Teasdale and Philip Barnard. *Cognition and Emotion*, **8**, 571–4.

Williams, R., Reeve, W., Ivison, D. and Kavanagh, D. (1987). Use of environmental manipulation and modified informal reality orientation with institutionalised confused elderly subjects: a replication. *Age and Ageing*, **16**, 315–18.

Wisner, E. and Green, M. (1986) Treatment of a demented patient's anger with cognitive behavioural strategies. *Psychological Reports*, **59**, 447–50.

Woods, R. T. (1999). *Psychological Problems of Ageing*. John Wiley and Sons Ltd, Chichester.

Woods, R. T. and McKiernan, F. (1995). Evaluating the impact of reminiscence on older people with dementia. In *The Art and Science of Reminiscing: Theory, Research, Methods and Applications* (Haught, B. K. and Webster, J., eds), pp. 233–42. Taylor and Francis, Washington, DC.

11 Cognitive therapy formulations and interventions for treating distress in dementia

Introduction

Cognitive therapy's Lamarckian progress is generally attributed to three key writers: Beck (1967), Ellis (rational–emotive therapy: Ellis and Whitley 1970) and Meichenbaum (self-instructional training: Meichenbaum 1977). Over recent years, the terms cognitive therapy (CT) and cognitive behavioural therapy (CBT) have become synonymous, with the addition of the term 'behavioural' emphasizing the importance of the behavioural component within the treatment. In this context, behavioural interventions are no longer based on the principles of classical and operant conditioning; rather, they are embedded within the cognitive rationale itself. CT is not a panacea for all psychiatric problems, but its empirical basis and testability have led to both a wealth of research and a desire for evidence-based practices. Currently it is recognized as the preferred psychological treatment for many of the affective disorders (Andrews 1996, Roth and Fonagy 1996).

Numerous researchers have found CT to be effective with the elderly (Woods and Roth 1996), with important work being done in both depression (Gallagher and Thompson 1982) and the anxiety disorders (Radley *et al.* 1997). More recently, CT formulations, and the related treatment strategies, have been applied to people with dementia in order to relieve distress (Teri and Gallagher-Thompson 1991, Grober *et al.* 1993, James 1999a,b, Kipling *et al.* 1999). This chapter examines this work, discussing issues of suitability for CT and showing how the approach needs to be adapted. The latter sections focus on using CT formulations with people with severe dementia. With this patient group, it is suggested that CT can help inform the therapist and staff about the experience of the person with dementia, highlighting appropriate intervention strategies. However, before discussing the latter work in detail, a brief review of CT theory is presented.

Summary of the theory

The theoretical framework outlined in this chapter is based on the work of Beck. However, relevant CT approaches have also been developed by Meichenbaum (1977) and Ellis (Ellis and Whitley 1970). Meichenbaum's self-instructional training (SIT) suggests that behaviour change can occur by the adoption of more adaptive self-talk. Ellis' rational–emotive therapy (RET; now termed rational–emotive behaviour therapy, or REBT) suggests that people's emotions and behaviours are the consequences (Cs) of beliefs (Bs), which are interpretations of activating events (As). Both of these approaches have been used in the past to help manage challenging behaviour in people with learning disabilities (Kroese *et al.* 1997) and have been particularly helpful in the treatment of aggression (Novaco 1994). However, despite addressing some aspects of these two models, this chapter principally outlines a Beckian perspective.

Beck defines CT, and its rationale, as follows:

> Cognitive therapy is based on the cognitive model, which hypothesizes that people's emotions and behaviours are influenced by their perceptions of events. It is not a situation in and of itself that determines what people feel but rather the way in which they construe a situation.
>
> *Beck J. (1995), p.14*

As outlined by Beck, CT theory suggests that mood is greatly influenced by the occurrence of negative cognitions (i.e. thoughts and images). These cognitions tend to pop into awareness without any conscious control and thus are termed 'automatic'. Owing to the negativity and the automaticity of these cognitions, depression and anxiety are often said to be characterized by negative automatic thoughts (NATs). The NATs associated with depression tend to have three major themes, concerning perception of the self, the world and the future (Beck 1976). People suffering from depression will typically think of themselves as being unworthy, inadequate or unlovable. They will see the world as punishing or unfulfilling, and have a sense that things will not improve over time (i.e. a sense of hopelessness). This tripartite relationship is known as the cognitive triad. A similar triad exists with respect to anxiety. For example, anxious people tend to view themselves as vulnerable, the world as threatening and their future as unpredictable. In addition, they do not feel that they have adequate resources to cope with their surroundings, and thus are prone to the various symptoms associated with anxiety (excessive arousal and alertness, poor concentration, lack of confidence, stress).

It is important to note that everybody has NATs, but over relatively short periods of time these negative cognitions are usually analysed rationally and evaluated effectively. However, during an episode of depression or anxiety, the NATs are not open to the normal corrective processes of logical thinking. In other words, a depressed person will be unable to rationally analyse her[1] NATs and therefore cannot re-

---

[1] In this chapter the person with dementia is discussed as an older woman. This has been done solely to improve the flow of the text.

evaluate them successfully. For example, when a depressed person meets a friend, and the friend fails to greet them as warmly as usual, this person may think that her friend does not like her any more. Being depressed, the person is unable to generate less negative alternative interpretations (e.g. their friend may have had something else on her mind).

One reason for not being able to assess thoughts objectively is an overwhelming tendency to bias and distort information. Some examples of these biases include:

- *Catastrophizing*, i.e. thinking the worst: 'Forgetting to turn off the oven means I've got dementia.'

- *Personalizing* (egocentric thinking), i.e. putting oneself forward as the reason/cause of any difficulties: 'My daughter doesn't visit me more often because I'm boring.'

- *Mind reading*, i.e. making negative assumptions regarding other people's thoughts: 'Everyone thinks I'm stupid.'

- *All-or-nothing thinking*, i.e. always thinking in extremes, and thus not being able to think in a balanced way: 'Unless I do it perfectly, there's no point in doing it at all.'

These biases are examples of the sorts of cognitive processing found in people with low affect. A great deal of research has examined the way in which people's processing of information changes when they are depressed and anxious. It appears that there is a marked negative impact on both their attributional style (Hollon *et al.* 1996) and their memory (Williams 1996a). For example, depression is associated with preferential retrieval of negative memories over positive ones (Williams 1999b). In addition, low affect makes memory over-general, so that recalling specific events is more difficult and problem-solving ability is reduced (Wahler and Afton 1980). Prospective memory (remembering plans) also appears to be negatively affected, leading to an increase in absent-mindedness. Evans *et al.* (1992), examining the impact of over-general memory phenomenon on interpersonal problem solving, found that depressed patients were more prone to using these less useful over-general memories as a 'database' to generate solutions to current interpersonal problems.

A dynamic way of representing the negative processing occurring in the affective states is illustrated via 'the fragile egg' (James 1997) (see Fig. 11.1). The egg's semi-permeable membrane functions as a filter with respect to the external data impinging on the individual. At the centre of the diagram is the depression triad, represented by a negative view of the self, environment and the future. This model represents how 'belief-consistent' information reinforces established cognitions (arrow 1), while inconsistent (i.e. positive) information is routinely ignored (arrow 2). Sometimes positive information can even be transformed negatively to become consistent with beliefs (arrow 3). The model highlights why depression and anxiety can be so devastating, because in these affective states, a person's mental and cognitive functioning are actively undermining her state of well-being, often leading to the

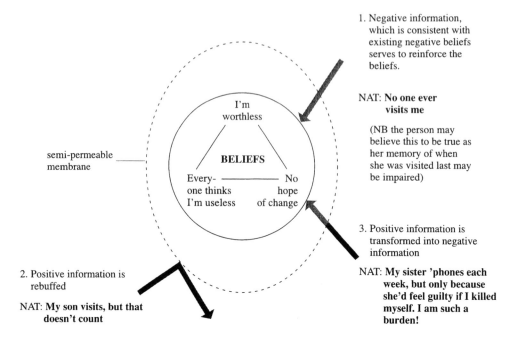

1. Negative information, which is consistent with existing negative beliefs serves to reinforce the beliefs.

NAT: **No one ever visits me**

(NB the person may believe this to be true as her memory of when she was visited last may be impaired)

semi-permeable membrane

I'm worthless

BELIEFS

Every- ——— No
one thinks   hope
I'm useless   of change

3. Positive information is transformed into negative information

NAT: **My sister 'phones each week, but only because she'd feel guilty if I killed myself. I am such a burden!**

2. Positive information is rebuffed

NAT: **My son visits, but that doesn't count**

Fig. 11.1   Representation of information processing in depression—the fragile egg.

development of mood-consistent behaviours. In depression this can result in withdrawal; in anxiety, one might observe avoidance strategies.

The NATs observed in this style of thinking may be regarded as the cognitive mediators, because they are believed to influence mood. They are also considered to interact with stable dysfunctional sets of beliefs the person holds about herself, as illustrated in the inner circle of Fig. 11.1. Such beliefs can take various forms, such as unconditional and conditional beliefs:

- *Unconditional beliefs* are rigid, inflexible and global descriptions of the self ('I am worthless, inadequate, a poor coper, vulnerable...'). CT theory suggests that these beliefs can lie dormant, remaining inactive until triggered by some specific event. Once activated, the person can be overwhelmed by the strength of the negative feelings associated with this belief.

- *Conditional beliefs* are rigid life-rules, which operate to guide the person's feelings, behaviours and decisions in day-to-day functioning. They are often represented by 'If ... then ....' constructions (e.g. 'If I can't do it perfectly, then I'm a failure'; 'If I do things for my daughter, then she will like me').

Some of these beliefs and rules will have had their genesis in early life experiences, or have been formed in adolescence or following a significant life event (e.g. divorce or retirement). The degree of credibility assigned to the beliefs may differ; however, it is the lack of flexibility within the belief that produces the major problems. The lack of flexibility becomes most evident when circumstances arise that require the person to adapt in some way. For example, consider Mrs P, who has recently become depressed. Despite obtaining insight into her problem via therapy, she is still having a great deal of difficulty relinquishing her dysfunctional network of beliefs.

Case example: Mrs P

Mrs P is a woman with a life-long underlying unconditional belief that she is worthless, but, perhaps surprisingly, no prior history of depression. It appears that over many years her self-esteem had been maintained through a conditional belief: 'If I do things for others, then I am worthwhile'. Therefore until recently she had been able to compensate for her unconditional belief via her conditional rule which involved her continually doing things for other people. For example, being the best daughter, most dutiful wife and most doting grandmother (cooking, shopping, babysitting, etc.). Unfortunately, this compensatory effect has now been neutralized, owing to the onset of mild cognitive difficulties. Indeed, as her family started to notice her difficulties, they began to withdraw and no longer trusted her to take good care of her grandchildren or to remember to get the correct shopping items. Because she is now unable to sustain her conditional belief of being worthwhile, her underlying vulnerability (i.e. a sense of worthlessness) is exposed.

At the moment Mrs P is unable to adapt her conditional belief appropriately, probably because for many years it functioned successfully to protect her from experiencing low self-esteem. Hence, this previously functional belief is now serving to increase her sense of worthlessness and feelings of rejection.

In order to demonstrate how the various features of the framework relate to each other, Mrs P's difficulties are formulated in Fig. 11.2, which summarizes how two different events, with different NATs, led to Mrs P feeling depressed. It is important to note that the model suggests that NATs need not always be the precursor to the mood; rather, the two features relate to each other within a vicious circle. This framework highlights the fact that certain situations, or events, trigger the underlying dysfunctional network of beliefs. The person is obviously unaware of the predisposing cognitive system, but is aware of the high levels of negative affect and physical discomfort produced. It is only through therapy that they are made aware of the NATs and the cognitions underlying them. In the present example, these experiences tend to result in Mrs P engaging in depressive forms of behaviour. Her cycle is self-perpetuating and is often labelled the 'vicious cycle' or 'depressive spiral'.

As demonstrated in the case of Mrs P, beliefs and biases are not dysfunctional all of the time, as their impact is often time- and situation-specific. Indeed, in many environments they may help the person cope well, and may even serve as a buffer to protect the person's self-esteem (as in the case of Mrs P, prior to the onset of dementia). It is therefore important to investigate the costs and benefits of a particular belief system when planning an intervention (James *et al.* 1999).

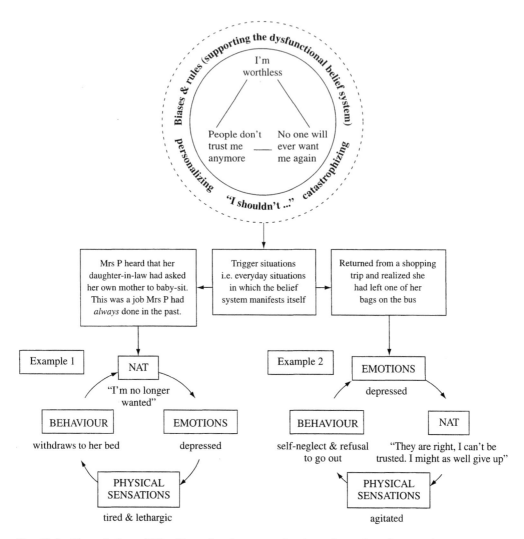

Fig. 11.2   Formulation of Mrs P's cycles, demonstrating how the various features interact.

Cognitive therapy interventions with older people

Standard CT aims to relieve the problematic emotions by identifying the associated NATs and biases and then contrasting them with the actual facts. Over time the person is helped to reassess her cognitive style in relation to factual information. Initially an assessment is carried out to provide a formulation of the person's difficulties; this involves collecting information about the person's emotions and associated NATs. A common strategy in CT is to ask the patient to monitor her NATs and emotions. The monitoring procedure often involves the use of a diary or work-sheet (see Table 11.1).

Such sheets help the patient to become more aware of the typical NATs and biases she engages in. The diaries also help the patient generate specific events rather than the more over-general versions, which are more common in depression (Williams 1996a). The patient is then helped to re-evaluate her cognitions by learning how to judge the dysfunctional cognitions against the factual evidence available to her (Table 11.2).

Thus the patient is given insight into the impact her thoughts have on her emotions and behaviours, and is assisted to collaborate with the therapist towards developing and implementing 'fact'-based perspectives and solutions. It usually takes a while for the patient to re-evaluate their NATs and beliefs effectively. Often the re-evaluation is initially more of an intellectual exercise, bringing little emotional relief. However, over a period of time, in which the patient is introduced to the re-evaluation process, one usually begins to see a positive shift in affect. There is a strong emphasis on behavioural work accompanying the cognitive features and therefore throughout therapy specific targets are both set and performed 'in' and 'outside' of the sessions; the latter are usually called homework assignments. While this technique may appear straightforward, it requires a high degree of competence in CT on the part of the therapist to yield an effective result. Applying CT techniques without clear understanding of their function will usually lead to poor outcome.

CT interventions have been adapted for different kinds of patient groups and disorders. For reviews of how to adapt CT for older people, see Gallagher-Thompson and Thompson (1991), Glantz (1989) and Morris and Morris (1991). The general consensus in this field is that the therapy must be goal-orientated, with high levels of structure and focus. Indeed, because older people show a decrease in their ability to shift between abstract concepts, a more concrete approach is advised (Church 1983). It is suggested that when working with people with cognitive impairment, the therapist should place less emphasis on cognitive restructuring (i.e. identifying and re-evaluating cognitive biases) and more on practical behavioural solutions. Obviously, the therapy must take account of physical and sensory difficulties and be paced accordingly. Despite such adaptations, it is important to remember that the

Table 11.1 Work sheet

Emotion	Describe the type of distress you were experiencing (depression, fear, anger, etc.).
Trigger situation	Describe what was happening to trigger the distress.
Thoughts	What thoughts or images went through your head during this event?
Physical sensations	What physical sensations were you experiencing (tension, heart-pounding, sweating, lack of energy)?
Behaviour	What did you do immediately after the event or as a result it (avoid friends, stay in bed)?

Table 11.2 Example of thought re-evaluation diary for Mrs P

Situation	Thoughts associated with the distressing emotion	Biases identified	Re-evaluation columns	
			factual details of episode that help re-evaluate the situation	alternative perspectives on the event
Left a bag on bus	'Everyone is right, I can't be trusted to do things right'	catastrophizing	'I remembered six of the bags and left only one'	'Just because I've made this mistake (one I've made before) does not mean my memory's gone completely. So I can be trusted, but need to slow down and rush less.'
	'I may as well give up'	all-or-nothing thinking	'I've left bags on the bus many times before'	'There are still many things I do well'

elderly population is made up of a hugely diverse group of people, and thus any recommendations must be treated with caution. For this reason, it is essential that the therapist treats each person as an individual, being guided by the unique formulation developed specifically for him/her.

Cognitive therapy and dementia

Standard psychological strategies generally require that patients have the ability to gain insight into their difficulties, learn alternative strategies (both cognitive and behavioural) and work collaboratively with the therapist. Safran and Segal (1990) have produced a 10-item scale to determine patient suitability for short-term CT (Table 11.3).

In truth, few patients, even those without cognitive impairment, score highly on all 10 criteria. Indeed, in an unpublished review of patients seen by people who had completed the Newcastle Cognitive Therapy Course, the mean score for patient suitability was 32 (out of 50), with a standard deviation of 6.5 (James 1998). As one might expect, many dementia sufferers do not possess many of the abilities outlined in Table 11.3, particularly in the later stages of the illness (Teri and Gallagher-Thompson 1991). Despite these reservations regarding suitability, CT is perceived to be appropriate for many people with dementia for the following reasons:

(1) It employs a structured format, in which an agenda is set collaboratively at the beginning of the session. The function of the agenda is to ensure that specific, relevant items are discussed within the session, and that the time is apportioned appropriately in relation to the perceived importance of the items. The therapist introduces the patient to this process early on in therapy, providing a sense of security and familiarity. Thus the predictable and structured format of CT is particularly helpful for those with attentional, concentration and executive ('frontal') difficulties.

Table 11.3   The suitability scale

Items 1-9: patient's ability to:
   1   access negative thoughts
   2   differentiate between different types of emotions (depression, anxiety, anger)
   3   accept responsibility for change
   4   work with the cognitive rationale
   5   display therapeutic alliance
   6   display out-of-session therapeutic alliance
   7   remain focused during therapy
   8   display optimism regarding the future
   9   avoid defensive and avoidant strategies
Item 10: the chronicity of the problem. The greater the chronicity, the less suitable is the patient for short-term CT.

(By Permission Safran J.D. and Sega Z.V. (1990). Interpersonal Processing in Cognitive Therapy Basic Books, New York.)

(2) It highlights the association between thoughts and feelings, requiring the patient to become aware of this link. This is particularly beneficial to those people experiencing high levels of emotional discomfort. By helping people to differentiate between different emotional states, and the NATs associated with them, people are able to obtain a better understanding of their discomfort.

(3) CT operates through an explicit conceptual model, and thus helps the person with dementia to quickly familiarize herself with the cognitive framework, the theory, educational components and intervention strategies. The formulation is developed collaboratively and thus the therapeutic framework is very explicit and structured; both of these elements are essential when working with a person who has cognitive difficulties.

(4) CT reinforces and encourages cognitive change through behavioural techniques. The behavioural tasks undertaken within the session, and as homework assignments, are designed to break the common cycles of withdrawal and inactivity. The tasks also help by (i) getting the person to re-engage in tasks that she previously found rewarding or pleasurable (Lewinsohn and Talkington 1979) and (ii) testing out hypotheses that have been developed within the therapy (for example, a therapist might say to a patient, 'From what you are saying, you seem less agitated when you go for a walk in the garden. Well, let's try it out.').

(5) It promotes an effective therapeutic relationship, placing a great emphasis on a positive, collaborative relationship. Rogers' core issues of trust, empathy and warmth are seen as crucial elements of the relationship in CT (Rogers 1957).

The structure, behavioural emphasis, collaboration and therapeutic relationship of CT hence make it beneficial for a person with dementia. Teri and Gallagher-Thompson (1991) have produced one of the few comprehensive CT treatment packages for people with dementia. The treatment strategies were designed for people with both mild and severe Alzheimer's disease. The people treated were generally seen as out-patients for periods of between 16 and 20 sessions. Family members were contacted to enlist their support for the treatment period. In this treatment approach, patients were provided with:

• a detailed explanation of the CT model of depression;

• an early introduction to the CT methodology, including the rationale for performing homework assignments; and

• the opportunity to present specific examples of the situations in which they felt depressed.

The patients' problematic situations were then recorded, together with the accompanying thoughts and feelings, using diaries. Having established a conceptual understanding of the problem, a number of thought re-evaluation techniques were used to produce more balanced styles of thinking. This was achieved by:

- examining the evidence for and against a specific cognition;
- listing the pros and cons of maintaining a specific idea in its current form;
- revising unhelpful rules; and
- encouraging patients to experiment with new attitudes and cognitions in stressful situations.

Many of the above interventions are presented in tabular form by Teri and Gallagher-Thompson (1991, p.415).

The following sections will examine some of the adaptations required to use CT with people with dementia.

Cognitive therapy with mild/moderate dementia

Grober *et al.* (1993) and Whitehouse (1994) provide a comprehensive list of problems that can be encountered by therapists when treating people with mild to moderate organic difficulties, including cognitive deficits, lack of awareness, concreteness, attentional deficits, hyper-arousal, aphasic problems, memory difficulties, aprosodia and physical limitations. Thus, the impact of the organic impairment is multi-factorial, often resulting in deficits in psychosocial and physical functioning (Prigatano and Fordyce 1986) and emotional processing (e.g. organic denial, in which the person displays an inability to be self-reflective). Grober *et al.* (1993) discuss how one can deal with some of these cognitive deficits in people who have experienced strokes; Whitehouse (1994) provides a similar description for those who have suffered head injuries. These strategies are summarized below, providing adaptations and recommendations for dementia in general.

Adaptations and recommendations for using cognitive therapy with people with dementia

(1) *Assess level of functioning and suitability*—the level of organic impairment should be assessed to determine the impact on patients' physical, cognitive and emotional functioning. The comprehensive assessment will lead to the development of a formulation, which includes details about the person's, history, personality, mental health status and environmental status (see Chapter 8).

(2) *Facilitate recognition of changes within emotional states*—the person with dementia should be encouraged to develop skills in identifying her various emotional states (e.g. 'Before I got angry and hit him, I felt really anxious'). Information about her state will help her and her therapist to understand her experience of the situation and the reasons for her actions. This understanding then helps target the interventions more effectively (i.e. treating both the anger and the anxiety). The ability to identify emotions is often a difficult skill to acquire as the person may now by more impulsive, reckless, apathetic or disinhibited.

(3) *Work on self-acceptance*—those people who retain insight into their losses often have difficulties coming to terms with the cognitive and physical changes that have occurred. This is because they have to deal with the dysfunctional beliefs associated with these changes (e.g. 'I am worthless, I'm not the person I used to be'; 'If I can't do the things the way I used to, then there's no point trying any more'). As part of the therapist's work, he must help the person with dementia to understand the difference between actual and perceived losses. Whitehouse (1994) suggests that this initially involves a mourning period, followed by an adjustment process whereby the person must come to terms with the things she perceives she has lost (see also Prigatano 1986). Thus the person is helped to accept potential changes in her identity, circumstances, personal goals and view of the world (i.e. helped to 'redefine the self'). The adjustment process is often difficult for someone with progressive dementia because the deterioration is ongoing.

(4) *Set realistic goals*—the goals set in therapy should be achievable, measurable, monitored and relevant for the person. They need to be appropriate for the type of disorder and its level of severity, and their impact should be assessed in relation to the environmental context. The goals also need to be planned and executed appropriately. For example, if a person has withdrawn and become chronically agoraphobic, merely walking to the supermarket will be far too frightening for her to accomplish. Thus in order to achieve such a goal, one needs to break it down into smaller, more manageable steps.

(5) *Foster a sense of realistic hope*—as outlined above, hopelessness is a key feature in determining and maintaining depression and therefore it is an important feature to target in treatment. In order to engender a sense of hope, it is important to reinforce therapeutic gains, no matter how small these might be.

(6) *Utilize the therapeutic alliance*—although standard CT emphasizes the importance of the therapeutic relationship, the therapist is required to place extra attention on this feature for people with dementia. This is because a greater number of ruptures in the relationship are possible, owing to the disinhibited or unfocused presentation of some patients. Transference issues are also crucial, often influencing the therapist's approach to the person. The person with dementia can come to represent many things to the therapist, such as her parent, grandparent or future self.

(7) *Work with carers*—owing to the relatively high levels of dependency in people with dementia, the therapist must invariably work with family members and paid carers. CT can be used to deal with care-givers affective problems or help them to re-evaluate thinking biases associated with dementia.

(8) *Use specific compensatory strategies for dealing with cognitive deficits*—Table 11.4 summarizes techniques therapists can use to deal with problems resulting from cognitive impairment in the person with dementia, such as memory problems and language difficulties.

Table 11.4 Compensatory strategies for dealing with cognitive deficits

Deficits	Compensatory strategies
Memory problems	Use diaries, checklists and notebooks. Record the sessions on audio or video tape. Use much feedback and repetition within session, and use highly structured formats.
Language difficulties	Receptive problems can be helped by using handouts, pictures, diagrams and audio aids. Expressive difficulties can be dealt with by using alternative communication strategies and appropriate writing, drawing or visual material.
Mental inflexibility (concreteness)	Use simple structured material with which the person can be easily socialized to the CT model. Use elicitation and two-way feedback; frequently asking the person to describe what the main themes of the therapy have been. Consolidate the sessional work through role-play and behavioural work.
Attentional problems	Set short-term, specific and highly relevant goals. Use sensitively paced therapy, with appropriate breaks within the session.

The recommendations outlined above are useful general tips, but specific adaptations are required when working with each of the different forms of dementia. Some of these issues are discussed below.

Special considerations for the different types of dementia

Each type of dementia (Alzheimer's disease, multi-infarct dementia and dementia with Lewy bodies) presents a different challenge for the cognitive therapist. For example, people with Alzheimer's disease are likely to have problems retaining information, while those with Lewy body dementia will have fluctuating abilities and present with executive problems, such as rigidity of thinking. In this section some of the specific problems and considerations with respect to the different forms of dementia will be outlined.

Alzheimer's disease

Alzheimer's disease is characterized by gradual global impairment with specific memory deficits. When engaging a person with alzheimer's in therapy it is necessary, therefore, to set, and constantly reinforce, small and appropriate goals. The specific cognitive difficulties of these people, especially their memory problems, must be supported by external cues (e.g. diaries, video recordings of the sessions, manualized sessions). It is estimated that 20–40% of Alzheimer patients have a major depressive disorder (Wragg and Jeste 1989). In a report of their CT treatment of depression in people with Alzheimer's disease, Teri and Gallagher-Thompson (1991) state that the therapy must be structured, and the problems be dealt with in a straightforward manner. They also suggest that cognitive-oriented interventions are particularly helpful when dealing with people with mild dementia who are catastrophizing about the effect of their cognitive impairment on their current status. In contrast, more behaviourally orientated interventions are useful when the '. . . abilities and level of activity [of the person with dementia] are compromised, causing a significant loss in pleasurable events' (Teri and Gallagher-Thompson 1991, p. 416).

Lewy body dementia

People with Lewy body dementia have executive difficulties, poor insight and vivid hallucinations and are prone to falls. This results in a rigid, apathetic presentation which is also characterized by problem-solving deficits. It is often necessary to engage such people in systemic work, as their poor motivation and lack of insight cause frequent conflicts between these people and their carers. Such conflicts are often exacerbated by the characteristic variability in cognitive difficulties, which makes the person's abilities appear to wax and wane. This feature is particularly difficult for the carer as it gives the impression that the person with dementia is deliberately not doing things or doing things incorrectly.

Multi-infarct dementia

People experiencing strokes are vulnerable to a number of problems in addition to their cognitive and motor difficulties. For a good overview of the effect of stroke and the use of CT interventions, see Grober *et al.* (1993). This review deals mainly with depression, however it is also very common to observe high levels of anxiety in this patients who have had strokes. The anxiety reactions may result from the initial circumstances of the stroke. For example, if the person's stroke left her unable to access help (e.g. lying immobile on her bedroom floor for 24 h), this may lead to symptoms of post-traumatic stress. The sudden onset of some strokes also tends to make it difficult for people to adjust to the change in their condition. Strokes can also produce changes in body image, resulting in people frequently exaggerating the extent of their level of impairment and disability. People who have had strokes are often over-anxious about their health, tending to misinterpret bodily sensations, identifying them as the potential onset of another stroke. In severe cases, particularly with older people who may have been living independently, the stroke may require them to relocate into a residential setting. Such moves often require careful handling by both staff and family in order to minimize the stressors associated with relocation (Danermark and Ekstrom 1990).

Parkinson's disease

Parkinson's disease is a complex disorder with neurological and psychiatric components. There are complex interactions between motor functions, affective features, cognitions and the effect of treatment. The psychiatric features (dementia, psychosis and anxiety) are common, but can be difficult to treat in people with advanced Parkinson's disease owing to the executive deficits, such as problems with memory, learning, reasoning and visuospatial awareness. In addition to the neuropsychological features, the physical symptoms (e.g. tremor, mask-like face, bradykinesia and salivation) cause frequent problems for the person. These can result in the person becoming socially embarrassed and anxious, often leading to the development of agoraphobic symptoms. The 'on' and 'off' phases of the disease can also produce major difficulties, owing to the dehabilitating effect of the 'off' phase in poorly controlled cases. During the 'off' phase, some people experience almost total rigidity with or without cognitive confusion. One patient described the feeling of the 'off' phase as being 'trapped inside a rusty metal frame, just waiting for the lubricant to work'. Such experiences often result in people experimenting with their medication in attempts to prolong the 'on' phase and reduce the 'off' phase. This experimenting may become dysfunctionally obsessive, becoming the major focus of the person's life.

The application of cognitive therapy to people with severe dementia

The formulation of distress

As outlined in Chapters 3 and 15, recent evidence suggests that neuroleptic agents, which are often used to treat agitated behaviours, may accelerate cognitive decline (McShane *et al.* 1997) and are associated with low levels of patient well-being (Ballard *et al.* 1999). Therefore, because of complications and side-effects of drugs, there is a strong need for the development of effective psychotherapeutic strategies that can be used both alongside, or independently of, pharmacological regimens. Effective therapy should aim to reduce levels of distress in the person with dementia as she interacts with her environment. Due to the severity of the impairment in this group, the interventions are likely to be more behavioural than intra-psychic (i.e. often behavioural and environmental modification strategies). It is important to note that the effect of the interventions is unlikely to generalize widely across different situations, and thus their goal is to provide pleasure and reduce stress during specific scenarios and events (O'Donovan 1996). However, if the level of ill-being is reduced across a broad range of specific situations, the person with dementia is likely to feel less distressed generally and enjoy a higher overall level of well-being.

As outlined earlier, in order to derive and target appropriate interventions, it is important that the therapist develops a suitable formulation. However, because the person with dementia is often unable to record thoughts and is less able to gain insight into her dysfunctional cognitive biases, some adaptation is required. Hence the formulation presented in Figure 11.3, which is based on the standard cognitive model (Beck 1976), places less emphasis on introspection and thought monitoring on the part of the patient. Nevertheless, in line with the standard model, the framework proposes that the person's perception of a given situation is the product of a complex set of interactive components (historical, environmental, etc.), and that cognitive processing is open to a number of personal (physiological, temperamental), societal and cultural influences (Kitwood 1997; see also Chapter 8).

To determine the nature of the distress of the person with dementia, the model uses Beck's cognitive triads (summarized above) to construct the formulation. For example, from our knowledge of the themes associated with the emotional triads, if a person with dementia is displaying anxiety, this would suggest she is experiencing a sense of vulnerability, within a context of perceived chaos and unpredictability. Table 11.5 summarizes the triadic and dyadic themes commonly associated with the emotions. Thus, by carefully examining the specific forms of distress (depression, anxiety, anger) and the features associated with them, insight into the experience and actions of the person with dementia can be gained and interventions planned.

Having ascertained the person's emotional experience and associated themes, the therapist examines the features responsible for the particular type of distress. As outlined in Figure 11.3, environmental, historical and contextual aspects are examined. It is important to note that in order to obtain the detailed information required, one will need to garner data from the various people who interact with the person with dementia. The next stage is to use the conceptual model to direct the treatment strategy used.

The application of this model is further illustrated through the case of Mrs S. She was a 82 year old widow, living in an EMI (elderly mentally ill) home. She was referred to the service when the staff in the home claimed that she had started to become 'stubborn' and 'aggressive'. The referral stated that this previously shy woman was displaying aggression towards staff members. As part of the assessment, an attempt was made to capture Mrs S's experience of one of her aggressive episodes. The following passage was constructed from her own description, together with information obtained from staff members who witnessed the event. The episode has been written in the first person to help appreciate the emotions experienced by Mrs S during the episode.

Table 11.5 Cognitive themes associated with emotional distress

Emotion	Themes
Triad	
depression	sense of self as worthless or inadequate, with negative view of world and future
anxiety	sense of vulnerability, perception of the environment as chaotic, and the future as unpredictable
anger	sense of personal injustice, perception of the environment as hostile, a need to act to protect self from future harm
Dyad	
shame	sense of self as an object of ridicule or humiliation as judged by others; shame is interpersonally driven (Gilbert 1994)
guilt	sense of the self as the source of harm or injury, with others suffering as a result of one's actions

Depression, anxiety and anger are represented by triadic relationships, whereas other emotions, such as shame and guilt are better described by dyadic relationships.

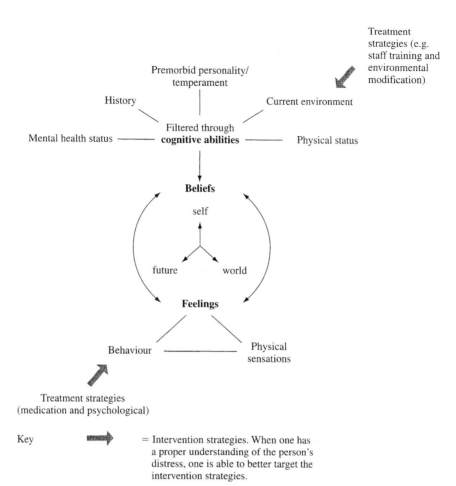

Fig. 11.3   Model of formulation of distress in dementia.

Case example: Mrs S

I know I must go to the toilet soon. I've been waiting ages for someone to ask me whether I need to go. I don't want to wet myself. What's become of me that I can't even remember where the toilet is? Last week I plucked up courage to try some of those doors, but I chose the wrong one and then got shouted at for walking into some kind of meeting.

Oh no, I've got to be quick! It's coming! I'll try this door: it's got a funny handle—that must mean something. Thank goodness for that, I'm right. But where is the light switch? Oh never mind, I'll just keep the door open a little bit to let some light in. I don't want the door closed anyway: tiny rooms frighten me.

Here comes one of the nurses. Why is she storming over like that? She's cross that I've left the door open. She's saying that she didn't think I was that sort of person. That hurts. She's embarrassing me in front of everyone, the whole room is looking at me. This nurse has got a cheek. If she had been doing her job properly, I wouldn't have got into this mess. Right, I'm going to give her a piece of my mind. She'll not do this again in a hurry.

Mrs S's ability to process information coherently had obviously been affected by her declining cognitive abilities. However, because she retained some insight, she was aware of her difficulties and inability to cope well and thus felt a heightened sense of anxiety. In this particular example, she was also experiencing a sense of shame, which quickly turned to anger as she began to perceive that she was being treated unfairly. A useful way of formulating these perceptions is via the cognitive triads and themes outlined in Figure 11.4. Thus, one can conceptualize Mrs S's initial anxiety, shame and the subsequent anger. Her behaviour appears to be consistent with her emotional state, and one can see that her anger was her way of attempting to regain some control in the situation and retain some self-esteem.

As can be seen from the above scenario, the reaction of carers and others to such behaviour will influence the level of distress and well-being experienced by the person with dementia. At times, practices that carers have developed to cope with the behaviours may serve to exacerbate the negative mood and behaviour (Chapter 13), so the carer's interaction needs to be taken into account. It is also important to remember that when the person with dementia is also suffering from anxiety and/or depression, this will further impoverish their thinking, because of irrational processing (negative thinking, catastrophizing and over-generalizing). These latter

Anxiety

The observed anxiety suggested that Mrs S was fearful, and unsure how she was going to cope in this confusing situation.

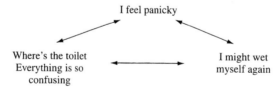

Shame

Mrs S felt humiliated, and the nurse (whom she perceived to be in a more powerful position) was recognized as the source of ridicule and humiliation.

Anger

The triad for anger suggests that Mrs S felt she had been treated badly

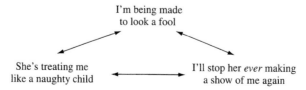

Fig. 11.4   Mrs S's triads.

features, interacting with the processing problems stemming from cortical impairment, often give overly negative impressions of the cognitive deficit. Thus when planning treatment, all these features need to be formulated appropriately.

Putting the model into practice

As outlined above, the first step in developing the conceptual model is to determine what emotion is being experienced in a particular situation. For example, if the emotion is anxiety, one should determine which aspects of the situation are making the person feel vulnerable. If the emotion is anger, one would examine what was making the person fell angry (does she think she is being maligned or patronized? Why?). The second step is to conduct a detailed assessment of the 'problem' behaviour using Figure 11.3 to generate a formulation of the person's distress. Hence one is trying to account for the behaviour using a person-centred perspective, by taking account of the person's history, environment, etc.

Once a thorough assessment has been conducted, appropriate interventions can be planned. Such strategies might involve a combination of medication and behaviour modification, with drugs perhaps used to calm the situation down and psychotherapy to eliminate the triggers and environmental reinforcing agents. Figure 11.5 illustrates this model in practice, detailing the formulation process and the intervention strategies with respect to Mrs S.

Formulating Mrs S's challenging behaviour

Mrs S was referred because of her aggressive outbursts towards staff. The problems occurred most often in the presence of two particular staff members. In order to examine Mrs S's difficulties in detail, a specific situation was chosen to illustrate the nature of her distress. In this case, the incident in the toilet was chosen as the key situation.

The model demonstrates the dynamic relationship between the triggers, emotions and cognitive themes. Because many people with dementia are unable to inform the therapist of their thinking, one uses the triadic and dyadic themes as templates to conceptualize the experience of the person with dementia. In the present example, the formulation suggested that the treatment should be targeted initially at the anxiety and fears associated with going to the toilet. Thus environmental disorientation was reduced by using clearer signs and better cueing devices. The traumatic fears stemming from the 'locked door' incident were treated using a systematic desensitization approach. Initially a staff member waited outside the door when Mrs S went into the toilet, periodically checking that she was all right through the closed door. Over a week, the nurse spoke less frequently, until eventually she was able to leave Mrs S to go to the toilet by herself. The training was done using one particular WC, which was the largest of the toilets; in this room the light was left permanently on. The latter features were designed to reduce confusion and enhance familiarity and predictability.

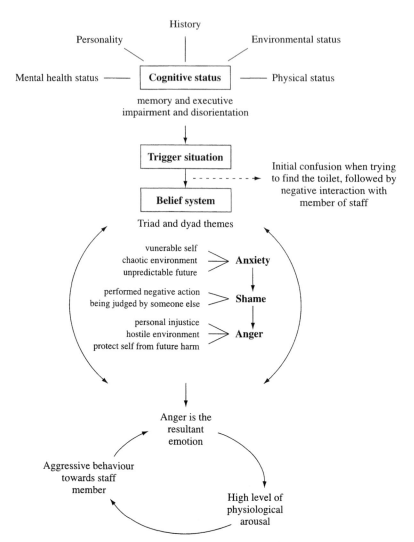

Fig. 11.5 Mrs S's formulation. **Personality**: Mrs S was described as confident and socially skilled. According to her daughter, she had 'quiet inner strength'. She rarely got angry, but got explosive when she lost her temper. **History**: Mrs S had been a housewife for most of her life, although before her marriage in 1947 she had been a personal assistant to a manager in the civil service. Her husband had owned two butcher's shops, and so they had lived comfortably. Her husband died 10 years ago. Her two daughters both live abroad. One daughter noted that, before moving into care, Mrs S had once accidentally locked herself in the bathroom, being unable to work out how to unlock the door. For a short while after this traumatic experience, Mrs S had disliked going into small rooms by herself. **Environmental status**: Mrs S had been living in the home for 3 years and was happy until recently but had become increasingly agitated over the last 6 months. The agitation was particularly noticeable in the presence of two particular staff members. **Mental health status**: apart from a period of post-natal depression in her late twenties, there was no evidence of previous difficulties. **Physical status**: Mrs S had arthritis (for which she was receiving analgesia) and shortness of breath.

   Work was also done with the staff to enhance their understanding of the experience of cognitive impairment and, more specifically, Mrs S's distress. The main
theme of the training was to help explain the types of staff interaction that were
resulting in dysfunctional triads. Specific work was done with those care staff who
had unintentionally provoked some of the triads and challenging behaviour. During
the training, one member of staff commented: 'I've never thought of it like that
before, I mean looking from her perspective: the way she is behaving is helping her
to respect herself.'

General discussion

In the above case, the aggressive action seemed to be a rather understandable
response to a provocative act. It is important to note, however, that aggression and
anger have numerous reinforcing consequences (the person with dementia often gets
what she wants), so these forms of response can become chronic. In such circumstances, the aggressive act may be become the dominant method of responding to
distress, and over time the person can lose the ability to select and engage in alternative behavioural coping strategies. In people displaying chronic aggression, one
frequently observes unrealistic and inflexible expectations, leading to hyperalertness
(vigilance, selective attention biases) for potential threats to their self-image (Black
et al. 1997). In addition to these cognitive elements, such people also tend to experience high levels of physiological arousal (cardiovascular, respiratory and muscular
activity), and this activity may be transferred from one situation to the next.
   Black *et al.* (1997, p. 35) comment that 'Pertinent to understanding chronic anger
problems, arousal that is prolonged by rumination can, when not fully dissipated,
transfer to subsequent situations of provocation. Zillmann (1983) has shown that
arousal residues from previous activation add to the arousal potency of new events,
a process that he has called "excitation transfer."'
   Such understanding regarding the features associated with the problem in its
chronic form will inform the therapist about the best strategy for tackling the
problem. In the case of a chronic condition, it would seem appropriate to devise
some strategies to deal with the high levels of arousal (relaxation work), as well as
helping the person to develop more functional (alternative) ways to deal with her
distress.
   In order to conduct successfully the various strategies outlined in the chapter, it is
imperative that staff and carers understand the strategies being employed. One of
the advantages of the CT approach is that the model can be readily appreciated by
the carers. Indeed, the approach emphasizes that in order to understand how the
person with dementia experiences a given situation, the carers merely need to reflect
on how they would think, feel and behave in that situation. Likewise, the carers can
be helped to appreciate that the memory and processing biases operating when they
are stressed (such as selective attention or absentmindedness) are also common for
people with dementia. This knowledge is often helpful in explaining why the person

with dementia sometimes appears able to motivate herself or understand things on one occasions, but not on another.

Conclusion

The CT framework is a useful model in helping to understand better the distress associated with having dementia. It provides a template that links feelings, thoughts and behaviour within a historical and environmental context. Adaptations to the model are required, even for people with mild dementia. However, people with dementia think and feel like everyone else, and the professional's ability to self-reflect can help them to understand the plight of the person with dementia.

The person with dementia is continually attempting to make sense of her world, and is using her remaining cognitive processes to do so. However, her view of the world is less coherent, her perceptions are degraded, things are no longer predictable and her life-long coping strategies are often unhelpful (James 1999b). As outlined above, it is believed that this experience can be effectively formulated using the cognitive triads (Table 11.5 and Figure 11.4). It is also suggested that many of the distressing behaviours observed in people with dementia (sometimes termed 'challenging behaviours') can be understood using the framework outlined in Figure 11.3. This model suggests that many of the challenging behaviours result from the person with dementia attempting to cope with their high levels of emotion.

The present discussion has focused on traditional cognitive perspectives and demonstrated how the field has begun to move away from reactive management strategies for people with dementia towards a more active therapeutic strategy. It is noteworthy that the discussions have not examined many of the recent CT information processing models, such as the interactive cognitive subsystem (Teasdale 1996) or the notion of modes (Beck 1996). These latter models are useful, offering some new insight into how to treat distress in people with dementia. Chapter 10 outlines some of the relevant features of Teasdale's model.

Acknowledgements

Thank you to Neil Sabin and F. Katharina Reichelt for their intellectual contributions to this work, and to Tricia Roe for her help in the preparation of the chapter.

REFERENCES

Andrews, G. (1996). Talk that works: The rise of cognitive behaviour therapy. *British Medical Journal*, **313**, 1501–2.
Ballard, C. G., Lana, M., Reichelt, K. (1999). Behavioural and psychological symptoms

amongst demetia sufferers in residential and nursing home care. (Abstract). Proceedings of the Ninth International Psychogeriatric Association Congress, Vancouver, August 1999.

Beck, A. T. (1967). *Depression: Clinical, Experimental and Theoretical Aspects.* Harper and Row, New York, NY.

Beck, A. T. (1976). *Cognitive Therapy and the Emotional Disorders.* International University Press, New York, NY.

Beck, A. T. (1996). Beyond belief: a theory of modes, personality and psychopathology. In *Frontiers of Cognitive Therapy* (Salkovskis, P. M., eds), pp. 1–25. Guilford Press, New York, NY.

Beck, J. (1995) *Cognitive Therapy: Basics and Beyond.* Guilford Press, New York, NY.

Black, L., Cullen, C. and Novaco, R. W. (1997). Anger assessment for people with mild learning disabilities in secure settings. In *Cognitive-Behaviour Therapy for People with Learning Disabilities* (Kroese, B. S., Dagnan, D. and Loumidis, K., eds), pp. 33–52. Routledge, London.

Church, M. (1983). Psychological therapy with elderly people. *Bulletin of the British Psychological Society*, **36**, 110–12.

Danermark, B. and Ekstrom, M. (1990). Relocation and health effects on the elderly. A comment and research review. *Journal of Sociology and Social Welfare*, **17**, 25–49.

Ellis, A. and Whitley, J. M. (1970). *Theoretical and Empirical Foundations of Rational-Emotive Therapy.* Basic Books, Monterey, CA.

Evans, J., Williams, J. M. G., O'Louglin, S. and Howells, K. (1992). Autobiographical memory and problem solving strategies of parasuicide patients. *Psychological Medicine*, **22**, 399–405.

Gallagher, D. and Thompson, L. W. (1982). Treatment of major depressive disorder in older adult out-patients with brief psychotherapies. *Psychotherapy, Theory and Research Practice*, **19**, 482–90.

Gallagher-Thompson, D. and Thompson, L. W. (1991). *Cognitive-Behavioural Therapy for Late-Life Depression: a Treatment Manual.* Department of Veterans Affairs Medical Center, Palo Alto, CA.

Gilbert, P. (1994) *Counselling for Depression.* Sage, London.

Glantz, M. D. (1989). Cognitive therapy with the elderly. In *Comprehensive Handbook of Cognitive Therapy* (Freeman, A., Simon, K., Beutler, Z. and Arowitz, H., eds), pp. 467–89. Plenum Press, New York, NY.

Grober, S., Hibbard, M. R., Gordon, W., Stein, P. N. and Freeman, A. (1993). The psycho-therapeutic treatment of post-stroke depression with cognitive-behavioural therapy. In *Advances in Stroke Rehabilitation* (Gordon, W., ed.), pp. 215–241. Butterworth-Heinemann.

Hollon, S. D., DeRubeis, R. J. and Evans, M. D. (1996). Cognitive therapy in the treatment and prevention of depression. In *Frontiers of Cognitive Therapy* (Salkovskis, P. M., ed.), pp. 293–317. Guilford Press, New York, NY.

James, I. A. (1997) Cognitive therapy and the elderly. Presentation at Newcastle Certificate Course in Cognitive Therapy, Newcastle-upon-Tyne, July 1997.

James, I. A. (1998) Moderators of trainee competence. Presented at a conference of the British Psychological Society, Napier College, Edinburgh. July.

James, I. A. (1999a). Using a cognitive rationale to conceptualise anxiety in people with dementia. *Behavioural Cognitive Psychotherapy*, **27**, 345–51.

James, I. A. (1999b). Cognitive conceptualisation of distress in dementia. *Clinical Psychology Forum*, **134**, 21–5.

James, I. A., Kendell, K. and Reichelt, F. K. (1999) Conceptualisation of depression in older people: the interaction of positive and negative beliefs. *Behavioural and Cognitive Psychotherapy*, **27**, 285–90.

Kipling, T., Bailey, M. and Charlesworth, G. (1999). The feasibility of a cognitive behavioural therapy group for men with mild/moderate cognitive impairment. *Behavioural and Cognitive Psychotherapy*, **27**, 189–93.

Kitwood, T. (1990). The dialectics of dementia: with particular reference to Alzheimer's disease. *Ageing and Society*, **10**, 177–96.

Kitwood, T. (1997). *Dementia Reconsidered*. Open University Press, Buckingham.

Kroese, B. S, Dagnan, D. and Loumidis, K. (1997). *Cognitive-Behaviour Therapy for People with Learning Disabilities*. Routledge, London.

Lewinsohn, P. M. and Talkington, J. (1979). Studies on the measurement of unpleasant events and relations with depression. *Applied Psychological Measurement*, **3**, 83–101.

McShane, R., Keene, J., Gedling, K., Fairburn, C., Jacoby, R. and Hope, T. (1997). Do neuro-leptic drugs hasten cognitive decline in dementia? Prospective study with necropsy follow up. *British Medical Journal*, **314**, 266–70.

Meichenbaum, D. (1977). *Cognitive-Behaviour Modification: an Interactive Approach*. Plenum Press, New York, NY.

Morris, R. G. and Morris, L. W (1991). Cognitive and behavioural approaches with the depressed elderly. *International Journal of Geriatric Psychiatry*, **6**, 407–13.

Novaco, R.W. (1994). Anger as a risk factor for violence among the mentally disordered. In *Violence and Mental Disorder: Development in Risk Assessment* (Monahand, J. and Steadman, H., eds), University of Chicago Press, Chicago, IL.

O'Donovan, S. (1996). A validation approach to severely demented clients. *Nursing Standard*, **11**, 48–52.

Prigatano, G.P. (1986). Psychotherapy after brain injury. In *Neuropsychological Rehabilitation After Brain Injury* (Prigatano, G. P., ed.), pp. 67–97. John Hopkins University Press, Baltimore, MD.

Prigatano, G. P. and Fordyce, D. J. (1986). Cognitive dysfunction and psychological adjustment. In *Neuropsychological Rehabilitation After Brain Injury* (Prigatano, G. P., ed.), pp. 1–17. John Hopkins University Press, Baltimore, MD.

Radley, M., Redston, C., Bates, F., Pontegrad, M. and Lindsay, J. (1997). Effectiveness of group anxiety management with elderly clients of a community psychogeriatric team. *International Journal of Geriatric Psychiatry*, **12**, 79–84.

Rogers, C. R. (1957). The necessary and sufficient conditions of therapeutic personality change. *Journal of Consulting Psychology*, **21**, 95–103.

Roth, A. and Fonagy, P. (1996). *What Works for Whom? A Critically Review of Psychotherapy Research*. Guilford Press, New York, NY.

Safran, J. D. and Segal, Z. V. (1990). *Interpersonal Processing in Cognitive Therapy*. Basic Books, New York, NY.

Teasdale, J. D. (1996). Clinically relevant theory: integrating clinical insight with cognitive science. In *Frontiers of Cognitive Therapy* (Salkovskis, P. M., ed.), pp. 26–47. Guilford Press, New York, NY.

Teri, L. and Gallagher-Thompson, D. (1991). Cognitive-behavioural interventions for treatment of depression in Alzheimer's patients. *Gerontologist*, **31**, 413–16.

Teri, L. and Reiffer B. V. (1987). Depression and dementia. In *Handbook of Clinical Gerontology* (Carstensen, L. L. and Edelstein B. A, eds), pp.112–19. Pergamon Press, New York, NY.

Wahler, R. J. and Afton, A. D. (1980). Attentional processes in insular and noninsular mothers: some differences in the summary reports about child problem behaviours. *Child Behaviour Therapy*, **2**, 25–41.

Whitehouse, A. M. (1994). Application of cognitive therapy with supervisors of head injury. *Journal of Cognitive Psychotherapy*, **8**, 141–60.

Williams, J. M. G. (1996a). Memory processes in psychotherapy. In *Frontiers of Cognitive Therapy* (Salkovskis, P.M., ed.), pp. 97–113. Guilford Press, New York, NY.

Williams, J. M. G. (1996b). Depression and the specificity of autobiographical memory. In *Remembering our Past: Studies in Autobiographical Memory* (Rubin, D. C., ed.), pp. 244–70. Cambridge University Press, Cambridge.

Woods, R. and Roth, A. (1996). Effectiveness of psychological interventions with older people. In *What Works for Whom? A Critical Review of Psychotherapy Research* (Roth, A. and Fonagy, P., eds), pp. 321–40. Guilford Press, New York, NY.

Wragg, R. E. and Jeste D. V. (1989) Overview of depression and psychosis in Alzheimer's disease. *American Journal of Psychiatry*, **146**, 577–87.

Zillmann, D. (1983) Arousal and aggression. In *Aggression: Theoretical and Empirical Reviews* (Green, R. G. and Donnerstein, E. I., eds), Academic Press, New York, NY.

12 Training carers in behavioural management skills

One of Florence Nightingale's (1859) major tenets was that good nurses did not arise through experience or inborn traits but through explicit teaching. Nurses needed to have knowledge in order to perform the functions and skills expected of them. Modern nursing continues to accept this principle, but its application in geriatric nursing has been minimal.

Wells (1980, p.29)

Introduction

This chapter examines the effectiveness of training programmes designed to enhance the standard of caregivers' emotional and psychological support for people with dementia. It will review the relevant literature regarding training schemes and provide details of effective models of human learning. The factors influencing the implementation of these training programmes are discussed, together with a review of assessment procedures. The main part of this chapter addresses the training of paid carers (i.e. staff), rather than interventions aimed at families. The material focuses on training in the delivery of good standards of care, and does not review programmes designed to reduce carer stress or burnout, as these are addressed in Chapter 13.

Background literature on training

Staff training is universally seen as a key feature in implementing and maintaining a good standard of care in nursing and residential homes. Therefore, it is important to identify examples of appropriate models of training that combine theory and practice in an effective manner. Over the last 20 years there have been many attempts to develop comprehensive training packages for these settings (see Alzheimer Disease Society 1995, Chapman and Fraser 1998, Innes 2000) and some have been aimed specifically at behavioural management (Cohn *et al.* 1990, Cohen-Mansfield *et al.* 1997, Chartok *et al.* 1988, Shah and De 1998). In addition to these rather formal packages, the need for training has precipitated the development of a multitude of short courses, seminars and information leaflets aimed at carers. Unfortunately, some of these developments have been of variable quality and a number have even increased carers' levels of confusion. For example, it has not been uncommon for presenters to highlight inadequate care provision, but fail to provide staff with examples of alternative strategies. In such situations, the staff are left feeling deskilled.

Despite the wealth of descriptive literature on delivering training in care settings, there is limited empirical evidence regarding a positive and sustained impact of training (Moniz-Cook et al. 1998). This is a common finding across specialisms and branches of applied psychology (Baldwin and Ford 1988; Hesketh 1997). Much of the quality research on training in residential homes has been conducted in the field of learning disabilities (see Milne and James 2000). For example, the time series study of Methot et al. (1996) monitored the effect of trainers' behaviours on the care staff, and the effect of staff on residents. That study provides a detailed description of training interventions, demonstrating how newly trained staff could go on to disseminate their new skills to fellow staff within their homes; the study demonstrated a 'pyramidal' or 'tiered' model of supervision. The results revealed a reduction in challenging behaviours (e.g. self-injurious behaviour, screaming, aggression) and an increase in 'desired' behaviours.

In the field of dementia there is a general paucity of controlled trials of training interventions aimed at improving psychosocial care, two major studies having been conducted in the USA (Smyer et al. 1992, Rovner et al. 1996) and two in the UK (Moniz-Cook et al. 1998, Proctor et al. 1999). These four studies are summarized in Table 12.1.

Moniz-Cook et al. (1998) examined the effect of a training package, which drew on the work of Stokes (1990, 1996). All staff from three EMI (elderly mentally ill) homes, including domestic staff, were required to attend the teaching sessions. Five weekly sessions, each lasting 3 h, were organized and their effect was assessed 3 months after training and followed up after 1 year. The initial results revealed no change in the number of problems in the homes, but an improvement in the management abilities of the staff in the two intervention groups. The ability of staff to manage residents' behaviour significantly worsened in the control group. Despite these encouraging initial findings, the improvements were not maintained at follow up.

Proctor et al. (1999) examined the effect on residents of a staff training/education programme. Staff and residents were selected from 12 matched residential and nursing homes, which were randomly allocated to the control group or intervention group. The study was conducted over a period of 6 months. The care staff in the intervention group received weekly visits from a psychiatric nurse and help in developing care plans; they also attended weekly seminars on psychosocial management of behavioural problems. Residents' depression and cognitive status improved in the intervention groups. The authors suggested that the findings supported the notion that regular supervision combined with formal teaching (seven 1 h seminars) from a hospital outreach team was an economically viable way of improving the quality care delivered by care staff.

Table 12.1 Summary of the designs for the controlled studies

Authors	Population	Design and aims	Type of training	Measures	Outcome
Moniz-Cook et al. (1998)	Residents/clients: 84 EMI patients; Staff: 83, all in contact with residents	Quasi-experimental design across three homes, one acting as control. Assessments were made at 3 months and 1 year follow up. The study examined the effect of a training programme for managing behavioural problems	A five-session model, based on person-centred theory. Formal talk, small group work.and help in developing care plans. Sessions lasted 3 h	Cognitive assessment scale; Clifton; Problem behaviour index.	Experimental homes displayed significant improvement in management of problem behaviours. These effects were not maintained at 1 year follow-up.
Proctor et al. (1999)	Residents/clients: n = 120 (60 intervention, 60 control); Staff: not stated	RCT to determine whether seminars and weekly visits from a psychiatric nurse over 6 months improved the well-being of residents in terms of depression, cognitive impairment and behavioural problems.	Training in management of behavioural problems. Seven 1 h seminars. Weekly visits for 6 months from psychiatric nurse, helping in the development of care plans.	AGECAT[a], Crichton Royal Behaviour Rating Scale; Barthel Activity of Daily Living Index; use of mental health resources measure.	Significant improvement in depression and cognitive impairment, but not on Crichton behaviour rating or Barthel index.
Rovner et al. (1996)	Residents/clients: 89; Staff: not stated	CT to determine whether structured activity, along with medication, reduced behaviour disorders to a greater extent than usual nursing home care.	AGE programme of dementia care (activities, education and guidelines for psychotropic medication).	Behaviour measures (Psycho-geriatric dependency rating scale and Cohen-Mansfield Agitation Inventory); MMSE; Resource Utilization Groups II; patient activity level; patient care reimbursement/costs.	AGE programme reduced prevalence of behaviour disorders, use of drugs and restraints.
Smyer et al. (1992)	Residents/clients: not stated; Staff: 193 staff (151 interventions, 42 control)	Multiple-treatment, non-equivalent control group design to determine the effects of two interventions, individually or combined.	Two training interventions were used, one designed to increase staff skill levels, the other to develop more appropriate roles (job re-design)	Behaviour knowledge questionnaire (adapted version); Job diagnostic questionnaire; Caregiver rating scale.	Experimental condition reported significant improvement in knowledge but not performance.

[a]Automatic Geriatric Examination for Computer-assisted Taxonomy. RCT Randomised Controlled trial

Rovner *et al.* (1996) conducted a study in a 250 bed community nursing home. Patients were screened for the presence of behavioural disturbance and dementia. The control group received treatment as usual, with normal nursing home care, while the intervention group received the AGE programme (activities, guidelines for psychotropic medication and education). As the name suggests, this involves designing activity programmes for the residents, reviewing their medication (discontinuing it, if necessary) and educating the staff in weekly 1 h sessions. The study was conducted over a period of 6 months and comparisons were made with baseline. The results showed that the AGE programme reduced the prevalence of behavioural problems, use of medication and use of restraints.

Smyer *et al.* (1992) employed a multiple treatment, non-equivalent, control group design. There were four conditions: (i) a skills training group, which involved five classes aimed at improving behavioural strategies in dealing with difficult behaviours; (ii) motivational training, which used a group problem-solving approach to investigate how changes in job design would enhance confidence and motivation; (iii) a combination of the two previous approaches (this third group was thus expected to yield more significant and lasting effects than the other conditions); and (iv) a control group. Knowledge, motivation and behaviour were assessed immediately after the interventions, and at 3 and 6 month follow-up. The results revealed improvement in knowledge across the test conditions only, with moderate changes in motivation and minimal changes in behavioural skills enhancement.

An interesting, although less rigorous, study was reported by Kihlgren *et al.* (1994), who achieved positive results when they trained 10 staff in 'integrity promoting care' with 28 residents. This programme was based on Erikson's (1982) theory of human development, where the staff were taught to achieve the highest levels of maturity possible in their interactions with residents with dementia (i.e. promoting trust, initiative, industry and integrity). The researchers also used Erikson's theory to develop a novel way of examining the dynamics of the care relationship, assisting the staff in gaining insight into the experience of dementia. This study is valuable because it showed how video recordings could be used to help analyse the interactions between the staff and residents. It also provided a welcome example of how theory and practice could be combined in both delivering good training and measuring its outcomes. As Kihlgren *et al.* (1994, p.316) pointed out:

> It is important to use theoretical frames for nursing which stress the patients' experience, as there is a considerable risk that severely demented patients are treated like objects (Athlin *et al.* 1990). The fact that it is difficult to find means to observe improvements in care should not refrain [*sic*] us from using elaborate theories, but should stimulate us to try harder to find means to make proper assessments.

The importance of using theory-led models to inform the approach will be discussed in a later section of this chapter (also see James 1999a). The next section reviews the designs of the studies that have been outlined above.

Design of the teaching package

Effective teaching requires the establishment of appropriate goals that meet the needs of staff and residents. Moniz-Cook *et al.* (1998) and Smyer *et al.* (1992) provide useful examples of needs-assessment procedures. Moniz-Cook *et al.* surveyed 60 staff (managers, nurses and nursing assistants) in order to identify problem behaviours that could be targeted for change, which led to the development of a 21-item measure termed the Problem Behaviour Index. In the Smyer study, the job-redesign intervention required a detailed assessment of the staff's perception of their roles.

None of the four controlled studies assessed the needs of their populations sufficiently thoroughly. Indeed, it could be suggested that the rather moderate effects perhaps testify to this: the importance of a good needs-assessment procedure should never be underestimated (Goldstein 1993). Having outlined some reservations about the assessment procedures, it is timely to examine the contents of the four studies presented in Table 12.1.

Study 1 (Moniz-Cook *et al.* 1998)

The programme consisted of five educational sessions:

(1) *Psychosocial basis of challenging behaviour*. In this session the staff examined the historical, cultural and social features that might underpin a challenging behaviour.

(2) *Neuropsychological and biogenic causation*. The role of neuropsychological impairment (memory loss, executive difficulties and apraxia) was discussed in terms of the origins of the difficult behaviour.

(3) *Communication with the resident*. The staff were asked to discuss and reflect on how to promote positive interactions with the person with dementia.

(4) *Quality of life and the effects of the physical environment*. This session investigated the role of the environment on behaviour and examined issues to do with quality of life.

(5) *Development of person-centred care plans*. The design of 'person-centred' care plans was discussed with the aim of preventing and managing challenging behaviours.

A standardized protocol was used for each of the 3 h sessions. The sessions included a formal talk by a psychologist or psychiatrist, group work undertaken by a community psychiatric nurse, small-group feedback sessions and homework assignments.

Study 2 (Proctor *et al.* 1999)

This training programme involved a series of seven 1 h sessions complemented by a 6 month period of outreach service support. The initial sessions covered areas for improvement identified by the staff (management of dementia, aggression and screaming). Basic information about all psychiatric disorders in old age and thera-peutic approaches was also provided. Following the training, an experienced psychiatric nurse went to each residential/nursing home on a weekly basis to give support in the development of appropriate goals and care plans. The strategies developed involved constructing a detailed formulation for the problems of each person with dementia, which built on the person's strengths and abilities.

Study 3 (Rovner et al. 1996)

This work involved using the AGE training programme in conjunction with a series of weekly 1 h educational rounds conducted by a psychiatrist. The AGE programme functioned as an activity scheduler within the nursing home. A creative artist engaged the residents in craft, music, exercise, relaxation and reminiscence activities (see Zgola 1987). The educational rounds involved engaging the staff in discussions about the predisposing factors of challenging behaviours (medical, psychological, social and environmental).

Study 4 (Smyer et al. 1992)

This employed two interventions, 'skills' and 'job redesign', either separately or in combination. The skills intervention involved staff attending five 90 min classes at monthly intervals. The classes focused on behavioural management strategies for dealing with depression, agitation, disturbance and disorientation. Each class con-tained three elements: (i) behavioural management principles; (ii) putting the prin-ciples into practice; and (iii) discussion and role-play of management steps. The work was supported with written protocols, notebooks and homework assignments. The job-redesign intervention also had three steps: (i) assessment of staff members' perception of their role; (ii) development of more appropriate roles; and (iii) imple-mentation of the redesigned post. This work was supported by a team of adminis-trators who used their experience and knowledge of the literature to devise the most suitable type and range of roles for the staff. A series of three meetings was held over 3 months to facilitate the assessment and implementation phases. Frequent com-munication by telephone supported the first 2-3 weeks of the implementation phase.

The contents, or designs, of these four studies showed a number of basic similarities. For example, they all employed an educational component, all supported theory with practical management strategies and provided support with respect to care plans and administration.

Preparation before training

The previous section outlined the contents of a number of successful programmes. However, despite good design and excellent teachers, many training schemes fail to achieve their goals, because they do not create the organizational conditions necessary for effective change to occur. This problem is well illustrated through the 'myth of the hero innovator' (Georgiades and Phillimore 1975), summarized by Milne (1999, p.224):

> The myth is that through training or other means we can create veritable knights in shining armour who will bring about changes in organisations at a stroke. As the authors [Georgiades and Phillimore] noted, such a view is oversimplistic: the fact of the matter is that large organisations, such as hospitals, will, like dragons, eat hero innovators for breakfast.

Hence effective trainers need to have a well-organized plan before entering the training forum. Such a plan should entail comprehensive knowledge of the staff, management and setting, including details of the strengths and needs of the organizational framework. Similarly, Innes (2000) advises that it is essential to engage in much preparatory work before implementing a training programme. She suggests that a trainer should plan the initial stages carefully and methodically, ensuring that the aims and objectives of the training are clear and obtainable. She emphasizes the importance of establishing good links with the various stakeholders, which should include examining the agendas of both management and care staff. The trainer should also become conversant with the politics and culture of the home. As a second phase, Innes recommends that the trainer become more intimately acquainted with the working environment. This would involve talking to staff and residents, observing the staff at work, auditing the establishment, and, where appropriate, working two shifts within the setting. According to Innes, these steps allow the trainer to gain awareness of what change is realistic in the particular setting.

McDonald (1991) reviewed the perceived conditions necessary for the delivery of effective staff training; this questionnaire study sampled 300 staff. Five factors were found to be important in the generalization of training:

(1) support of the administration (facilitation of good communication between trainers, trainees and management, and appropriate support and supervision from within the organization);

(2) the perceived relevance and credibility of the training as assessed by agencies working in the field;

(3) work incentives;

(4) personal attributes of staff; and

(5) self-perceived competence of staff.

This study demonstrates that when trying to implement a training programme, it is vital to consider the interaction of staff and systems. It is also worth noting that management and organizational features were perceived to be the most important features in terms of success. Therefore it is suggested that a failure to recognize the influence of organizational features, and their interactive effects, is a flaw in the design of any training programme.

Having outlined the design of effective training regimes, and discussed organizational issues, we focus in the next section on teaching style, drawing on learning theory principles and the literature on change processes in psychotherapy.

Implementation: developing effective models of training

Training, like therapy, involves creating environments that help change people's perspectives and behaviours. Thus when developing effective models of training, one should ideally undertake a detailed analysis of human learning and change. Literature from educationalists and clinicians, who have investigated the factors involved in promoting effective change, provide a useful insight (Kolb 1984, Whisman 1993, Hayes *et al.* 1996). These insights are detailed below.

Teaching style: carer-centred change

A crucial element when developing an effective training programme is the teaching style. The following section suggests a model for change, emphasizing the role of the trainer with respect to the training experience of the staff. Traditional didactic teaching methods are generally concerned with giving instructions. Teaching in this framework is seen as the acquisition and transfer of knowledge and skills theory (Schlesinger 1996). However, as Knowles (1970) points out, an adult learners' experience should be a movement from being dependent to becoming more self-directed. A useful self-directed model was developed by Kolb (1984), who drew from previous work by Piaget (1926) and others. He suggested that human learning and change occur through an interactive cycle involving the learner 'reflecting on', 'experiencing', 'experimenting with' and 'conceptualizing' the new information. It is Kolb's contention that the learner needs to move between all four of these different modes for an optimal learning experience. In terms of developing a programme of training for staff, this model would suggest the need to:

- promote *reflection* on their current practices;
- understand the staff's *experience* of their role;
- help them to *experiment* with new forms of practice and behaviour; and
- help them *re-conceptualize* their roles and interactions with the residents.

Over the last 4 years, Kolb's model has been used as a framework for teaching competence in therapists (Milne *et al.* 1999). During this time it has undergone further revisions. The revised version, a 3-D conceptual cycle promoting change and learning, is summarized in Figure 12.1.

This 3-D model suggests it is crucial to address factors supporting people's belief systems (i.e. intellectual, affective, physiological and behavioural components) when promoting effective change and learning. When someone's belief system is stable, new information is less likely to be assimilated, unless it is congruent with the existing beliefs. Stability generally occurs when (i) new information is consistent with the way one thinks about, and behaves in relation to, a topic; (ii) one is confident that

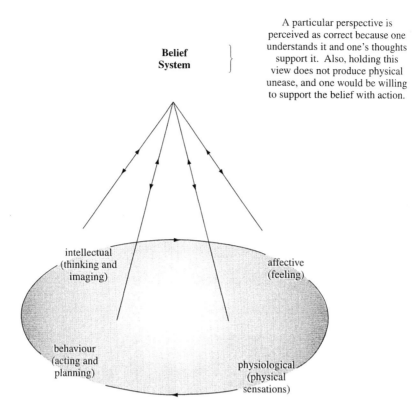

A particular perspective is perceived as correct because one understands it and one's thoughts support it. Also, holding this view does not produce physical unease, and one would be willing to support the belief with action.

Belief System

intellectual (thinking and imaging)

affective (feeling)

behaviour (acting and planning)

physiological (physical sensations)

Fig. 12.1   The 3–D change/learning cycle

one's views are correct; and (iii) one feels secure (i.e. neither anxious nor physiologically upset) by holding this perspective. Therefore, in order to create change, training must first produce instability within the existing conceptual model and then generate an alternative stable framework that incorporates the new learning.

In the past, training packages have mainly used change mechanisms based on didactic teaching methodologies. These have attempted to produce conceptual shifts via intellectual methods alone (i.e. mostly lectures). However, Kolb (1984) noted that in order to obtain any lasting shift in staff attitudes, it is necessary to achieve intellectual shift with behavioural tasks (such as role play), which help to reinforce the change in perspective. It is also important to provide material and scenarios that motivate the staff without making them feel overwhelmed (i.e. too stressed or deskilled). Thus, it is suggested that to ensure effective learning takes place, a trainer should lead learners round the 3-D cycle several times to achieve change in the belief system.

Table 12.2 examines the sorts of question a trainer might ask him/herself regarding his trainees when using the 3-D cycle. In the example presented in the table, the

Table 12.2 Typical issues and questions associated with using the 3-D cycle

Component of the change cycle	Aim of the trainer with respect to this component	To achieve this aim the trainer will need to ask himself
Issues to do with the belief system (conceptual issues)	To understand the staff's beliefs about their roles and their understanding of how to communicate best with someone with dementia.	Do staff believe it is useful to talk with the residents? Do they perceive that good-quality communication is important in enhancing people's lives? Have they got a template of what would be regarded as good practice?
Intellectual issues	To get the staff to reflect on what they are doing when they speak to a resident, and brainstorm how the interaction could be improved. Thus this feature involves using intellectual discussion, information and instructions to promote change.	Have staff received sufficient theory and education? Do they need any specific information about the person with dementia to help them to improve their communication skills (eg. impact of poor memory, perseveration, etc.)? Do staff reflect on the effect of their current practice? Have they thought through the problems and benefits of changing the way they interact with the residents? What pressures within their job (organizational, resources, cultural) will prevent effective change?
Affective issues	To help staff feel motivated to change from unhelpful ways of communicating with the residents to more appropriate ways. Help them to feel confident in their ability to make this change, and reduce any commensurate anxiety.	How can these be overcome (see Behaviour/planning)? How do they feel about altering their practices? Are they motivated to change? Are they confident in adopting a new approach? Will they get anxious?
Physiological issues	To reduce excessive physiological arousal, as this will disrupt the staff's learning and performance. It is important to try to achieve the optimum level of arousal (not too high or too low) for effective learning to take place.	How will staff cope with the nervous arousal that accompanies change? Will the physiological discomfort be an obstacle to change? Ensure that staff not too aggressive or forceful in their style of communicating.
Behaviour/planning issues	To help staff plan their actions before executing them; theory needs to be supported with action. Observations of the staff's planning abilities and performance is an important way to determine whether the new style of communicating can be carried out in practice.	What is the best way to implement the change? What are the specific steps? How can problems and obstacles best be dealt with? Can staff demonstrate how to use the new approach via role-play? How well do they perform?
Re-conceptualization of belief system	To help the staff to integrate all of the above information (theory, details from performance, experiences, etc.) in order to promote a more positive way of communicating with the residents	What feedback is required to improve their performance further? Has the experience of engaging in the new approach altered the staff's belief system? How can any positive changes be maintained?

trainer is attempting to introduce a revised model of communication, designed to improve the quality of the interaction between staff and residents.

The 3-D model provides a learner-centred framework, which ensures that an holistic learning experience occurs. It guarantees that the relevant theory can be demonstrated behaviourally, and it draws attention to the important experiential features of the learning process. However, like all effective learning programmes, the training must be delivered appropriately. Therefore the teaching should be presented in a structured, credible manner, being paced adequately for the needs of the trainees. Likewise, the trainer should display the relevant interpersonal skills, work collaboratively with the carers and provide appropriate levels of feedback. Smyer *et al.* (1992) provided a good example of how theory can be consolidated by behavioural strategies and role play.

In addition to the importance of an effective teaching style, the features both predicting and leading to change (i.e. moderators and mediators) need to be addressed.

Moderators and mediators

Another important way to plan effective training is to distinguish between moderators and mediators. A 'moderator' variable is one that predicts both the direction and the degree of change (e.g. characteristics of the resident and trainee, such as gender, intellect or profession). A 'mediator' variable is the mechanism through which change takes place (e.g. increased knowledge; improvement in coping style; skills enhancement). Thus mediators are generally the features that are altered via the intervention or training. Table 12.3 describes some of the relevant features influencing effective change. In the following section, some of the mediators and moderators outlined in Table 12.3 will be discussed in more detail, to see how they might effect the training experience.

Moderators

Professions and qualifications
In residential care settings, a major distinction is made between qualified and unqualified staff (Workman 1996, Chang and Lam 1998). Unqualified staff are mainly engaged in the more 'basic' care tasks (e.g. hygiene, nutrition, toileting and mobility), while qualified staff are engaged in professional duties. The majority of the unqualified staff are care assistants, whom Jaques and Innes (1998) describe as

Table 12.3 Moderators and mediators of training programmes

Moderators	*trainer & trainee(s)*: profession, experience, gender, age, qualifications, intelligence, motivation, personality, previous training, psychological health *other features*: staffing levels, environment, training method
Mediators	staff's knowledge base, skill base, attitude, coping style, attributional style, confidence

an undervalued and neglected population (see also Hockey 1990, Lee-Treweek 1997). It is suggested that care assistants are often in a paradoxical situation, whereby they wield an enormous amount of practical power, but have little formal authority and status (Jacques and Innes 1998). It has been suggested that although this situation is fraught with problems, it is inevitable as necessary resources need to be freed up to allow the qualified nursing staff to undertake 'professional level' care activities (Chang and Lam 1998).

Thus, qualifications form the basis for numerous distinctions in nursing homes, including role demarcations, decision-making powers, wages and respect (both self and societal, Hepburn 1998). These distinctions can sometimes produce unhealthy tensions during the delivery of a training programme. Thus, while some studies (e.g. Moniz-Cook *et al.* 1998) have encouraged all staff to undertake training together, others have suggested running different programmes for each population. Indeed, in a recent trial in Newcastle (James 1999b), it was decided to run two separate programmes for trained and untrained staff. Whether this arrangement turns out to be appropriate remains to be seen. Whichever programme is designed, it is imperative that the trainers have an understanding of the different staffing groups' unique experience of caring. Jacques and Innes (1998, p.36), speaking up for care assistants, point out:

> Until we have an understanding and hear many more accounts of what it is like to be a care assistant—the difficulties and frustrations as well as the motivations and satisfactions—it is going to be difficult to 'tap into' their world and find psychosocial interventions with which care assistants will be happy to work.

Gender

The issue of gender is often neglected within training programmes, but numerous studies inform us that the gender of the person with dementia influences the nature of the interaction with the staff. For example, Lindsay and Skea (1996) found that both male and female carers tended to initiate more actions with male residents. Evers (1981) found that female patients were more likely to be subjected to various forms of oppression and to be labelled as 'difficult'. It has been suggested that these biases can be attributed to cultural stereotypes of women and men; women being seen as 'providers of care' while men are 'to be cared for'. Having been made aware of these tendencies, it is important that these issues are debated within the training forum. This insight should be supported with role play and simulations in the training sessions.

Health status

Chapter 13 highlights the high incidence of affective problems in staff. People with such affective problems are likely to have reduced learning capacity and poor motivation to change. It is essential to take account of these cognitive and emotional features during training. Stress caused by a demanding job can lead to impoverished problem-solving (Reason 1984, Williams 1996). Hence, stressed carers might appear to be locked in inflexible routines and even display some cognitive problems (e.g.

rigidity of thinking, poor problem-solving), which will need to be considered when planning a teaching session.

In order to deal with these issues, one should first examine the major stressors in the carers' environment and reduce them where feasible. Another strategy is to consider whether the role of staff members within the home could be redesigned to reduce their burden (Hackman and Oldham 1975). Examples of this are combining tasks into meaningful sequences, forming cohesive work units and improving communication (Smyer *et al.* 1992).

Staffing levels

A common problem when organizing training programmes is insufficient staffing. Smyer *et al.* (1992) attempted to overcome some of the problems of staff attendance by presenting identical workshops over 2 days. To support the changes further, during the implementation phase of their interventions, the administrators kept in close contact with the staff by telephone. The manner in which the training is organized and presented is a key issue. For example, if the training is presented as an opportunity to learn new skills, collaborating with a team of facilitators to improve job satisfaction, this may be received with enthusiasm and motivation. However, if the staff are given no choice and are required to undertake a compulsory programme in their own time, it might not be received so well. Another problem is the lack of staffing resources available to allow effective implementation of the new training techniques. Thus while in many homes a significant percentage of staff may never have attended training sessions, even those that did may not have the time to implement what they have learnt.

It is interesting to note, however, that Sixsmith *et al.* (1993) failed to find an association between staffing levels and evidence of 'positive care' in EMI nursing homes. They investigated the quality of care in three highly resourced homes and compared them with three control homes. The three experimental homes were specifically set up following an initiative by the Department of Health in the UK to explore new ways of caring for EMI people. All homes were designed to provide homely living environments, individualized patterns of care and a high quality of life. The interpretation of the results, although somewhat controversial, suggested that employing more staff with generic roles did not lead to higher levels of psychosocial care, rather it led to 'an even cleaner, tidier and fresher-smelling home'. (Sixsmith *et al.* 1993, p.411). Hence, they advised that in order to improve the level of care and well-being in homes, one needs 'to employ staff with this specific function, and no other' (p.411).

Setting and environment

Moniz-Cook *et al.* (1997) noted that homes differ widely in terms of their *milieu*, while Moos (1981) suggested that each home has its own unique 'personality'. In order to intervene successfully in a home, one must understand its unique character and work with its strengths. It is also important to assess homes more than once, as their character is dynamic and will change over time.

Mediators

Mediators are the mechanisms through which change takes place. Whisman (1993) suggested that change can be implemented competently when the trainer applies appropriate knowledge both skilfully and in an interpersonally effective manner. Some of these features are outlined below.

Knowledge enhancement

As outlined above, knowledge and insight are crucial aspects of the educational process. Indeed, all the above designs included an educational component. However, it is important to note that the work must be pitched at the right level.

Improvement of skills

Proctor *et al.* (1999) suggested that their training programme had greatly improved the staff's assessment and care planning abilities. The staff were specifically trained to select the most relevant, achievable and appropriate goals to bring about effective change (Barrowclough and Flemming 1986a,b). Smyer *et al.* (1992) also placed great emphasis on the teaching of practical skills. Their staff were supervised closely, engaging in role play and receiving guidance from written protocols with respect to their behavioural management strategies.

Interpersonal effectiveness

A by-product of the increased awareness achieved by improved knowledge is greater insight into the experience of having dementia (Kitwood 1997). Kitwood suggests that such awareness helps to improve the quality of the staff-resident interaction. There are numerous components to this interaction, some verbal (e.g. speech content, tone, intonation) and some non-verbal (e.g. body posture, facial expression). Bohling (1991), for example, claimed that good listening skills helped to prevent anxiety building up in people with dementia. Numerous other studies have placed equal emphasis on improving communication and interactional skills. Indeed, it is often believed that effective communication is an essential way of improving the well-being of people with dementia and raising their threshold of distress (Helen 1998).

The latter sections of this chapter have addressed design and teaching style; while these guidelines are likely to promote effective training, it is essential to evaluate the effect of the interventions appropriately. The issues associated with assessment and evaluation are discussed below.

Assessment and measures

Evaluation is an essential element of the training package because it helps one to determine objectively the effects of the teaching intervention on staff and residents. It can also help to determine the long-term impact of an intervention, and the reasons why a package might not have fulfilled its goals. The setting of achievable goals is important in devising a good assessment method. Ideally, these goals should be clear, specific, relevant, measurable and realistic. Having defined the goals, it is important to select appropriate ways of assessing the extent to which an intervention has achieved these goals. Indeed, poor results are often not due to ineffective interventions, but rather to the use of inappropriate (e.g. off-the-shelf) measures, which do not assess the aims of the training.

Choosing the most appropriate measures

Table 12.4 outlines some considerations that are important when deciding which measures to use. An example of goal setting is to clarify initially which behaviours one needs to change in order to produce the desired effect. For example, if one wants to improve the level of well-being of the residents via staff education, it makes sense to use measures for both the residents and staff. Indeed, one would want to know whether any change in the residents (or lack of change) can be attributed to the factors associated with changes in the staff.

It is also relevant to examine the nature of the effect on the target populations. For example, one might find that the training increased staff's level of motivation and knowledge, but failed to influence their actions.

Different measures provide different forms of insight into the nature of change; for example, process measures (which assess the mechanism of change) are good for examining mediating factors. By establishing a working hypothesis of the likely mechanisms of change, one can use the most appropriate measure to examine this feature. For example, one might hypothesize that residents' mood would improve as a result of better staff-resident interaction; to test such a hypothesis one would have to measure each of these features, i.e. mood and interaction. This particular hypothesis would also predict that there would be a lag, with improvement in interaction occurring before the shift in mood. It would be easy to measure this lag, and demonstrating that it occurred would greatly enhance the credibility of the interpretation of outcomes.

In order to examine these process features, one would need to use a continuous monitoring procedure or a time sampling technique. Time-sampling methods are often preferred because one can observe both staff and resident behaviour over a short period of time using moderate resources. Data collected using time sampling

Table 12.4 Relevant questions determining selection of measures

	For example:
What are the target groups to be assessed?	trainees; residents; management
What features are to be targeted for change?	attitude and motivation; knowledge; behaviour
How does the effect of the intervention generalize?	between people or places; across time or behaviours
What is the proposed mechanism of change (i.e. working hypothesis)?	
What are the proposed mediators of change (e.g. increase in knowledge base or staff attitude)	
What are the criteria for recognizing change?	statistically significant change (quantitative/ qualitative); clinically significant change
What is the most appropriate sampling procedure?	before vs after; continuous; time-sampling

have been shown to be representative (Alevizos *et al.* 1978, Saudargas and Zanolli 1990) and this method has been widely used within elderly residential settings (Moos *et al.* 1984, Burgio and Burgio 1990).

One should also pay attention to the generalization effect of a study. It is worth assessing whether the effect of the training can be observed at some time in the future, across different settings, or even within the attitudes and behaviours of the workmates of those who were trained. Without such generalization it is arguable that training is pointless.

The final issue to be discussed when deciding the suitability of an instrument is the use of an appropriate criterion for judging change. Statistical techniques are often used to assess pre and post aspects of change, or to discover structural patterns within a data profile. However, many researchers suggest using clinical significance (see Jacobson *et al.* 1986). In testing clinical significance, widely accepted norms and cut-off points are used to assessing levels of 'relevant' change. Thus, one can determine how many people move from a 'clinically abnormal' range to a 'clinically normal' range, which might be a more appropriate measure of success. After all, with statistically significant change one never knows whether patients have moved into a range that most clinicians would deem 'functional'. In terms of residents, clinical change might be a movement from a state of ill-being to one of well-being. In terms of staff, this would suggest a movement from a state of incompetence to competence.

Having outlined some of the relevant questions that need to be asked when developing measures, let us examine some of the instruments routinely used.

Common measures used

The following list has drawn heavily from the recent reviews by Woods (1999) and Burns *et al.* (1999) in this area.

Measures of resident functioning

Scales for screening for level of cognitive impairment
- *Clinical Dementia Rating Scale* (CDR, Hughes *et al.* 1982)—clinician rated scale, taking into account memory, orientation, daily functioning and other features;
- *Mini-mental* state examination (MMSE, Folstein *et al.* 1975)—assesses orientation to time and place, mental calculation, immediate and delayed recall, praxis, expression and mental control;
- *CAMCOG* (Roth *et al.* 1988)—the cognitive section of CAMDEX, indicating cognitive strengths and weaknesses;
- other tools: Middlesex Elderly Assessment of Mental State (Golding 1989), Geriatric Mental State (GMS; Copeland *et al.* 1976) and a host of other screening tests, which are reviewed by Burns *et al.* (1999).

Scales for assessing mood
- *Cornell Scale for Depression in Dementia* (Alexopoulos *et al.* 1988)—a 19-item observer-rated scale for depression in dementia, using semi-structured interviews with resident and carer;
- *Dementia Mood Assessment Scale* (Sunderland *et al.* 1988)—a 17-item scale rated on the basis of an observation and a semi-structured interview with the resident;
- *Geriatric Depression Scale* (Brink *et al.* 1982, Ott and Fogel 1992)—a self-report measure, suitable for mild dementia (30- and 15-item versions);
- *AGECAT* (Dewey *et al.* 1992—assesses the effect of resident's organic-based and depression symptoms in terms of a symptom profile using a five-point scale.

Scales for assessing behavioural abilities and self-care skills
- *Crichton Royal Behavioural Rating Scale* (CRBRS; Robinson, 1961)—assesses behavioural characteristics in terms of physical disability, communication difficulties, apathy and social disturbance and is particularly useful as a screening tool;
- *Clifton Assessment Procedures for the Elderly* (CAPE; Pattie and Gilleard 1979);
- *Barthel Activity of Daily Living Index* (Mahoney and Barthel 1965)—assesses the level of physical disability (where 0 means dependent and 20 independent, but not necessarily normal);
- other tools include Behavioural Assessment Scale of Later Life (BASOLL; Brooker 1998), Index of Activities of Daily Living (ADL; Katz *et al.* 1963), Physical Self-Maintenance Scale (PSMS; Lawton and Brody 1969), Functional Activities Questionnaire (Pfeffer *et al.* 1982), Instrumental Activities of Daily Living Scale (Lawton and Brody 1969) and Functional Dementia Scale (Moore *et al.* 1983)

Scales for assessing presence of challenging behaviour
- Rating of Aggressive Behaviour in the Elderly (RAGE; Patel and Hope 1992);
- *Caretaker Obstreperous Behaviour Rating Assessment* (COBRA, Drachman *et al.* 1992)—a 30-item scale for the assessment of difficult and troublesome behaviours in dementia;
- *Cohen-Mansfield Agitation Inventory* (CMAI; Cohen-Mansfield 1986)—this inventory is based on carer information and looks at the frequency of agitated behaviour in people with cognitive impairment;
- *Present Behavioural Examination* (Hope and Fairburn 1992)—a well-defined and very detailed tool for assessing behavioural disturbance;
- *Agitation Scale* (Whall 1999)—a scale used by nursing aides to identify the onset and rate of agitation;
- other tools include the Behavioural and Mood Disturbance Scale (Greene *et al.* 1982) and the Problem Check-list (Gilleard 1984), two user-friendly tests that can be used by relatives.

Scales for assessing needs and resources
- *Revised Memory and Behavior Problems Checklist* (Teri *et al.* 1992)—a 24-item caregiver checklist, which assesses behavioural problems in people with dementia;
- *Caregiver Activity Survey* (CAS; Davis *et al.* 1997)—measures caregivers' time spent caring; it is a tool for assessing the economic impact of dementia;
- other tools include the Camberwell Assessment of Need (Slade *et al.* 1996) and Care Needs Assessment Pack for Dementia (Carenap-D; McWalter *et al.* 1998)

Ecologically valid scales of performance in everyday life
- *Patient Behaviour Observation Instrument* (Bowie and Mountain 1993);
- *Quality of Interactions Schedule* (QUIS; Dean *et al.* 1993);
- *Dementia Care Mapping* (DCM; Kitwood and Bredin 1992);
- *Positive Response Schedule for Severe Dementia* (PRS; Perrin 1997);
- *Psychogeriatric Dependency Rating Scale* (PGDRS; Wilkinson and Graham-White 1980)—assesses dependency attributable to behaviour disorders, disorientation and functional impairment;
- *Neuropsychiatric Inventory* (NPI; Cummings *et al.* 1994)—examines 12 features, ranging from delusions, agitation and anxiety to sleep and appetite.

Staff and interaction measures

Scales for assessing levels of mood and stress in caregivers
- *Behavioural and Instrumental Stressors in Dementia* (BISID; Keady and Nolan 1996)—assesses caregiving burden in terms of behavioural aspects, ADL and continence;
- *Caregiver Strain Index* (Robinson 1983)—a 13-item observer-rated scale, which is useful for assessing strain resulting from the physical effects of caring;
- *Care-giving Burden Scale* (Gerristen and van der Ende 1994)—a 13-item scale examining the personal consequences of caring on the relationships between the carer and recipient;
- *Caregiver Burden Inventory* (Novak and Guest 1989)—a multi-dimensional scale measuring burden on five different subscales (physical, time-dependence, social, emotional and developmental);
- *General Health Questionnaire* (Goldberg 1978, Goldberg and Hillier 1979)—a self-administered questionnaire examining diagnosable psychiatric disorder (not specifically developed for carer population);
- *Beck Depression Inventory* (Beck *et al.* 1963)—a 21-item self-report scale aimed at assessing severity of depression.

Scale for assessing caregiver knowledge
- *Dementia Knowledge Questionnaire* (Graham *et al.* 1997).

Scales for assessing caregiver management skills
- *Dementia Care Mapping* (DCM; Kitwood and Bredin 1992)—a time-sampling measure which assesses levels of well-being in people with dementia during their normal activities of daily living, and also assesses the quality of interactions with staff;
- *Quality of Interactions Schedule* (Dean *et al.* 1993)—an observer measure of interactions between residents and care staff, coding interactions in terms of positive social, positive care, neutral, negative protective and negative restrictive;
- *Multi-phasic Environmental Assessment Procedure* (MEAP; Moos and Lemke 1980).

Conclusion

There is a large literature on the subject of staff training, but there are only a few quality studies in the area of dementia care. In the present chapter, four controlled trials have been examined, which, despite positive results, showed that the impact of training is variable and often short lived. Many local training and education packages currently being delivered into homes may be ineffective because the designs are inappropriate or because they are delivered inadequately. In addition, training often fails to take account of the structure and dynamics of the trainee populations. Innes (2000, p.14) refers to this issue in terms of 'student-centred' learning:

> Thus, just as in recent years there has been a move towards person-centred care for people with dementia, there is now a growing recognition that for person-centred care to be achieved the personhood of staff also needs to be recognised. If staff are to partici-pate in training that facilitates the move towards delivering person-centred care it follows that the training must be similarly person-centred; this is known in the education world as student-centred learning.

To overcome ineffective training, interventions should be aimed at the levels of the individual and the organization (Corrigan and McCracken 1997). Such an approach favours a holistic perspective, encouraging the development of strategies that simul-taneously address changes directed at both the staff (attitudes, skills and know-ledge), and the organizational and management structures. This chapter has outlined the importance of selecting appropriate measures: measures must be specific and relevant, and must address the goals of the training. These issues were illustrated above through a number of questions aimed at helping the reader to make a judge-ment about the suitability of the various assessment tools routinely used within this area.

In preparing this chapter, it became evident that good work is being done in the field of training, but that it is dispersed between many different areas and dis-ciplines. For example, this chapter has examined models from learning disability, education, psychotherapy and organizational psychology. It is therefore evident that one needs to cast one's net widely when planning to work in this field. While the rewards can be great, one needs to invest a lot of time, resources and energy to achieve an effective training package.

Acknowledgements

Thank you to Derek Milne and F. Katharina Reichelt for their intellectual contributions to this work, and to Tricia Roe for her help in preparing the chapter.

REFERENCES

Alevizos, P., DeRisi, W., Liberman, R. Eckman, T. and Callahan, E. (1978). The behaviour observation instrument: a method of direct observation for program evaluation. *Journal of Applied Behaviour Analysis*, **11**, 243–57.

Alexopoulos, G. S., Abrams, R. C., Young, R. C. and Shamoian, C. A. (1988). Cornell scale for depression in dementia. *Biological Psychiatry*, **23**, 271–84.

Alzheimer's Disease Society (1995). *Care to Make a Difference*. Alzheimer's Disease Society, Gordon House, 10 Greencoat Place, London, SW1P 1PH.

Athlin, E., Norberg, A. and Asplund, K. (1990). Caregiver's perceptions and interpretations of severely demented patients during feeding in a task assignment system. *Scandinavian Journal of Caring Sciences*, **4**, 147–55.

Baldwin, T. T. and Ford, J. K. (1988). Transfer of training: a review of directions for future research. *Personnel Psychology*, **41**, 63–105.

Barrowclough, C. and Fleming, I. (1986a). *Goal Planning with Elderly People: Making Plans to Meet Individual Needs: A Manual of Instruction*. Manchester University Press, Manchester.

Barrowclough, C. and Fleming, I. (1986b). Training and direct care staff in goal planning with elderly people. *Behaviour of Psychotherapy*, **14**, 192–209.

Beck, A. T., Ward, C. H., Mendelson, K., Mock, J. E. and Erbaugh, J. K. (1963). An inventory for measuring depression. *Archives of General Psychiatry*, **4**, 561–71.

Bird, M., Alexopoulus, P. and Adamowicz, J. (1995). Success and failure in five studies: use of cued recall to ameliorate behaviour problems in senile dementia. *International Journal of Geriatric Psychiatry*, **10**, 305–11.

Bohling, H. R. (1991). Communication with Alzheimer's patients: an analysis of caregiver listening patterns. *International Journal of Ageing and Human Development*, **33**, 249–67.

Bowie, P. and Mountain, G. (1993). Using direct observation to record the behaviour of long-stay patients with dementia. *International Journal of Geriatric Psychiatry*, **8**, 857–64.

Brink, T. L., Yesavage, J. A., Lum, O., Heersema, P., Adey, K. *et al.* (1982). Screening tests for geriatric depression. *Clinical Gerontologist*, **2**, 60–61.

Brooker. D. (1998). *BASOLL—Behavioural Assessment Scale of Later Life*. Winslow, Bicester

Burgio, L. D. and Burgio, K. L. (1990). Institutional staff training and management: a review of the literature and a model for geriatric, long-term care facilities. *International Journal of Aging and Human Development*, **30**, 287–302.

Burns, A., Lawlor, B. and Craig, S. (1999). *Assessment Scales in Old Age Psychiatry*. Dunitz, London

Chang, A. N. and Lam, L. (1998). Can health care assistants replace student nurses? *Journal of Advanced Nursing*, **27**, 399–405.

Chapman, A. and Fraser, M. (1998). *Dementia: a Self Study Pack*. Dementia Services Development Centre, University of Stirling, Stirling.

Chartock, P., Nevins, A., Rzetelny, H. and Gilberto, P. (1988). A mental health training programme in nursing homes. *Gerontologist*, **28**, 503–7.

Cohen-Mansfield, J. (1986) Agitated behaviours in the elderly. II. Preliminary results in the cognitively deteriorated. *Journal of the American Geriatrics Society*, **34**, 722–7.

Cohen-Mansfield, J., Werner, P., Culpepper, W. J. and Barkley, D. (1997). Evaluation of an in-service training programme on dementia and wandering. *Journal of Gerontological Nursing*, **23**, 40–47.

Cohn, M. D., Horgas, A. L. and Marsiske, M. (1990). Evaluation of a behaviour management training programme for nursing home caregivers. *Journal of Gerontological Nursing*, **16**, 21–5.

Copeland, J. R. M., Kelleher, M. J., Kellett, J. M. *et al.* (1976). A semi-structured clinical interview for the assessment of diagnosis and mental state in the elderly. The geriatric mental state schedule. I: Development. *Psychological Medicine*, **6**, 439–49.

Corrigan, P. W. and McCracken, S. J. (1997). *Interactive Staff-training*. Plenum Press, New York, NY.

Cummings, J. L., Mega, M., Gray, K., Rosenberg-Thompson, S., Carusi, D. A. and Gornbein, J. (1994). The Neuropsychiatric Inventory: comprehensive assessment of psychopathology in dementia. *Neurology*, **44**, 2308–14.

Davis, K., Mann, D. B., Kane, R., Patrick, D., Peskind, E. R., Raskind, M. A. and Puder, K. L. (1997). The Caregiver Activity Survey (CAS): development and validation of new measure for caregivers of persons with Alzheimer's disease. *International Journal of Geriatric Psychiatry*, **12**, 978–88.

Dean, R., Proudfoot, R. and Lindesay, J. (1993). The Quality of Interactions Schedule (QUIS): development, reliability, and use in the evaluation of two domus units. *International Journal of Geriatric Psychiatry*, **8**, 819–26.

Dewey, M. E., Copeland, J. R. M., Lobo, A., Saz, P. and Dia, J. L. (1992). Computerised diagnosis from a standardised history schedule: a preliminary communication about the organic section of the HAS-AGECAT system. *International Journal of Geriatric Psychiatry*, **7**, 443–6.

Drachman, D. A., Swearer, J. M., O'Donnell, B. F., Mitchell, A. L. and Maloon, A. (1992). The Caretaker Obstreperous-Behavior Rating Assessment (COBRA) Scale. *Journal of the American Geriatrics Society*, **40**, 463–70.

Erikson, E. H. (1982). *The Life Completed*. W.W. Norton, New York, NY.

Evers, H. (1981). Care of custody? experience of women patients in long stay geriatric wards. In *Controlling Women* (Hutter, B. and Williams, G., eds), Croom Helm, London.

Folstein, M. F., Folstein, S. E. and McHugh, P. R. (1975). "Mini-Mental State": a practical method for grading the cognitive state of patients for the clinician. *Journal of Psychiatric Research*, **12**, 189–98.

Georgiades, N. J. and Phillimore, L. (1975). The myth of the hero-innovator and alternative strategies for organisational change. In *Behaviour Modification with the Severely Retarded* (Kierman, C. C. and Woodford, F. P., eds), Associated Scientific Publishers, London.

Gerritsen, J. D. and van der Ende, P.C. (1994). The development of a care-giving burden scale. *Age and Ageing*, **23**, 483–91.

Gilleard, C. J. (1984). *Living with Dementia*. Croom Helm, Beckenham.

Goldberg, D. (1978). *Manual of the General Health Questionnaire*. NFER-Nelson, Windsor.

Goldberg, D. P. and Hillier, V. F. (1979). A scaled version of the General Health Questionnaire. *Psychological Medicine*, **9**, 139–45.

Golding, E. (1989). *Middlesex Elderly Assessment of Mental State.* Thames Valley Test Company, Titchfield.

Goldstein, I. L. (1993). *Training in Organizations: Needs Assessment, Development and Evaluations.* Brooks/Cole, Pacific Grove, CA.

Graham, C., Ballard, C. and Sham, P. (1997). Carers' knowledge of dementia, their coping strategies and morbidity. *International Journal of Geriatric Psychiatry*, **12**, 931–6.

Greene, J. G., Smith, R., Gardiner, M. and Timbury, G. C. (1982). Measuring behavioural disturbance of elderly demented patients in the community and its effect on relatives: a factor analytic study. *Age and Ageing*, **11**, 121–6.

Hackman, J. R. and Oldman, G. R. (1975) Development of the job diagnostic survey. *Journal of Applied Psychology*, **60**, 159–70.

Hayes, A., Goldfried, M. and Castonguay, M. (1996). The study of change in psychotherapy: a re-examination of the process outcome correlation paradigm. Comment on Stiles and Shapiro 1994. *Journal of Consulting Clinical Psychology*, **64**, 909–14.

Helen, C. R. (1998). Communication: understanding and being understood. In *Alzheimer's Disease: Activity-focused Care* (Helen, C. R., ed.), pp. 67–86. Butterworth-Heinemann, Woburn.

Hepburn, A. (1998). Worth a lot more than stifled titters. *Journal of Dementia Care*, **6**, 8.

Hesketh, B. (1997). Dilemmas in training for transfer and retention. *Applied Psychology: an International Review*, **46**, 317–86.

Hockey, J. (1990). *Experiences of Death.* Edinburgh University Press, Edinburgh.

Hope, R. A. and Fairburn, C. G. (1992). The present behavioural examination (PBE): the development of an interview to measure current behavioural abnormalities. *Psychological Medicine*, **22**, 223–30.

Hughes, C. P., Berg, L., Danziger, W. L., Coben, L. A. and Martin, R. L. (1982). A new clinical-scale for the staging of dementia. *British Journal of Psychiatry*, **140**, 566–72.

Innes, A. (2000) *Training and Development for Dementia Care Workers.* Jessica Kingsley, London.

Jacobson, N. S., Follette, W. C. and Revenstorf, D. (1986). Toward a standard definition of clinically significant change. *Behaviour Therapy*, **17**, 308–11.

James, I. A. (1999a) A cognitive conceptualisation of distress in people with dementia. *Clinical Psychology Forum*, **134**, 21–5.

James, I. A. (1999b) Training carers in nursing homes. Workshop presented at UK Dementia Forum, Newcastle upon Tyne.

Jaques, I. and Innes, A. (1998). Who cares about care assistant work? *Journal of Dementia Care*, **6**, 33–7.

Katz, S., Ford, A. B., Moskowitz, R. W., Jackson, R. A. and Jaffe, M. W. (1963). Studies of illness in the aged: the index of ADL. *Journal of the American Medical Association*, **185**, 914–19.

Keady, J. and Nolan, M. (1996). Behavioural and Instrumental Stressors in Dementia (BISID): refocusing the assessment of caregiver need in dementia. *Journal of Psychiatric and Mental Health Nursing*, **3**, 163–72.

Kihlgren, M., Hallgren, A., Norberg, A. and Karlsson, I. (1994). Integrity promoting care of demented patients: pattern of interaction during morning care. *Journal of Ageing and Human Development.* **39**, 303–19.

Kitwood, T. (1997). *Dementia Reconsidered.* Open University Press, Buckingham.

Kitwood, T. and Bredin, K. (1992). A new approach to the evaluation of dementia care. *Journal of Advances in Health and Nursing Care*, **1**, 41–60.

Knowles, M. (1970). *The Modern Practice of Adult Education*. Association Press, New York, NY.

Kolb, D. A. (1984). *Experiential Learning: Experience as the Source of Learning and Development*. Prentice-Hall, Englewood Cliffs, NJ.

Lawton, M. P. and Brody, E. (1969). Assessment of older people: self-maintaining and instrumental activities of daily living. *Gerontologist*, **9**, 179–86.

Lee-Treweek, G. (1997). Emotion work, order and emotional power in care assistant work. In *The Sociology of Health and the Emotions* (James, N., ed.), Blackwell, Oxford.

Lindsay, J. and Skea, D. (1997). Gender and interactions between care staff and elderly nursing home residents with dementia. *International Journal of Geriatric Psychiatry*, **12**, 344–8.

Mahoney, F. I. and Barthel, D. W. (1965). Functional assessment in dementia: the Barthel index. *Maryland Medical Journal*, **14**, 61–5.

McDonald, R. M. (1991). Assessment of organisational context: a missing component in evaluations of training programmes. *Evaluation and Programme Planning*, **14**, 273–9.

McWalter, G., Toner, H., McWalter, A., Eastwood, J., Marshall, M. and Turvey, T. (1998). A community needs assessment: the care needs assessment pack for dementia (Carenap-D)—its development, reliability and validity. *International Journal of Geriatric Psychiatry*, **13**, 16–22.

Methot, L. L., Williams, L., Cummings, A. and Bradshaw, B. (1996). Measuring the effects of a manager—supervisor training programme through the generalised performance of managers, supervisors, front-line staff and clients in a human service setting. *Journal of Organisational Behavioural Management*, **16**, 3–34.

Milne, D. (1999). *Social Therapy*. John Wiley and Sons, Chichester.

Milne, D. and James, I. (2000). A systematic review of effective cognitive-behavioural supervision. *British Journal of Clinical Psychology* **39**, 111–27.

Milne, D., Baker, C., Blackburn, I. M., James, I. and Reichelt, K. (1999). Effectiveness of cognitive therapy training. *Journal of Behavior Therapy and Experimental Psychiatry*, **30**, 81–92.

Monaghan, D. J. (1991). Staff perceptions of behavioural problems in nursing home residents with dementia: the role of nursing. *Education Gerontology* **19**, 683–94.

Moniz-Cook, E., Millington, D. and Silver, M. (1997). Residential care for older people: job satisfaction and psychological health in care staff. *Health Society Care Community*, **5**, 124–33.

Moniz-Cook, E., Agar, S., Silver, M., Woods, R., Wang, M., Elston, C. and Win, T. (1998) Can staff training reduce carer stress and behavioural disturbance in the elderly mentally ill? *International Journal of Geriatric Psychiatry*, **13**, 149–58.

Moore, J. T., Bobula, J. A., Short, T. B. and Mischel, M. (1983). A functional dementia scale. *Journal of Family Practice*, **16**, 499–503.

Moos, R. H. (1981). *Work Environment Scale Manual*. Consulting Psychologists Press, Palo Alto, CA.

Moos, R. and Lemke, S. (1980). Assessing the physical and architectural features of sheltered care settings. *Journal of Gerontology*, **35**, 571–83.

Moos, R. H., David, T., Lemke, S. and Postle, E. (1984). Coping with intra-institutional relocation: change in resident and staff behaviour patterns. *Gerontologist*, **24**, 495–502.

Nightingale, F. (1859). *Notes on Nursing*. London, Duckworth.

Novak, M. and Guest, C. (1989). Application of a Multidimensional Caregiver Burden Inventory. *Gerontological Society of America*, **29**, 798–803.

Ott, B. R. and Fogl, B. S. (1992). Measurement of depression in dementia—self vs clinician rating, *International Journal of Geriatric Psychiatry*, **7**, 899–904.

Patel, V. and Hope, R. A. (1992). A rating scale for aggressive behaviour in the elderly. *Psychological Medicine*, **22**, 211–21.

Pattie, A. H. and Gilleard, C. J. (1979). Manual for the Clifton Assessment Procedures for the Elderly. In *Psychological Assessment of the Elderly* (Wattis J. P. and Hindmarch I., eds), pp. 61-80. Churchill Livingstone, Edinburgh.

Perrin, T. (1997). The positive response schedule for severe dementia. *Aging and Mental Health*, **1**, 184–91.

Pfeffer, R. I., Kurosaki, T. T., Harrah, C. H., Chance, J. M. and Filos, S. (1982). Measurement of functional activities in older adults in the community. *Journal of Gerontology*, **37**, 323–9.

Piaget, J. (1926). *The Language and Thought of the Child*. Harcourt-Brace, New York, NY.

Proctor, R., Burns, A., Powell, H. S., Tarrier, N., Faragher, B., Richardson, G., Davies, L. and South, B. (1999). Behavioural management in nursing and residential homes: a randomised control trial. *Lancet*, **354**, 26–9.

Reason, J. T. (1984). Absent-mindedness and cognitive control. In *Everyday Memory, Actions and Absent-mindedness* (Harris, J. E. and Morris, P. E., eds), pp. 113–32. Academic Press, London.

Robinson, B. C. (1983). Validation of a caregiver strain index. *Journal of Gerontology*, **38**, 344–8.

Robinson, R. A. (1961) Some problems of clinical trials in elderly people. *Gerontologia Clinica*, **3**, 247–57.

Robinson, R.A. (1977). Differential diagnosis and assessment in brain failure. *Age and Ageing*, **6** (Suppl.), 42–9.

Roth, M., Huppert, F. A., Tym, E. and Mountjoy, C. Q. (1988). *CAMDEX—Cambridge Examination for Mental Disorders of the Elderly*. Cambridge University Press, Cambridge.

Rovner, B. W., Steele, C. D., Shmuely, Y. and Folstein, N. F. (1996). A randomised trial of dementia care in nursing homes. *General American Geriatric Society*, **44**, 7–13.

Saudargas, R. and Zanolli, K. (1990) Momentary time sampling as an estimate of percentage time: a field validation. *Journal of Applied Behaviour Analysis*, **23**, 533–7.

Schlesinger, E. (1996) Why learning is not a cycle. I: Discovering pattern. *Industrial and Commercial Training*, **28**, 30–35.

Shah, A. and De, T. (1998). The effect of an educational intervention package about aggressive behaviour directed at the nursing staff on a continuing care psychogeriatric ward. *International Journal of Geriatric Psychiatry*, **13**, 35–40.

Sixsmith, A., Hawley, C., Stilwell, J. and Copeland, J. (1993). Delivering 'positive care' in nursing homes. *International Journal of Geriatric Psychiatry*, **8**, 407–12.

Slade, M., Phelan, M., Thornicroft, G. and Parkman, S. (1996). The Camberwell Assessment of Need (CAN): comparison of assessments by staff and patients of the needs of the severely mentally ill. *Social Psychiatry and Psychiatric Epidemiology*, **31**, 108–13.

Smyer, M., Brannon, D. and Cohn, M. (1992). Improving nursing-home care through training and job re-design. *Gerontologist*, **32**, 327–33.

Stokes, G. (1990). Controlling disruptive and demanding behaviours. In *Working with Dementia* (Stokes, G. and Goudie, F., eds), Winslow Press, Bicester.

Stokes, G. (1996). Challenging behaviour in dementia. In *Handbook of Clinical Psychology of Ageing* (Woods, R. T., ed.), pp. 601–28. Wiley, Chichester.

Sunderland, T., Alterman, I. S, Yount, D., Hill, J. I., Tariot, P. N., Newhouse, P. A., Mueller, E. A., Mellow, A. M. and Cohen, R. M. (1988). A new scale for the assessment of depressed mood in demented patients. *American Journal of Psychiatry*, **145**, 955–9.

Teri, L., Truax, P., Logsdon, R., Uomoto, J., Zarit, S. and Vitaliano, P. P. (1992). Assessment of behavioral problems in dementia: the revised memory and behavior problems checklist. *Psychology and Aging*, **7**, 622–31.

Wells, T. J. (1980). *Problems in Geriatric Nursing Care*. Churchill Livingstone.

Whall, A. L. (1999). The measurement of need-driven dementia-comprised behaviour. Achieving higher levels of interrate reliability *Journal of Gerontological Nursing*, **25**,(9) 33–7.

Whisman, M. A. (1993). Mediators and moderators of change in cognitive therapy of depression. *Psychological Bulletin*, **114**, 248–65.

Wilkinson, I. M. and Graham-White, J. (1980). Psychogeriatric dependency rating scales (PGDRS). A method of assessment for use by nurses. *British Journal of Psychiatry*, **137**, 558–65.

Williams, G. M. (1996) Memory processes in psychotherapy. In *Frontiers of Cognitive Therapy* (Salkovskis, P., ed.), pp. 97–113. Guilford Press, New York, NY.

Woods, R.T. (1999). Psychological assessment of older people. In *Psychological Problems of Ageing* (Woods, R. T., ed.), pp. 219–52. John Wiley and Sons, Chichester.

Workman, B. (1996). An investigation into how the health care assistants perceive their role as support workers to the qualified staff. *Journal of Advanced Nursing*, **23**, 612–19.

Zgola, J. M. (1987). *Doing Things: A Guide to Programming Activities for Persons with Alzheimer's Disease and Related Disorders*. John Hopkins University Press, Baltimore, MD.

13 Managing carers' psychological needs

Caregivers looking after a person with dementia are often highly stressed, and frequently experience clinically significant depression. Behavioural and psychological symptoms in dementia (BPSD) are a major trigger of both increased burden and depression amongst caregivers (Donaldson *et al.* 1997). BPSD also accelerate admission to institutional care (Steele *et al.* 1990), probably largely as a result of the additional strain that they place upon caregivers. Treatment issues, such as developing more effective management strategies for the spectrum of BPSD symptoms, and specific treatment interventions for caregivers are of prime importance.

The need to support and help caregivers is widely recognized, with many health and social care organizations and voluntary bodies providing caregiver support groups. In routine practice, these groups may take the form of a time limited closed group, often with education about dementia as a primary focus. This is often delivered as a series of didactic presentations about important aspects of the dementia process, with opportunities for questions afterwards; or as a longer-term rolling group which enables caregivers to provide advice and empathy to each other, under the guidance of a facilitator. Whilst both types of group are appreciated by caregivers, there is very little empirical evidence for their value. Many studies have evaluated the effectiveness of educational groups. Although the majority of individual studies have failed to demonstrate a significant benefit, a meta-analysis (Knight *et al.* 1993) did demonstrate some limited improvements in improving coping strategies and reducing burden. Many of these studies have focused the education around a very medical model of illness and treatment, and important issues such as the availability of practical help, such as a sitter service; what benefits people may be entitled to and how to access these benefits or services are often not addressed. The value of longer-term support groups has not been systematically evaluated. Although caregivers clearly have a high level of need, providing labour-intensive, expensive and often ineffective interventions is not an acceptable option. Because of the variable success of carer intervention programmes, auditing the effectiveness of an intervention is an essential part of any treatment provided within a clinical service setting.

'Family' or 'caregivers'?

Many of the people that would be considered by health and social service professionals to be 'caregivers' dislike this term, and prefer to consider themselves as partners, children, siblings or friends. There is a potentially important issue, as the term 'caregiver' carries with it certain inherent implications about the nature of the relationship. For example, the 'caregiver' gives whilst the person with dementia receives; the relationship is hence no longer considered to be mutual within this model, and the implication is that the person with dementia has little to offer the relationship. Usage of this terminology hence has a subtle, but discernable effect in changing the nature of the relationship, and perhaps the tolerability threshold of the 'caregiver'. It is probably best to listen to the person's own perception of their role, and work within their own model, whether it is as a partner, child or caregiver.

Evidence-based practice

Few studies have demonstrated significant benefit from caregiver intervention studies. Perhaps the most promising approach has been based upon a cognitive behavioural therapy model. Donaldson *et al.* (1998) have shown that whilst caregivers attribute cognitive deficits and impairments of activities of daily living to the dementia process, they often see BPSD symptoms as 'deliberate bad behaviour' or 'being manipulative'. This has an important effect upon the way in which a caregiver responds to a particular behaviour. Other work suggests that caregivers with more assertive coping strategies and a more internal locus of control are less likely to become depressed (Saad *et al.* 1995). This literature provides a theoretical background to suggest that a cognitive behaviour therapy approach, which tackles attributions and coping strategies, may be helpful. Preliminary studies of this kind have been encouraging. Marriott *et al.* (2000), using a manual based upon the work of Donaldson *et al.*, delivered a package of individual cognitive behaviour therapy to 19 caregivers, who each received 14 sessions of therapy from a clinical psychologist. The intervention significantly reduced caregiver depression and altered attributional style. Seymour (1999) used a group cognitive therapy approach delivered by a consultant psychiatrist with training in psychotherapy for 72 caregivers. Again a significant reduction in caregiver depression was reported. A recently completed study, currently in preparation, from our own centre, also used a group cognitive behaviour therapy approach, although the treatment was of shorter duration (six sessions), focused specifically upon caregivers looking after people with clinically significant BPSD and was delivered by a psychiatric nurse with a diploma in cognitive behaviour therapy, under the supervision of a clinical psychologist. The intervention did not reduce caregiver depression, although there was a significant reduction in the amount of distress caregivers experienced in response to the BPSD, and there was a mean six-point reduction in the Neuropsychiatric Inventory scores of the people with dementia. Although each of these studies was small, and each used a slightly different approach, the results are certainly encouraging. Further work needs to:

(1) develop a cost-effective cognitive behaviour therapy intervention that may be suitable for use in routine clinical practice;

(2) evaluate whether the beneficial effects upon the caregivers are maintained; and

(3) determine whether interventions of this kind can delay admission to institutional care.

The other approach that has been shown to be effective involves carer training (Brodaty and Gresham 1989, Brodaty *et al.* 1993, 1997). Brodaty and colleagues randomized caregivers into three groups: an intensive carer training group, a delayed training group (waiting-list control) and a memory retraining group (a control condition). This intensive training package was undertaken over 10 days in a hospital setting, with a parallel programme for people with dementia. The training had a number of different elements, including management of distress, developing new ways of thinking and new coping skills, coping with problem behaviours and advice about using local community services. The package, which incorporates many elements of cognitive behaviour therapy interventions, is very labour intensive and expensive, but significantly reduces psychiatric morbidity amongst caregivers and has significantly delayed admission to institutional care at 3, 5 and 8 year follow-up. Despite the resources required, the clear demonstration of long-term benefits makes this an important intervention model. If these advantages can be replicated in other settings, the initial investment in this type of training package will be more than offset by savings from delaying the need for care facilities.

Pharmacotherapy has received very little attention among dementia caregivers. Despite the high frequency of depression, only a minority of caregivers are prescribed antidepressant medication (Coope *et al.* 1995). This is perhaps in some ways a reflection of the terminology used in the literature, where 'burden', although a useful concept, deflects attention from the fact that many caregivers are suffering from clinically significant depression. Depression does affect perceived abilities, one's sense of helplessness or hopelessness, an individual's energy level and their irritability. Hence depression can have a profound effect upon coping skills. There is no reason why caregivers with depression should respond any differently to antidepressant pharmacotherapy than any other group of individuals with depression, particularly when considering that individuals with depression in response to a severe life event, such as a bereavement, experience significant improvements with antidepressant treatment. However, studies are needed to examine the effects on coping skills and perceived burden as well as psychiatric morbidity.

Only one of these studies has focused specifically upon caregivers looking after people with clinically significant BPSD, although most of the treatment packages that were used included elements that focused upon coping strategies in general, and specific approaches for managing BPSD. Further work specifically examining the effect on the caregiver and person with dementia in a cohort of dementia sufferers with BPSD would be informative, especially with regard to the potential to delay institutional placement in this group of 'high-risk' individuals.

An individual approach

While it is very important to develop effective group interventions for caregivers, which can be delivered in a cost-effective manner, this does not detract from the importance of a detailed and individualized needs assessment for each dementia sufferer and their caregiver. Although BPSD are an important stressor, their impact will be greater in the absence of a care package that does not meet the other core needs. For example, a caregiver who struggles for 2 h every morning to lift their immobile partner with dementia out of bed and to help them get dressed is far less likely to deal with verbal aggression in a calm and responsive manner if they have no assistance and are already approaching their maximum tolerability threshold. If, on the other hand, a care worker is coming to assist, the whole process is likely to be far less stressful for the caregiver. In addition, if a support network of sitters and day centre attendance allows a caregiver some time each week to complete household tasks, shopping and perhaps have some time for relaxation or social interaction; they are likely to deal far more effectively with difficult situations as they arise. The best way of providing support will depend very much on the individual situation. The most important principle is to listen to what the needs are, and not to try and 'fit' people into a limited array of generally available options.

The assessment of an individual situation may make it easier to select appropriate additional treatment options (e.g. pharmacotherapy, carer training or cognitive behaviour therapy) and provides the opportunity to inform people about the services that are available locally, how these can be accessed and about entitlements to benefits. A system for monitoring a situation, such as a contact person and telephone number, or regular follow-up visits can also be introduced as appropriate.

Conclusion

Providing for the needs of caregivers is an important part of managing a person with dementia suffering from BPSD. This will include a detailed individualized assessment to provide a tailored care package, and might include specific interventions such as a carer training group or pharmacotherapy. However great the needs of these individuals, expensive and ineffective treatments should not be an option, and any locally provided carer intervention should be audited for its effectiveness. This suggested approach to management issues can be summarized as follows:

(1) Determine how people see their own role. If people do not consider themselves to be caregivers, then do not label them as such.

(2) An appropriate, flexible, individualized approach to planning care and the support package is important.

(3) It is important to provide information about locally available services: medical, social services and voluntary sector provisions.

(4) Carers' training groups or cognitive behaviour therapy can be helpful. However, interventions should be delivered according to an established manual, and efficacy should be evaluated.

(5) If carers are clinically depressed, pharmacotherapy may be helpful.

Case example

> Mr X is an 86 year old man, living at home with his wife. He has been suffering from dementia for the last 2 years. Mr and Mrs X have been referred to a specialist old-age psychiatry team because Mr X tends to follow Mrs X around the house, which she finds extremely stressful. In addition, Mr X is a little unsteady on his feet and Mrs X worries that if he walks outside he may fall. This is problematic, as Mr X becomes very frightened if his wife tries to leave him at home while she goes shopping. After an appointment with the consultant psychiatrist, arrangements are made for Mr X to attend a local day centre three times a week. The bus comes to pick him up between 10 and 11 a.m., and returns him home between 2 and 3 p.m.

Mr X has been channelled into a locally available resource. While this might be very helpful for some people with different needs, it has not really addressed the problems for Mr and Mrs X. Mr X has been a keen sportsman most of his life, and used to enjoy meeting his friends at the local bar for a drink. He finds the day centre a very stressful social environment because of the predominance of females there: he has always felt less comfortable in the company of women. In addition, as he does not want to leave Mrs X, he becomes very restless when the bus arrives to collect him. At the day centre he spends most of the day in an anxious state, walking about and constantly asking staff members where his wife is. When he returns home, for 2–3 h he feels even more insecure about the whereabouts of Mrs X, and will not let her go into a different room.

The management plan has not been particularly helpful for Mrs X either. Because of the unpredictable times of the return transport, Mrs X has to be back at the house by 2 p.m. This means that by the time she has arrived in town, she has only 45 min to complete the shopping at a busy time of day. She also has the additional stress of rushing back and knowing that the situation will be difficult for her to cope with for the first few hours after Mr X returns.

> At a subsequent visit to the hospital, a conference was organized between the different members of the multidisciplinary team and Mr and Mrs X to try to plan a more effective care package. It was decided that a care worker would come to the house twice a week for 4 h. Mrs X could then use one afternoon to complete the shopping and the other to visit a friend. Mr X expressed a preference for a male care worker, with whom he could play cards. After the conference, the social worker met with Mr and Mrs X to make sure that they knew about their benefit entitlements and to give information about

locally available services. Mrs X felt that it would be helpful to speak to someone else with experience of looking after someone with dementia, and was given a contact number for the Alzheimer's Disease Society.

Initially Mr X still felt very anxious when Mrs X left the house. However, the strategy of Mrs X staying there for the first few visitsworked very well. Once Mr X got to know the care worker, he felt much more relaxed when Mrs X went out and enjoyed the afternoon talking about football and playing cards. In addition, Mrs X had sufficient time to complete the shopping without rushing and had the additional benefit of maintaining social contact with a friend and confidante. This much more individualized care package was no more expensive than attendance at a day centre, but was much more successful in meeting the needs of Mr and Mrs X.

> The new support package was working well, but Mrs X was still finding the situation stressful, particularly the limited opportunities to have some time to herself while she was in the house. Over 2 months she started feeling low in mood, becoming tearful and feeling very irritable with Mr X. A community psychiatric nurse visited, and helped Mrs X by teaching her some anxiety management techniques and discussing some strategies to help reduce the effect of Mr X's trailing. Over a few weeks, Mrs X tried to implement this advice, but felt that she wasn't really 'doing it right', that she was useless as a caregiver and was finding it difficult to find the energy to keep trying. At this point the consultant psychiatrist prescribed an antidepressant, which over 8 weeks improved Mrs X's mood markedly. However, she was still finding the trailing very stressful and felt that she needed some more intensive training to help her manage the situation more effectively. The community psychiatric nurse, who had a diploma in cognitive behaviour therapy, offered a formal 8 week cognitive behaviour therapy intervention, supervised by a clinical psychologist. The team used a standard approach to therapy based upon a treatment manual. The treatment helped Mrs X manage her own anxiety about leaving Mr X unattended. Through rehearsing problem-solving strategies, Mrs X developed an approach based upon giving Mr X a clear explanation of what she was doing when she left the room, and how long she would be. This was reinforced by returning to the room every 15 min if she was engaged in a task lasting longer than this, to reiterate the explanation of what she was doing. She also began to ask Mr X to undertake simple household tasks.

Once Mrs X's depression had resolved, she was able to use the operationalized cognitive behaviour therapy intervention very effectively to reduce her own anxiety and to develop a management approach that reduced the 'trailing' and made Mr X feel more valuable and able to contribute.

REFERENCES

Brodaty, H. and Gresham, M. (1989). Effects of a training programme to reduce stress in the carers of patients with dementia. *British Medical Journal*, **299**, 1375–9.

Brodaty, H., McGilchrist, C., Harris, L. and Peters, K. (1993). Time until institutionalization and death in patients with dementia. *Archives of Neurology*, **50**, 643–50.

Brodaty, H., Gresham, M. and Luscombe, G. (1997). The Prince Henry Hospital dementia caregivers' training programme. *International Journal of Geriatric Psychiatry*, **12**, 183–92.

Coope, B., Ballard, C., Saad, K., Patel, A., Bentham, P., Bannister, C., Graham, C. and Wilcock, G. (1995). The prevalence of depression in the carers of dementia sufferers. *International Journal of Geriatric Psychiatry*, **10**, 237–42.

Donaldson, C., Tarrier, N. and Burns, A. (1997). The impact of the symptoms of dementia on caregivers. *British Journal of Psychiatry*, **170**, 62–8.

Donaldson, C., Tarrier, N. and Burns, A. (1998). Determinants of carer stress in Alzheimer's disease. *International Journal of Geriatric Psychiatry*, **13**, 248–56.

Knight, B. G., Lutzky, S. M. and Macofsky-Urban, F. (1993). A meta-analytic review of interventions for caregiver distress: recommendations for future research. *Gerontology*, **33**, 240–48.

Marriott, A., Donaldson, C., Tarrier, N. and Burns, A. (2000). Effectiveness of Cognitive-Behavioural family intervention in reducing the burden of care in care of patients with Alzheimer's disease. *British Journal of Psychiatry*, **176**, 557–62.

Saad, K., Hartman, J., Ballard, C., Kurian, M., Graham, C. and Wilcock, G. (1995). Coping by the carers of dementia sufferers. *Age and Ageing*, **24**, 495–8.

Seymour, J. (1999). Group cognitive behaviour therapy for dementia caregivers. Abstract presented at UK Dementia Research Group Congress.

Steele, C., Rovner, B., Chase, G. A. and Folstein, M. (1990). Psychiatric symptoms and nursing home placement of patients with Alzheimer's disease. *American Journal of Psychiatry*, **147**, 1049–51.

14 Alternative therapies: other non-pharmacological therapies

Introduction

Whether or not a person has cognitive impairment, he/she will have needs. These will include physiological (food, water, shelter) and psychological features (security, activity, companionship, stimulation). It is suggested that people with dementia retain their desire to have needs fulfilled, but become less able to communicate and obtain them. Therefore it is not unusual for a person with dementia to be energized by a need and to become distressed when it is not met. In such circumstances, the energy may be expressed in terms of feelings and emotionally driven activities (shouting, aggression), and thus trigger a challenging behaviour.

This perspective is in keeping with the view of Stokes (1996), who describes dementia as a time of *feeling* rather than *knowing*. He suggests that, as the condition progresses, a person with dementia is less able to solve problems and communicate rationally, and instead becomes more likely to signal his/her needs through emotions. Unfortunately, the ability of a person with dementia to express these emotions is also affected: 'When emotions are expressed they can be gross, immediate and un-restrained. They may also be of short duration and alternate rapidly from one emotional state to another.' (Stokes, 1996, p.619)

The form of emotionality can be explained partially in terms of frustration and psychological ill-being (Kitwood 1997a,b), but organic changes also play an important role in how feelings are expressed. Sometimes the person's emotionality can be expressed in subtle or indirect ways. For example, when a person continually asks to go home, or asks about his/her family, this can be conceptualized as communicating an emotional need for security or warmth. Miesen (1993) claimed that the phenomenon of 'parent fixation' (fictitiously seeing a parent; mistaking some-one for a member of the family) is another aspect of the need for security. Miesen found that this feature was evident in 60% of Alzheimer's disease patients and was most common in those with severe dementia. It was suggested that those with poorer cognitive functioning were less able to bond with the outside world, and parent fix-ation was interpreted as an aspect of attachment and bonding difficulties.

The present discussion has highlighted the fact that a person with dementia, like everyone else, requires his/her needs to be fulfilled in order to maintain a sense of well-being and worth. Unfortunately, he/she is often less able to express and access these desired goals. In addition, owing to organic features and to the low affective states associated with dementia, the person with dementia is unable to use previous coping and compensatory strategies to deal with the lack of fulfilment.

The function of challenging behaviour may be to highlight distress (e.g. by shouting, which may have the underlying message 'I'm in pain!') or to obtain a desired goal directly (e.g. by striking out, which may have the underlying message 'Get away from me! I don't want you to undress me'). This chapter discusses interventions that have been devised to enable the person to deal with their emotions better, whether they are expressed overtly or covertly (as fear, anger or depression). The work discusses art and music therapy, showing how the person with dementia can be encouraged to express needs in non-language-based ways. Activity therapy, and its use as a way to help channel emotional and physical energy appropriately, is also outlined. The potential benefits of the sensory therapies, aromatherapy and *Snoezelen*, are also summarized.

As revealed in the various discussions, the evidence underpinning many of the approaches is poor. Nevertheless, the interactive cognitive subsystem model (Teasdale 1996) described in Chapter 10 provides a good conceptual model that can account for the potential benefits derived from these various therapeutic approaches (see p.133).

The therapies

Art therapy

This first section discusses art in terms of drawing, painting and visual appreciation; music therapy and activity therapy (dance and drama) are reviewed in separate sections. Participation in art activities can provide people with dementia with meaningful stimulation, improve levels of social interaction and boost self-esteem (Wald 1983, Killick and Allan 1999a). It is believed that drawing and painting can provide the person with dementia with the opportunity to express him/herself both physically and emotionally. He/she can explore textures and colour combinations and engage in activities without the need for achieving an end product (i.e. a coherent piece of artwork). During the work, the person with dementia can also exercise choice in terms of the themes and media through which to express ideas (e.g. line drawings, painting or sculpture).

It has been demonstrated that art therapy also benefits the staff, because it engages them in joint activities with the residents. In addition, it can provide staff with insight into the remaining abilities of the residents. For example, because art tends to engage procedural rather than declarative memory, it frequently highlights abilities that have been spared during the dementing process. Indeed, it is often the case that a person with dementia can produce a good piece of artwork but be unable to comment on or describe any detail of that artwork.

In determining the usefulness of art with people with dementia, it is relevant to distinguish between its use as an activity and a therapy. To date, most art has been used as a form of activity in which the person with dementia benefits by achieving a greater sense of enjoyment and well-being (e.g. Sterritt and Pokorny 1994). However, a number of researchers have used art as a form of therapy (Jensen 1997, Kahn-Denis 1997, Shore 1997, Waller 1999). In order to qualify as therapy, the work should ideally be underpinned by a theoretical model, and this model serves to guide both the assessment and intervention phases. In addition, the goals of the work need to be specifically targeted to cure or alleviate a particular aspect of the condition (e.g. depression, confusion, aggression).

Kahn-Denis (1997) provides examples of how art therapy can assist in the diagnosis and assessment of dementia. She discusses its role as a psychosocial tool and as a method for facilitating communication and enjoyment. A key message in her descriptive paper is that art is capable of rekindling the identity of a person with dementia, a feature often thought to be lost during the course of the dementing process. Shore (1997) discusses the use of art therapy with two individuals, in which Erikson's developmental perspective was used to help interpret the artwork (Erikson 1982). In her work, Shore used Erikson's notion of life-span conflicts (integrity versus despair; trust versus mistrust) to identify both how a person with dementia is experiencing his/her condition and the type of emotional resolution required to improve mental health. In one of the few controlled studies in the area, Sheppard (1998) reported the benefits of art therapy over a group that did not receive art therapy. Levels of depression among those who received therapy were lower after treatment. However, the findings have to be viewed with caution as the study had several methodological shortcomings.

In addition to the production of artwork, people with dementia usually retain some ability to make choices and express preferences regarding art. In a project conducted in a residential home by Foster and McMorland (1993), residents were encouraged to help select new prints and encouraged to comment on existing ones. This work provides a good example of resident–staff collaboration and is an illustration of resident-centred care.

Music therapy

Despite there being a long association between music and health (Bunt 1994), the widespread use of music as a therapy only began after the Second World War. Since then, like art therapy, music therapy has been divided into two broad camps. One group is concerned with the investigation of music as therapy and the other has promoted the use of music within therapy (Pavlicevic 1991, Killick and Allan 1999a). Clearly there is a lot of overlap between these two approaches, but the former is far keener to establish itself as an academic discipline and thus promotes empirical research. Some of the projects that have been conducted using music therapy in the field of dementia are listed below (see also Bright 1992 and Killick and Alan 1999b for comprehensive reviews). Music, and associated musical activities, can:

- relieve stress and aid relaxation (Guzzetta 1989);
- reduce physiological arousal (Norberg *et al.* 1986);
- aid sleep, leading to a reduction in the need for medication (Momhimweg and Voignier 1995);
- promote socialization and motor activity (Ford *et al.* 1987, Braben 1992, Lindsay 1993);
- facilitate communication, particularly for those with poor language abilities (Gaebler and Hemsley 1991, Mapp 1995, Walker 1996, Ishizuka 1998);
- trigger memory and aid reminiscence (McCloskey 1990, Brooker 1991, Lipe 1992).

While the above studies have reported the positive effect of music therapy on people with dementia, the quality of the research in this area is generally poor. The designs are often inadequate and the methodological rigour lax. Typically, populations are small and assessment procedures usually inappropriate and subjective. One of the few exceptions to this criticism is the work of Lord and Garner (1993) with people with mild/moderate dementia. In their study, groups of 20 nursing home residents were stimulated using three different methods to determine the effect on their well-being (i.e. perceived enjoyment and social interaction). The three conditions, administered in 30 min recreational periods over 6 months, were music (big band music), puzzle exercises and standard recreational activities (television, drawing). People in the music group showed higher levels of well-being, better social interaction and improvements in autobiographical memory compared with those in the other two groups.

In addition to the studies outlined above, music has been successfully used with people displaying challenging behaviours, including agitation and arousal (Norberg *et al.* 1986, Gerdner and Swanson 1993, Brotons and Pickett-Copper 1996), excessive vocalizing (Casby and Holm 1994) and wandering (Fitzgerald-Cloutier 1993). While these studies have generally obtained positive effects, they were again of poor quality. It is noteworthy that many studies carry the proviso that the music must be carefully selected to meet the needs of the listener. For example, Norberg *et al.* (1986), studying people displaying challenging behaviours, observed fewer challenging behaviours when familiar music from the past was played as opposed to music that was either unfamiliar or non-relaxing. This finding was confirmed by Casby and Holm (1994), who noted a significant decrease in repetitive disruptive vocalizations in two people with Alzheimer's disease after familiar music was played.

An intriguing set of recent observations by Miller *et al.* (1998) suggests that certain forms of dementia may enhance artistic talent. These authors propose, from observations of five patients with frontotemporal dementia, that preservation of dorsolateral prefrontal cortex in conjunction of loss of function in the anterior temporal lobes may lead to the enhancement of artistic skills. Miller *et al.* put forward an excitatory/inhibitory processing mechanism to explain the emergence of this talent. They contrast these findings with the poor artistic skills found in people with Alzheimer's disease. The decline is accounted for by the early loss of visuo-constructive abilities together with loss of function in posterior parietal and posterior temporal regions (Miller *et al.* 1996).

To improve the quality of research in this area, two assessment tools have been developed: the Music Therapy Assessment Tool (MTAT, Glynn 1992) and the Residual Music Skills Test (RMST, York 1994). The MTAT aims to quantify the interplay of biopsychosocial dimensions of Alzheimer's patients within their environments, while the RMST assesses 'music behaviours' of people with dementia.

Music is a flexible medium that has broad applicability across a variety of settings. It can be used with individuals and in group settings, with individuals as either listeners or active participants. However, as Morrison (1997) notes, music should be used judiciously, and the person listening should be given control over its presence and volume whenever possible. If used unsympathetically it can become a source of 'noise pollution', leading to further distress. Finally, music is capable of having immediate positive effects on many people when used both sensitively and in keeping with the needs of the individual. It generally has few side-effects, places few cognitive demands on people, and is a cost-effective intervention. This view was supported by the US Senate Special Committee on Aging, who claimed in 1991 that music therapy showed much promise. Indeed, the committee advocated that further clinical research needed to be done with this form of therapy.

Activity therapy

Regular physical exercise can have major health benefits for people with dementia. For example, King *et al.* (1997) note that regular exercise helps prevent falls, improves mental health status and aids sleep. Activity also helps prevent 'disability, immobility and isolation' (Dinan 1998, p.22) and benefits people's confidence and mood (Young and Dinan 1994). In her recent review of the use of exercise with people with dementia, Dinan (1998) provides advice on appropriate forms of activity. She stresses the need to enlist the help of appropriately trained professionals when devising exercise programmes for individuals. In addition to the benefits described above, activities have also been found to be helpful when dealing with disruptive behaviour in people with dementia. For example, a recent study by Alessi *et al.* (1999) revealed that physical activity during the day helped reduce daytime agitation and night-time restlessness. In this controlled study, 29 nursing home residents were randomly assigned to either an intervention programme of increased activity (exercise, walking) and reduced night noise, or a control group. A comparison with the control group, who only received the night-time intervention, showed a marked reduction in both daytime sleeping and agitation for the intervention group.

Two specific forms of activity therapy are drama and dance therapy. Drama therapy has often been used with people with dementia (Huddleston 1989, Casson 1994, Batson 1998), although empirical support for its effectiveness is limited. This form of therapy uses a number of different activities, such as mime, storymaking, role play, movement, games and play. Batson (1998) provides a useful non-technical account of his work as a drama therapist with people with dementia. In his group approach, he uses props, such as hats and common household items, to cue people into mime and storytelling exercises. He suggests that it is often necessary to offer a great deal of structure initially, but over time (as members grow in confidence) the group generates is own momentum. Indeed, he claims that through storytelling, members of the group may be given the opportunity to 'express hopes and fears, recognising within them that we are not alone in what we think and feel.' (Baston 1998, p.21). Wilkinson *et al.* (1989) performed one of the few controlled studies in this field. While this 12 week programme of movement and drama showed inconclusive results and the participants reported benefits.

In recent years there have been a number of informative articles on dance therapy (Crichton 1997, Perrin 1998, Donald and Hall 1999, Hill 1999). For example, Perrin (1998) provided a readable article describing group dance sessions for people with dementia. In this work, she demonstrated the benefits of the approach in both qualitative and statistical terms, monitoring the improvements in people's well-being through the use of dementia care mapping and positive response scheduling. The form of dance employed by Perrin was jabadao (Crichton 1997), a technique designed to promote communication and social interaction. There are no specific steps or prescribed activities in this method, people are merely encouraged to engage in interactive movements with each other. For example, Crichton (1997) describes Amy, a resident prone to aggression, who loved to be waltzed to the toilet. Other residents in Crichton's care benefited from the use of simple ball games, and interactive sessions involving the wafting of ribbons and scarves. Donald and Hall (1999) have used a more structured approach termed dance movement therapy. In their article, they report on a 10 week group therapy programme designed to 'integrate the cognitive, emotional and physical well-being of an individual' (p.25). They observed that this particular programme had four discrete phases: (i) socialization and acclimatization; (ii) formation of group identity; (iii) emergence of an issue; and (iv) resolution. The work employs a loose psychotherapeutic framework, endeavouring to allow significant issues to emerge during the performance of the exercises (movement, dance, mime, body mirroring, prop work). In the resolution phase, the participants are encouraged to express their feelings through emotionally congruent exercises (e.g. the release of tension and anger by throwing a sponge ball vigorously to one another).

Dance therapy appears to be promising. It provides exercise and enjoyment, engaging many senses simultaneously. It can be used as a vehicle for physical contact, allowing the sharing of body warmth in a non-sexual way; a feature that many people with dementia find soothing. As well as stimulating interaction and conversation, dance can also be a mechanism for self-expression in its own right, as noted by Critchton (1997, p.16):

The overwhelming feelings of loss, confusion, frustration and powerlessness caused by dementia often flow too deep for words. Dance can speak volumes. The approach gives clear structures to contain the expression of these strong, often uncomfortable emotions.

Sensory therapies

Aromatherapy has been used for 'healing' since 3000 BC. Knowledge of the distillation of essential oils and perfumes was brought to Europe in the tenth century and aromatic oils have been used there for the treatment of a wide variety of ailments ever since. Although acquired knowledge has been passed on through herbalist texts, there has been very little formal testing of aromatherapy treatments using clinical trial methodology.

In the context of dementia, aromatherapy has a number of potential advantages over traditional pharmacotherapy. It is generally perceived positively, facilitates interaction and offers a sensory experience. In addition, the commonly used pharmacological approaches for the treatment of behavioural and psychological symptoms in dementia (BPSD) are often very poorly tolerated by people with dementia, especially in the later stages of the illness. Therefore, if efficacious, aromatherapy could offer a safer and more pleasant alternative.

Aromatherapy can be administered in a number of different ways: by inhaling oils through vaporization, by bathing or massage, as a compress or by applying the oil in a cream or aqueous solution. The best technique of application for someone with dementia will probably depend upon the individual situation. For example, for some people touch can be very relaxing and reassuring (Montague 1971), but for others it can result in distress or anxiety. In addition, someone with severe agitation or marked restlessness may be unwilling or unable to remain still for long enough for a massage to be completed. Bathing or infusing an aroma into an environment may provide an alternative. Applying the treatment in a cream may have several advantages, as it ensures a fairly consistent exposure to the essential oils over the course of a day.

The putative mechanisms of action are unclear, but a number of possibilities exist:

(1) The act of massage accompanying the aromatherapy may be the effective component (Fraser and Kerr 1993), or providing a massage may improve the mood of the person applying the massage or promote enjoyable social interaction, hence leading to non-specific additional benefits.

(2) The essential oil may evoke particular memories or the mood associated with particular types of environment. Tengen *et al.* (1973) have demonstrated that olfactory memory is stronger than visual memory, whilst Vernet-Maury *et al.* (1999) have shown the strong relationship between olfactory stimulus and mood. This does provide a possible explanation for a therapeutic effect; for example, an essential oil derived from a meadow flower may evoke the pleasant and relaxed mood that someone may feel in a quiet country field, or may induce a specific mood. However, this suggested mode of action is not altogether

straightforward in dementia, as the sense of smell is usually lost early in the course of the disease. Even someone with very early Alzheimer's disease may have severe difficulties distinguishing different smells, and may even have problems identifying the presence of an odour at all (Vance 1999). Several smells, such as coffee, lemon and lavender, can, however, be detected by many people at later stages of the illness, so it is interesting that lavender and melissa (which has a lemon odour) are the two oils that have been suggested to be beneficial for people with dementia.

(3) The remaining hypothesis is that any therapeutic effect is mediated through a direct chemical effect. Essential oils contain many terpenes, which are rapidly absorbed through the lungs, cross the blood–brain barrier and are psychoactive (Perry 1996); many have cholinergic activity.

It is likely that improvements result from a combination of these different elements, contributing to different extents depending upon the individual circumstance.

What symptoms and what treatments?

Most of the limited work with people suffering from dementia has been undertaken with the aim of reducing agitation, anxiety or distress; rather than focusing upon cognitive enhancement. These BPSD are frequent, and often distressing, particularly in people with moderate or severe dementia. Given the severe side effects and modest efficacy of traditional pharmacological treatments in this group of people, alternatives such as aromatherapy require careful consideration, although evidence of their benefit is required. So far, only a limited number of intervention studies have been completed, many of which are single case reports (e.g. West and Brockman 1994, MacMahon and Kermode 1998), or small open case series (e.g. Fraser and Kerr 1993, Brooker *et al.* 1997).

Melissa and lavender

Essential oils extracted from both melissa balm and lavender have been used in herbal medicine and aromatherapy for many years because of their reputed calming properties and effect upon symptoms such as anxiety, restlessness, excitability and depression (Worwood 1995). Although safety has been well established (Price and Price 1995), there are few formal efficacy trials, particularly among people with dementia. In one small placebo-controlled trial of 12 dementia patients, improvements were seen in cooperation and communication for people receiving a combination of lavender and melissa balm aromatherapy, although the small numbers precluded formal statistical analysis (Mitchell 1993). The level of evidence is currently inadequate to recommend widespread usage, but the advantages of aromatherapy in terms of safety and tolerability, and the current case series literature, make further placebo-controlled trials imperative.

Bright light therapy

An accumulating literature describes alterations in diurnal patterns of activity and an altered sleep–wake cycle in people with dementia. These disturbances, thought to underlie specific disorders of restlessness such as the 'sundowning' syndrome (Chapter x), have been linked to changes in the diurnal rhythm of melatonin (Mishima *et al.* 1999). These observations led to the hypothesis, now tested in a number of controlled trials, that bright light may improve certain dysfunctions of diurnal rhythm. There is certainly some evidence (reviewed in more detail in Chapter x) that bright light treatment may reduce sleep disturbance (Koyama *et al.* 1999) and agitation (Mishima *et al.* 1998, Lyketos *et al.* 1999).

Multisensory environments

A literature emerged in the 1950s highlighting the 'sensory deprivation' experienced by many people with dementia and learning difficulties (Liederman *et al.* 1958) and proposing sensory therapies as a potential therapeutic opportunity (Bower 1967). One of the most widely used forms of sensory stimulation has been *Snoezelen*. The term originates from work conducted at the Haarendael Institution in Holland (Hulsegge and Verheul 1987), based upon the tradition of a *Snoezel* room or 'sensory cafeteria' (Cleland and Clarke 1966). The treatment usually occurs in a specifically designed multisensory room which can contain a variety of materials to stimulate different senses. Usually the central feature is a fibre-optic system with flashing lights of various colours, which provides visual and tactile features. Additional tactile sensations are often provided with a range of different textured materials, and specific aromas may be introduced into the environment. Sound can also be an important constituent, and can include music or recordings of traditionally relaxing sounds such as a stream, bird song or the sea. There is no overall specified combination of sensory stimuli, and the exact constitution may be tailored to the needs of a particular group of people within a particular setting, or to the needs of a particular individual.

In the context of dementia, *Snoezelen* has predominantly been used for people with severe cognitive impairment, either to provide sensory stimulation and interaction for individuals who have difficulty responding to more general environmental stimuli and social interaction, or with the aim of promoting relaxation among people who are experiencing restlessness or agitation. Although the *Snoezelen* method has good face validity and has the advantage of providing a framework where carers and people with dementia can interact in a safe and rewarding environment (Bloemhard 1992), there have been very few studies to quantify or evaluate any potential benefits vigorously. Anecdotal clinical impressions (Morrisey and Biela 1997) and several small case series have highlighted potential benefits in a variety of parameters including mood, engagement and relaxation (Long and Haig 1992, Pinkney and Barker 1994, Pinkney 1997). Two larger crossover studies (Holtkamp *et al.* 1997, Kragt *et al.* 1997), althoug modest in size with 16 and 17 participants respectively, demonstrated significant improvement in well-being and a reduction in behavioural problems among people with severe dementia during the multi-sensory treatment period, although it was not clear whether any of the gains persisted after the treatment session. One double-blind study focusing upon people with learning disability did indicate that benefits did not persist after the session (Martin *et al.* 1998), although in a comparative study of two groups of eight patients with dementia attending a day hospital, the socially disturbed behaviour of people receiving *Snoezelen* treatment was reduced more than in those participating in an activity group. Given the small sample size, the results did not reach statistical significance, but there were indications that the improvement continued in period immediately after treatment (Baker *et al.* 1997).

Clearly *Snoezelen* has not been adequately assessed as a possible treatment intervention, and placebo-controlled trials are required. In addition, further consensus is required to address issues such as the ideal length of each treatment session and the number of treatments that constitute an adequate intervention. Most studies have evaluated the therapy over eight or nine 20 min sessions. The goals of treatment also need to be clarified: is the aim to determine whether improvement is experienced during the session or whether the treatment may be of more general benefit? What is the therapeutic goal: to improve interaction, promote well-being or to reduce disturbed behaviour? If treatment durations and the constituents of the sensory environment are tailored to each individual, this should follow operationalized guidelines, so that the procedure can be replicated. Procedures for the selection of suitable participants, and the style of interaction between the carer and the participant, also need to be standardized, possibly involving a brief training programme for care staff. While *Snoezelen* is potentially helpful for a group of people where few other 'non-harmful' treatment options exist, a great deal of further work is required to address these key issues.

Addressing the concerns discussed in the previous paragraph is an essential part of determining the potential value of *Snoezelen* therapy, and these issues are even more important in routine care practice. Often therapies are implemented without adequate planning of the multisensory environment, and many of the care staff involved in the treatment process do not have sufficient skills to enable the participant to benefit from the experience. It is also a worry that failing to pay adequate attention to patient selection may result in the treatment being offered to people who become distressed, frightened or agitated. Some of the materials used in multi-sensory environments, such as fibre-optic systems, are expensive and it is unlikely that they can be used effectively without adequate training in care facilities. Although the current level of evidence does not yet support the routine use of *Snoezelen* for people with severe dementia, if it is already being used within care environments, it is important that specialist teams provide advice and training to optimize and monitor the therapeutic approach.

Conclusion

This chapter has outlined the use of a number of alternative therapies currently used with people with dementia. When evaluating their impact, one must be cautious in drawing conclusions about their efficacy without evidence from controlled trials. Indeed, any intervention involving increased personal attention to residents is likely to result in improvement in well-being, irrespective of the content of the intervention. Hence, although there are some positive indicators within the various fields, the jury will remain out until controlled studies have been done.

Despite the misgivings expressed above, the therapies discussed in this chapter offer face valid approaches for the care of people with dementia. It is also worth pointing out that, although research evidence of benefit is lacking, many of the approaches are currently being used in care-settings to good effect (Ellis and Thorn, 2000). On occasion they are used singularly, but more often they are employed in some form of combination. For example, an approach called SONAS (Threadgold 1995) combines a number of features from the different therapies. SONAS consists of a 45 min audio-tape programme for groups; it uses song, keep-fit exercises, music, dancing and reminiscence. Like much of the other work in this field, recent uncontrolled studies have found benefits of this package in terms of relative well-being (Linehan and Birkbeck 1996), but more conclusive empirical findings are awaited.

Over the next few years it is likely that there will be further growth within the area of alternative therapies for people with cognitive impairment. It is anticipated that this will lead to the development of more quality research into the active ingredients of their effect. The combination of theory and practice will surely be positive, seeing the growth of sound empirically tested person-centred therapies that meet the needs of both the residents and the staff.

REFERENCES

Alessi, C. A., Yoon, E. J., Schnelle, J. F., Al Samarrai, N. R. and Cruise, P. A. (1999). A randomized trial of a combined physical activity and environment intervention in nursing home residents: do sleep and agitation improve? *Journal of the American Geriatrics Society*, **47**, 784–91.

Baker, R., Dowling, Z., Wareing, L. A., Dawson, J. and Assey, J. (1997). Snoezelen: its long term and short term effects on older people with dementia. *British Journal of Occupational Therapy*, **60**, 213–18.

Batson, P. (1998). Drama as therapy: bringing memories to life. *Journal of Dementia Care*, **6**, 19–21.

Bower, H. (1967). Sensory stimulation and the treatment of senile dementia. *Medical Journal of Australia*, **22**, 1113–19.

Braben, L. A. (1992). A song for Mrs Smith. *Nursing Times*, **88**, 54.

Bright, R. (1992). Music therapy in the management of dementia. In *Caregiving in Dementia Research and Application* (Miesen, B. and Jones, G.), pp. 000–000. Routledge, London.

Brooker, D. J., Snape, M., Johnson, E., Ward, D. and Payne, M. (1997). Single case evaluation of the effects of aromatherapy and massage on disturbed behaviour in severe dementia. *British Journal of Clinical Psychology*, **36**, 287–96.

Brooker, E. (1991). Just a song at twilight. *Nursing Times*, **87**, 32–5.

Brotons, M. and Pickett-Cooper, P. K. (1996). The effects of music therapy intervention on agitation behaviours of Alzheimer's disease patients. *Journal of Music Therapy*, **33**, 2–18.

Bunt, L. (1994). *Music Therapy: An Art Beyond Words*. Routledge, London.

Casby, J. A. and Holm, M. B. (1994). The effect of music on repetitive disruptive vocalizations of persons with dementia. *American Journal of Occupational Therapy*, **48**, 883–9.

Casson, J. (1994). Flying towards Neverland. *Dramatherapy*, **16**, 2–7.

Cleland, C. G. and Clark, C. (1966). Sensory deprivation and aberrant behaviour among idiots. *American Journal of Mental Deficiency*, **71**, 213–93.

Crichton, S. (1997). Moving is the language I use, communication is my Goal. *Journal of Dementia Care*, **5**, 16–17.

Dinan, S. (1998). Fit for life: why exercise is vital for everyone. *Journal of Dementia Care*, **6**, 22–5.

Donald, J. and Hall, S. (1999). Dance: the getting there group. *Journal of Dementia Care*, **7**, 25–7.

Ellis, J. and Thorn, T. (2000). Sensory stimulation: where do we go from here? *Journal of Dementia Care*, **8**, 33–7.

Erikson, E. H. (1982). *The Life Completed*. W. W. Norton, New York, NY.

Fitzgerald-Cloutier, M. L. (1993). The use of music to decrease wandering: an alternative to restraints. *Music Therapy Perspectives*, **11**, 32–5.

Ford, M., Fox, J., Fitch, S. and Donovan, V. (1987). Psychiatric skills: light in the darkness: the environment of patients with Alzheimer's disease. *Nursing Times*, **83**, 26–9.

Foster, K. and McMorland, A. (1993). *Art Prints in Residential Homes*. DSDC, University of Stirling, Stirling.

Fraser, J. and Kerr, J. R. (1993). Psychophysiological effects of back massage on elderly institutionalised patients. *Journal of Advanced Nursing*, **18**, 238–45.

Gaebler, H. C. and Hemsley, D. R. (1991). The assessment and short-term manipulation of affect in the severely demented. *Behavioural Psychotherapy*, **19**, 145–56.

Gerdner, L. A. and Swanson, A. (1993). Effects of individualised music on confused and agitated elderly patients. *Archives of Psychiatric Nursing*, **7**, 284–91.

Glynn, N. J. (1992). The music therapy assessment tool in Alzheimer's patients. *Journal of Gerontological Nursing*, **18**, 3–9.

Guzzetta, C. (1989). Psychological aspects of critical care. *Heart and Lung*, **18**, 609–16.

Hill, H. (1999). Dance therapy and communication in dementia. *Signpost*, **4**, 13–14.

Holtkamp, C. C., Kragt, K., van Dongen, M. C., van Rossum, E. and Salentijn, C. (1997). Effect of Snoezelen on the behaviour of demented elderly. *Tijdschrift Voor Gerontologie en Geriatrie*, **28**, 124–8.

Huddleston, R. (1989). Drama with elderly people. *British Journal of Occupational Therapy*, **52**, 298–300.

Hulsegge, J. and Verheul, A. (1987). *Snoezelen*. ROMPA, Chesterfield.

Ishizuka, O. (1998). Between words and music: creative music therapy as verbal and nonverbal communication with people with dementia. Master's thesis. Available from Nordoff–Robbins Music Therapy Centre, 2 Lissenden Gardens, London NW5 1PP.

Jensen, S. M. (1997). Multiple pathways to self: a multisensory art experience. *Art Therapy: Journal of the American Art Therapy Association,* **14**, 178–86.

Kahn-Denis, K. B. (1997). Art therapy with geriatric dementia clients. *Art Therapy: Journal of the American Art Therapy Association,* **14**, 194–9.

Killick, J. and Alan, K. (1999a). The arts in dementia care: tapping a rich resource. *Journal of Dementia Care,* **7**, 35–8.

Killick, J. and Alan, K. (1999b). The arts in dementia care: touching the human spirit. *Journal of Dementia Care,* **7**, 33–7.

King, A. C., Oman, R. F., Brassington, G. S., Bliwise, D. L. and Haskell, W. L. (1997). Moderate-intensity exercise and self-rated quality of sleep in older adults. A randomized controlled trial. *Journal of the American Medical Association,* **277**, 32–7.

Kitwood, T. (1997a). *Dementia Reconsidered.* Open University Press, Buckingham.

Kitwood, T. (1997b). The uniqueness of persons with dementia. In *State of the Art in Dementia Care* (Marshall, M., ed.), Centre for Policy on Ageing, London.

Koyama, E., Matsubara H. and Nakano, T. (1999). Bright light treatment for sleep–wake disturbances in aged individuals with dementia. *Psychiatry and Clinical Neurosciences,* **53**, 227–9.

Kragt, K., Holtkamp, C. C., van Dongen, M. C., van Rossum, E. and Salentijn, C. (1997). The effect of sensory stimulation in the sensory stimulation room on the well-being of demented elderly. A cross-over trial in residents of the R.C. Care Center Bernardus in Amsterdam. *Verpleegkunde,* **12**, 227–36.

Liederman, P. H., Mendelson, J., Wexler, D. and Solomon, P. (1958). Sensory deprivation, clinical aspects. *Archives of International Medicine,* **101**, 389.

Lindsay, S. (1993). Music in hospitals. *British Journal of Hospital Medicine,* **50**, 660–62.

Linehan, C. and Birkbeck, (1996). *An Evaluation of SONAS APC: a Multisensorial Approach to Activate the Potential of Communication in the Elderly.* National Research Agency.

Lipe, A. (1992). Musical debate. *Journal of Gerontological Nursing,* **18**, 3.

Long, A. P. and Haig, L. (1992). How do clients benefit from Snoezelen? An exploratory study. *British Journal of Occupational Therapy,* **55**, 103–6.

Lord, T. R. and Garner, J. E. (1993). Effects of music on Alzheimer patients. *Perceptual and Motor Skills,* **76**, 451–5.

Lyketsos, C. G., Lindell Veiel, L., Baker, A. and Steele, C. (1999). A randomized, controlled trial of bright light therapy for agitated behaviors in dementia patients residing in long-term care. *International Journal of Geriatric Psychiatry,* **14**, 520–5.

MacMahon, S. and Kermode, S. (1998). A clinical trial of the effect of aromatherapy on motivational behaviour in a dementia care setting using a single subject design. *Australian Journal of Holistic Nursing,* **5**, 47–9.

Mapp, S. (1995). Thanks for the memory. *Community Care,* 26 October, 10.

Martin, N. T., Gaffan, E. A. and Williams, T. (1998). Behavioural effects of long-term multisensory stimulation. *British Journal of Clinical Psychology,* **37**, 69–82.

McCloskey, L. J. (1990). The silent heart sings. *Generations,* Winter, 63–5.

Miesen, B. M. L. (1993). Alzheimer's disease, the phenomenon of parent fixation and Bowlby attachment theory. *International Journal of Geriatric Psychiatry,* **8**, 147–53.

Miller, B. L., Ponton, M., Benson, D. F., Cummings, J. L. and Mena, I. (1996). Enhanced artistic creativity with temporal lobe degeneration. *Lancet,* **348**, 1744–55.

Miller, B. L., Cummings, J., Mishkin, F., Boone, K., Prince, F., Ponton, M. and Cotman, C. (1998). Emergence of artistic talent in frontotemporal dementia. *Neurology,* **51**, 978–82.

Mishima, K., Hishikawa, Y. and Okawa, M. (1998). Randomized, dim light controlled, crossover test of morning bright light therapy for rest–activity rhythm disorders in patients with vascular dementia and dementia of Alzheimer's type. *Chronobiology International*, **15**, 647–54.

Mishima, K., Tozawa, T., Satoh, K., Matsumoto, Y., Hishikawa, Y. and Okawa, M. (1999). Melatonin secretion rhythm disorders in patients with senile dementia of Alzheimer's type with disturbed sleep–waking. *Biological Psychiatry*, **45**, 417–21.

Mitchell, S. (1993). Aromatherapy's effectiveness in disorders associated with dementia. *International Journal of Aromatherapy*, **5**, 20–24.

Momhinweg, G. C. and Voignier, R. R. (1995). Music for sleep disturbance in the elderly. *Journal of Holistic Nursing*, **13**, 248–54.

Montague, A. (1971). *Touching: the Human Significance of the Skin*. Columbia University Press.

Morrisey, M. and Biela, C. (1997). Snoezelen: benefits for nursing older clients. *Nursing Standard*, **12**, 38–40.

Morrison, J. (1997). It is music to their ears? *Journal of Dementia Care*, **5**, 18–19.

Norberg, A., Melin, E. and Asplund, K. (1986). Reactions to music, touch and object presentation in the final stage of dementia: an exploratory study. *International Journal of Nursing Studies*, **23**, 315–23.

Pavlicevic, M. (1991). Music therapy in Scotland. *Health Bulletin*, **49**, 191–4.

Pearce, J. The power of touch. *Nursing Times*, **84**, 24.

Perrin, T. (1998). Lifted into a world of rhythm and melody. *Journal of Dementia Care*, **6**, 22–24.

Perry, N. (1996). Cholinergic transmitteractivities in European herbs: potential in dementia therapy. *International Journal of Geriatric Psychiatry*, **11**, 1063–9.

Pinkney, L. (1997). A comparison of the Snoezelen environment and a music relaxation group on the mood and behaviour of patients with senile dementia. *British Journal of Occupational Therapy*, **60**, 209–12.

Pinkney, L. and Barker, P. (1994). Snoezelen: an evaluation of a sensory environment used by people who are elderly confused. In *Sensations and Disability* (Hutchinson, R. and Kerwin, J., eds), ROMPA, Chesterfield.

Price, S. and Price, L. (1995). *Aromatherapy for Healthcare Professionals*. Churchill Livingstone, Edinburgh.

Sheppard, L. and Clive, B. (1998). Evaluating the use of art therapy for people with dementia: a control group study. Department of Experimental Psychology, School of Biological Sciences, University of Sussex, Brighton BN1 9QG.

Shore, A. (1997). Promoting wisdom: The role of art therapy in geriatric settings. *Art Therapy: Journal of the American Art Therapy Association*, **14**, 172–7.

Sterritt, P. F. and Pokorny, M. E. (1994). Art activities for patients with Alzheimer's disease and the role of the American art therapy association. *Geriatric Nursing*, **22**, 57–64.

Stokes, G. (1996). Challenging behaviours in dementia: a psychological approach. In *Handbook of the Clinical Psychology of Ageing* (Woods, R. T., eds), pp. 601–28. Wiley, Chichester.

Teasdale, J. D. (1996). Clinical relevant theory: integrating clinical insight with cognitive science. In *Frontiers of Cognitive Therapy* (Salkovskis, P. M., ed.), pp. 26–41. Guilford Press, New York, NY.

Tengen, ?. (1973). Long term memory of odours with and without verbal descriptions. *Journal of Experimental Psychology*, **100**, 221–7.

Threadgold, M. (1995). Touching the soul through the senses. *Journal of Dementia Care*, **3**, 18–20.

Vance, D. (1999). Considering olfactory stimulation for adults with age-related dementia. *Perceptual and Motor Skills*, **88**, 398–400.

Vernet-Maury, E., Alaoui-Ismaili, O., Dittmar, A., Delhomme, G. and Chanel, J. (1999). Basic emotions induced by odorants: a new approach based on autonomic pattern results. *Journal of the Autonomic Nervous System*, **75**, 176–83.

Wald, J. (1983). Alzheimer's disease and the role of art-therapy in its treatment. *American Journal of Art Therapy*, **22**, 57–64

Walker, O. (1996). Music vibrates in the memory. *Journal of Dementia Care*, **4**, 16–17.

Waller, D. (1999). Art therapy: a channel to express sadness and loss. *Journal of Dementia Care*, **7**, 16–17.

West, B. and Brockman, S. (1994). The calming power of aromatherapy. *Journal of Dementia Care*, **94**, 20–23.

Wilkinson, N., Srikumar, S., Shaw, K. and Orrell, M. (1998). Drama and movement therapy in dementia: a pilot study. *The Arts in Psychotherapy*, **25**, 195–201.

Worwood, V. A. (1995). *The Fragrant Mind: Aromatherapy for Mind, Mood and Emotion.* Transworld Publishers, London.

York, E. (1994). The development of quantitative music skills test for patients with Alzheimer's disease. *Journal of Music Therapy*, **31**, 280–96.

Young, A. and Dinan, S. (1994). ABC of sports medicine. Fitness for older people. *British Medical Journal*, **309**, 331–4.

15 Side effects of psychotropic medication

Introduction

Before discussing individual classes of drugs and specific compounds, it is important to make some general observations regarding pharmacotherapy in the elderly and, in particular, those with dementia. Although changes in normal ageing are often complex (for example, a decline in a neurotransmitter may be accompanied by a compensatory increase in its receptors) and controversial, decreases in dopaminergic, noradrenergic, cholinergic and serotonergic neurones and/or neurotransmitter have been described in association with normal ageing (Blennow and Gottfries 1998). It is, therefore, not surprising that psychotropic drugs that primarily affect these neurotransmitter systems often have greater adverse effects in the elderly. Changes in these neurotransmitter systems are even more pronounced in those with dementia. For example, Alzheimer's disease and dementia with Lewy bodies are associated with profound cholinergic loss (Perry *et al.* 1992, 1994), while dementia with Lewy bodies is also associated with disturbances in dopaminergic function (Piggott *et al.* 1999). Serotonergic and noradrenergic loss has been described in Alzheimer's disease and other dementias, particularly when these disorders are complicated by depression and behavioural disturbance (Chen *et al.* 1996, Esiri 1996). Again, it is unsurprising that patients with dementia are even more sensitive to the adverse affects of psychotropic medication than the normal elderly.

Other general pharmacokinetic and pharmacodynamic factors will affect both efficacy and side-effect profile of psychotropic medication. Pharmacokinetic changes with ageing include reduced hepatic and renal clearance, reduced hepatic metabolism, an increase in fat:lean ratio, changes (usually a decrease) in absorption and a reduction in plasma proteins such as albumin, which affects protein binding; these may all have an effect on blood concentrations of drugs. The net effect of different changes (for example, perhaps a decrease in absorption combined with a decrease in metabolism) may be difficult to predict, though in general the net effect of these changes is either an increase or no change (rather than a decrease) in drug concentrations as a result of ageing. In addition, it is important to remember that elderly patients, particularly those with dementia, are far more likely to suffer other concurrent illnesses (for example, hepatic and renal problems), which may influence plasma drug concentrations, and they may also be on other medications which may have important interactions with pscyhotropic medication.

Therefore, it is clear that extreme caution is needed with regard to pharmacotherapy of elderly patients with dementia. There may be pharmacokinetic changes that result in a given dose of a drug producing a much higher blood concentration in elderly patients with dementia than in younger subjects. There may be neurochemical deficits that make such patients far more likely to suffer adverse effects from a drug given the same blood concentrations. Finally, concurrent illnesses mean that the effects of these illnesses on body systems and the potential for drug interactions are much higher. Hence a cautious approach is required. The old adage of 'start low, go slow' regarding pharmacotherapy in elderly dementia patients could never be more appropriate.

Antidepressant drugs

These can broadly be divided into tricyclic and related antidepressants, monoamine oxidase inhibitors, selective serotonin re-uptake inhibitors and other antidepressant drugs. Each has a characteristic side-effect profile, which depends on the neurotransmitter system(s) affected by the drug.

Tricyclic and related antidepressant drugs

These are often divided into sedative antidepressants, such as amitriptyline, clomipramine, dothiepin and trazodone, and those with less sedative properties such as imipramine, lofepramine and nortriptyline. Lofepramine is usually included in this category as a modified tricyclic and, though it is often thought to have a slightly more benign side-effect profile, it should be noted that its main metabolite, desipramine, is a tricyclic. The therapeutic effects of tricyclics are generally attributed to their pharmacological action in blocking reuptake of norepinephrine and/or serotonin combined with the actions of some in blocking post-synaptic receptors. It is always important to explain to patients and carers that while therapeutic effects of antidepressants take a minimum of 2–3 weeks to appear, and sometimes twice as long in the elderly, side effects are immediately apparent. Side effects of tricyclics can best be understood by the effects they have on different transmitter systems:

- antimuscarinic effects, e.g. dry mouth, blurred vision, constipation, urinary retention, drowsiness and confusion;
- anti-adrenergic effects, e.g. postural hypotension;
- antihistaminic effects, e.g. sedation;
- serotonergic effects, e.g. sexual dysfunction.

Other side effects of this class are problems such as arrhythmias and heart block, hepatic and haematological reactions, hyponatraemia, rash and, very rarely, neuroleptic malignant syndrome. Current CSM advice warns particularly that:

Hyponatraemia (usually in the elderly and possibly due to inappropriate secretion of anti-diuretic hormone) has been associated with all types of antidepressants and should be considered in all patients who develop drowsiness, confusion or convulsions while taking an antidepressant.

BNF (1999)

This problem appears to be particularly common in the elderly (Liu *et al.* 1996, Sharma and Pompei 1996) and may be most pronounced with the selective serotonin reuptake inhibitors (SSRIs) (Pollock 1999), which are discussed below. While median time from starting treatment to hyponatraemia is about 2 weeks, wide variations (from 3 days to 4 months) have been reported (Liu *et al.* 1996). When inappropriate anti-diuretic hormone secretion is suspected, it can be easily diagnosed by blood urea and electrolytes and analysing blood and urine samples for osmolality.

Drug interactions

Most tricyclic antidepressants have several interactions and it is wise to check the current edition of publications such as the *British National Formulary* (BNF 1999) for details. Some common interactions of this class are illustrated in Table 15.1. However, it is important to realize that the presence of a possible interaction does not always preclude co-prescription (except in particular cases, listed in the BNF), though clearly extreme caution will be needed with careful clinical monitoring and, perhaps, close monitoring of plasma concentrations of drugs (for example, in the case of anti-epileptic medication).

Monoamine oxidase inhibitors

Monoamine oxidase inhibitors include irreversible inhibitors such as phenelzine and isocarboxazid and reversal monoamine oxidase inhibitors such as moclobemide (a reversible inhibitor of monoamine oxidase type A (RIMA)). It is now difficult to envisage a situation when older monoamine oxidase inhibitors will be prescribed to patients with dementia. Side effects include severe interactions with tyramine-containing foods (cheese, pickled herring, broad bean pods, yeast extract such as

Table 15.1   Some common drug interactions with tricyclic antidepressants

Drug	Effect
Alcohol	enhanced sedative effect
Anti-arrhythmics e.g. amiodarone	risk of ventricular arrhythmia
Antidepressants	CNS excitation, hypertension, particularly with monoamine inhibitors
Anti-epileptics	antagonism because of lowered convulsive threshold
Anti-hypertensives	enhanced hypertensive effect
Cimetidine	increased plasma concentrations of tricyclic
Diuretics	increased risk of postural hypertension

Bovril and Marmite, soya bean extracts) which can lead to a dangerous rise in blood pressure (an early warning symptom of which is a throbbing headache). Other major side effects of this class include postural hypotension, dizziness, drowsiness, insomnia, headache, dry mouth, agitation, tremor and hepatic problems. Moclobemide, a reversible inhibitor of the enzyme, causes less potentiation of the pressor effect (i.e. increased blood pressure) of tyramine. However, patients should still avoid consuming large quantities of tyramine-rich foods and also need to avoid sympathomimetics such as ephedrine and pseudo-ephedrine, which are often contained in proprietary cold remedies (as do patients taking irreversible monoamine oxidase inhibitors). The main side effects of moclobemide include dizziness, gastrointestinal problems, sleep disturbance, headache, dry mouth, restlessness and agitation.

Drug interactions

Apart from their potentially lethal interaction with tyramine-containing foods, irreversible monoamine oxidase inhibitors interact with a number of other drugs, including alcohol, other antidepressants, antihypertensives, anti-epileptics, anti-psychotics, barbiturates, sympathomimetics and anaesthetics. The reversible monoamine inhibitor moclobemide has many fewer interactions (these are shown in Table 15.2), though as with irreversible monamine oxidase inhibitors co-prescription of moclobemide and other antidepressants should be avoided.

Selective serotonin re-uptake inhibitors (SSRIs)

This group includes citalopram, fluoxetine, fluvoxamine, paroxetine and sertraline and is so named because these compounds selectively inhibit the uptake of serotonin (5-HT). This contrasts with the effects of tricyclics which also inhibit the re-uptake of norepinephrine. In general, SSRIs are less sedating and have fewer anti-muscarinic and cardiotoxic effects than tricyclics and are often better tolerated by elderly people. However, it is important to note that their side-effect profile is different, rather than absent, and there some patients cannot tolerate SSRIs. Because of the possibility of interactions, it is important not to start an SSRI until 2 weeks after stopping a monoamine oxidase inhibitor (except moclobemide, see above) and conversely a monoamine oxidase inhibitor should not be started until at least 1 week

Table 15.2   Some drug interactions of moclobemide

Drug	Effect
Analgesics, e.g. codeine and pethidine	CNS excitation or depression
Levodopa	hypertensive crisis (selegiline should be avoided)
5-HT1 agonists	CNS toxicity
Sympathomimetics	hypertensive crisis
Ulcer healing drugs, e.g. cimetidine	increased concentrations of moclobemide because of inhibition of metabolism (give half dose of moclobemide)

after an SSRI has been stopped (2 weeks for paroxetine and sertraline and 5 weeks for fluoxetine). Because of its short half-life and reversible mechanism of action, no treatment-free period is required after stopping moclobemide before prescribing an SSRI.

The main side effects of SSRIs include gastrointestinal disturbance (nausea, vomiting, diarrhoea and abdominal pain), anorexia, weight loss, headache, tremor, dizziness, dry mouth, insomnia, sexual dysfunction and sweating. As with tricyclics, hyponatraemia may develop.

Drug interactions

Drug interactions for SSRIs differ considerably between the different SSRIs. Interested readers are referred to the BNF (1999) and other reviews (Pollock 1998). These differences are largely due to the effect SSRIs have on inhibiting different sub-types of the cytochrome P450 system. By inhibiting the cytochrome P450 hepatic enzyme system, the pharmacokinetics of other hepatically oxidized drugs can be affected. For example, most SSRIs (especially paroxetine and fluoxetine) are potent inhibitors of the cytochrome P450 CYP 2D6, which can affect other drugs metabolized by this system, including tricyclic antidepressants and trazodone, neuroleptics, lipophilic beta-blockers, some antiarrhythmics, and other drugs such as codeine. Some drugs inhibit the P450 enzyme that is responsible for their own metabolism (e.g. fluoxetine and paroxetine and the 2D6 system), leading to non-linear kinetics with increasing drug dose. Some 5–10% of the population genetically lack the CYP 2D6 enzyme. This means that they are poor metabolizers of drugs oxidized by this pathway, though equally they are unaffected by problems caused by compounds that inhibit this system. Fluvoxamine, fluoxetine and sertraline are inhibitors of the P450 CYP 2C19 and 2C9 isoenzymes which are important in the metabolism of warfarin, diazepam and some anticonvulsants (e.g. phenytoin). Because of the potential for such interactions, prescription of an antidepressant always requires careful consideration of what other medication the patient is on and, though such interactions do not necessarily preclude co-prescription, they do indicate the need for increased caution and more careful clinical monitoring. The practice of co-prescription of a tricyclic and an SSRI, something that was becoming fashionable before newer agents such as venlafaxine were available, is not recommended by the authors because of the risk of toxic concentrations of tricyclics occurring. Elderly patients with dementia, who often have associated co-morbid physical illnesses, are frequently on other medications, making the frequency and nature of drug interactions an important consideration.

Antidepressant withdrawal reactions

There has recently been great interest in the syndrome of withdrawal reactions on cessation of antidepressants and, in particular, SSRIs (Haddad 1998). These have been particularly associated with SSRIs, such as paroxetine, that have a relatively short half-life, rather than those, such as fluoxetine, that have a long half-life and so may be less likely to cause withdrawal, though half-life is not the only factor involved (Drugs and Therapeutics Bulletin 1999). However, this is a complex area as all antidepressants (including newer ones such as venlafaxine) have been associated with withdrawal reactions. In the light of this, current advice is to avoid abrupt withdrawal of any antidepressant unless absolutely necessary (e.g. because of a severe reaction to drug) and to taper withdrawal over a period as long as 6–8 weeks (Drugs and Therapeutics Bulletin 1999), particularly when dealing with a compound with a relatively short half-life, such as paroxetine.

Other antidepressant drugs

These include compounds such as mirtazepine (a pre-synaptic α_2 antagonist thought to increase noradrenergic and serotonergic neurotransmission), venlafaxine (a selective serotonin and norepinephrine re-uptake inhibitor, or SNRI), nefazodone (an inhibitor of serotonin re-uptake and a 5-HT2 blocker) and reboxetine, a selective inhibitor of norepinephrine re-uptake. Mirtazepine has few antimuscarinic affects but can cause sedation (paradoxically in low rather than high doses) as well as postural hypotension, weight gain and tremor. The side-effect profile of nefazodone is similar to the SSRIs but its 5-HT2 blocking effect makes sexual dysfunction less likely. Venlafaxine generally lacks the sedative and antimuscarinic properties of the tricyclics but it can still cause nausea, headache, insomnia, dry mouth, constipation and hypertension (though it can also cause hypotension). Trazodone is often used for the control of behavioural disturbance in dementia. It has similar side effects to the tricyclics but causes fewer antimuscarinic cardiovascular effects, though it can be associated with priapism, sedation and postural hypotension.

Antipsychotic drugs

These are also known as neuroleptics or major tranquillizers. The latter term is not to be recommended because of confusion with minor tranquillizers such as benzodiazepines and because the main effects of antipsychotics are not to tranquillize. The main classes of antipsychotics are:

- phenothiazines, e.g. chlorpromazine and thioridazine;
- butyrophenones, e.g. haloperidol;
- thioxanthenes, e.g. zuclopenthixol;
- substituted benzamides, e.g. amisulpiride; and
- new 'atypical' antipsychotics, which include risperidone, olanzepine, quitiapine and clozapine.

For the purposes of side effects, it would be most helpful to divide drugs into typical and atypical antipsychotics.

Typical antipsychotics

The main side effects associated with this group are motor disturbances. These include acute dystonia (severe muscle spasms seen most commonly in young men), akathisia (a restlessness common soon after starting the drug), parkinsonism (tremor, bradykinesia and rigidity, which usually develops after several weeks) and tardive dyskinesia (dyskinetic oral facial movements commonly occurring with prolonged therapy). Other side effects include headache, drowsiness, dry mouth, constipation, difficulty with micturition, hypotension, tachycardia, convulsions, weight gain, haematological disturbances and depression. Extrapyramidal problems such as parkinsonism are more common with a drug such as haloperidol (which has little intrinsic anticholinergic activity) than thioridazine (which has significant antimuscarinic activity). This is because the anticholinergic activity partially counteracts the parkinsonism induced by blockade of dopamine (particularly D2) receptors. However, conversely, drugs with antimuscarinic activity are the most likely to cause confusion and cannot be recommended in patients with dementia who are known to already have severely compromised cholinergic function.

Extrapyramidal side effects are of particular concern in patients with dementia, particularly in those with dementia with Lewy bodies who already have compromised dopaminergic function. It is for this reason that current CSM advice is to use antipsychotics with great caution in elderly patients with dementia. About 60% of patients with dementia with Lewy bodies who are treated with an antipsychotic experience a severe sensitivity reaction that has some resemblance to the neuroleptic malignant syndrome (McKeith *et al.* 1992). Patients exhibit severe extrapyradmidal problems, decreased levels of consciousness and increasing confusion; these reactions often result in precipitive cognitive decline and early death.

Neuroleptic malignant syndrome is a rare but potentially fatal side effect of antipsychotics and has also been reported with some other compounds such as antidepressants and lithium. It usually occurs shortly after starting a drug, or after an increase in dose, and is characterized by hypothermia, muscular rigidity, autonomic dysfunction (tachycardia, labile blood pressure, sweating) and a fluctuating level of consciousness. Such a clinical picture may mimic many other severe illnesses (such as encephalitis) but other physical causes for the clinical picture are absent and plasma CPK is characteristically elevated. Emergency treatment is needed, including immediate cessation of the antipsychotic, supportive treatment (e.g. fluid replacement and nursing care) and, possibly, the use of agents such as bromocriptine and dantrolene.

One possible problem of antipsychotics which is of great concern is the recent observation that patients with dementia treated with these drugs have a greatly accelerated cognitive decline compared with those not on medication (McShane *et al.* 1997). This effect needs to be confirmed as a true drug effect in randomized controlled trials but is yet another reason why judicious use of these agents would seem prudent.

Drug interactions of antipsychotics are varied and very dependent on the actual drug involved. Readers are advised to consult the *British National Formulary* or similar publications for details.

Atypical antipsychotics

This group includes amisulpiride, clozapine, olanzepine, quetiepine and risperidone. These drugs are better tolerated, particularly in the elderly patients with dementia, because they tend to cause fewer extrapyramidal side effects, hence the term 'atypical'. Clozapine is only indicated for patients with schizophrenia unresponsive to or intolerant of conventional antipsychotics, and though it has been used to good effect in patients with Parkinson's disease (Anonymous 1999) and in those with dementia, this can only be undertaken under specialist supervision. There is a regular monitoring system involving weekly blood tests for the first 18 weeks for patients prescribed clozapine because of the risk of life-threatening neutropaenia.

The main side effects of risperidone include headache, drowsiness, insomnia, agitation, constipation, and nausea and vomiting. Olanzepine can be associated with mild antimuscarinic effects, drowsiness, increased appetite and weight gain, and occasional blood dyscrasias. Quetiapine has a similar side-effect profile and may prolong QT interval; it needs to be used with severe caution in those with cardiovascular disease. Once again, drug interactions depend on the specific compound but can include interactions with alcohol, analgesics, anti-arrhythmics, antidepressants, antidiabetics, anti-epileptics, antihistamines, antihypertensives, antimuscarinics, beta-blockers, diuretics and anxiolytics. Unfortunately, atypical antipsychotics can still cause severe sensitivity reactions in patients with dementia with Lewy bodies (McKeith *et al.* 1995).

Hypnotics and anxiolytics

There is considerable overlap between these two classes. A hypnotic is really an anxiolytic with a short half-life. Hypnotics should be prescribed with great caution in patients with dementia. As with all subjects, current CSM advice is that benzodiazepines are only indicated for short-term (2–4 weeks) relief of anxiety or insomnia and only when this is severe. Because of the tendency of benzodiazepines to accumulate and their tendency to be poorly tolerated and cause withdrawal reactions, their use in elderly patients with dementia is hardly ever justified. The main side effects of all these compounds include drowsiness and light-headedness on the day after treatment, confusion, ataxia and dependence. Zopiclone and zolpidem are short-acting hypnotics with little hangover effect. Chlormethiazole also has limited hangover effects but can cause dependence and is associated with side effects such as headache, increased nasal congestion and irritation, and gastrointestinal disturbances.

Psychotropics and falls

Falls are such an important problem in elderly patients, with potentially disastrous consequences in terms of morbidity and mortality from hip and other fractures, that they deserve specific comment. Falls are particularly common in elderly patients with dementia, especially those with dementia with Lewy bodies, where they are so frequent as to be included as supportive features in the current consensus clinical diagnostic criteria (McKeith *et al.* 1996). A landmark study (Ray *et al.* 1987) showed that antidepressants, antipsychotics and long-acting anxiolytics and hypnotics were all strongly associated with the risk of hip fracture in the elderly, with an odds ratio of about 2. This finding has been confirmed in several subsequent studies (Tune *et al.* 1991, Ruthazer and Lipsitz 1993; Yip and Cumming 1994, Mustard and Mayer 1997, Liu *et al.* 1998). While some have suggested that newer agents, whether antipsychotic or antidepressant, may be less likely to cause falls, a recent case–control study of antidepressants suggested that SSRIs were as likely to be associated with hip fractures as older antidepressants (Liu *et al.* 1998). However, such results are difficult to interpret as there may be selection biases, because those most likely to be at risk of fractures (frail elderly patients with dementia and cardiovascular disorder) are often put on SSRIs rather than tricyclics. There is, as yet, insufficient evidence to judge whether the newer antidepressants and atypical antipsychotics are less likely to cause falls and be associated with hip fractures than older drugs. The important message for management of those with dementia is that all psychotropics may be associated with an increased risk of falls and hip fractures and this is yet another reason why extreme caution is needed before prescribing psychotropics in the elderly with dementia.

Carbamazepine

Carbamazepine has been shown to be useful for the control of behavioural disturbance, particularly aggression, in dementia (Tariot *et al.* 1998). Its main side effects are drowsiness, headache, nausea and vomiting, confusion, diplopia, rash, gastrointestinal disturbance and leucopenia. Hepatic problems and hyponatraemia may also occur. It has several important drug interactions, some of which are illustrated in Table 15.3.

Cholinesterase inhibitors

Three cholinesterase inhibitors are currently licensed in the UK, namely donepezil, rivastigmine and galantamine. They are licensed for use in mild to moderate Alzheimer's disease. As their name suggests, their pharmacological action is to inhibit the naturally occurring enzyme acetylcholinesterase and so prolong the action of endogenously released acetycholine, the transmitter that shows the greatest depletion in Alzheimer's disease and dementia with Lewy bodies. These

Table 15.3   Some drug interactions of carbamazepine

Drug	Effect
Anti-bacterials	carbamazepine concentrations can be increased (e.g. by erythromycin) or decreased (e.g. by rifabutin)
Anticoagulants	warfarin concentrations reduced
Antidepressants	metabolism of tricyclics accelerated; carbamazepine concentrations increased by fluoxetine and fluvoxamine
Other anti-epileptics	increased sedation, reduced plasma concentrations
Antipsychotics	metabolism of some antipsychotics (e.g. risperidone, olanzepine, haloperidol) increased
Corticosteroids	reduced steroid concentrations
Diuretics	increased risk of hyponatraemia
Thyroxine	increased metabolism (may need to increase dose of thyroxine)
Theophylline	concentrations decreased
Cimetidine	increased carbamazepine concentrations

drugs are effective in improving both cognitive and non-cognitive features (Rogers and Friedhoff 1996, Cummings and Back 1998, Rogers *et al.* 1998, Burns *et al.* 1999, Rosler *et al.* 1999) and are generally well tolerated but caution is needed in patients with sick sinus syndrome or supraventricular induction problems and those at risk of developing ulcers or obstructive airways disease including asthma. The main side effects include gastrointestinal disturbance (nausea, vomiting, diarrhoea), fatigue, insomnia, muscle cramps and, less commonly, bradychardia, convulsions and bladder outflow obstruction. The most important drug interaction of donepezil and rivastigmine is with muscle relaxants: they enhance the muscle relaxant suxamethonium but antagonize the effect of non-depolarizing muscle relaxants. It is, therefore, essential that the use of such drugs is highlighted when anaesthetic is considered.

Lithium

Lithium as an adjunct to antidepressants in the treatment of depression in patients with dementia, or as prophylaxis for those with recurrent depressive episodes, should only be used when recommended by specialists. The main side effects of lithium include gastrointestinal disturbances, fine tremor, polyuria and excessive thirst as well as weight gain and oedema. There is a very narrow therapeutic index, as therapeutic levels are only 50% of toxic levels. Lithium toxicity may be recognized by coarsening of tremor, blurred vision, increasing nausea and vomiting, ataxia, drowsiness and confusion. In severe cases, hyperreflexia, convulsions, coma and death may occur. Serum lithium levels must be monitiored regularly (weekly until stabilized, then every 3 months). Longer-term problems such as hypothyroidism and renal problems can develop. This necessitates regular (6 monthly) monitoring of urea and electrolytes, thyroid function tests, blood pressure and weight in all patients on lithium. Overdose is particularly dangerous and may require dialysis.

Conclusion

In chapter, broad principles regarding the side effects of psychotropic medication are summarized and some of the more common side effects and interactions of commonly prescribed psychotropic medication in patients with dementia are illustrated. It clearly has not been possible to describe every side effect or interaction, and prescribers are recommended to consult appropriate comprehensive text (such as the *British National Formulary*) for full and further details. Once again, it is important to emphasize the increased vulnerability of elderly patients with dementia to both pharmacokinetic and pharmacodynamic problems associated with pharmacotherapy, to advise caution whenever prescribing medication for such patients and, perhaps most importantly of all, to ensure that appropriate mechanisms are in place for the monitoring any new treatment or change in dose so that any interactions or adverse effects can be detected early.

REFERENCES

Anonymous (1999). Low-dose clozapine for the treatment of drug-induced psychosis in Parkinson's disease. The Parkinson Study Group. *New England Journal of Medicine*, **340**, 757–63.

Blennow, K. and Gottfries, C. (1998). Neurochemistry of aging. In *Geriatric Psychopharmacology* (Nelson, J. C., ed.), pp. 1–25. Marcel Dekker, New York, NY.

BNF (1999). *British National Formulary*. Pharmaceutical Press, Wallingford.

Burns, A., Rossor, M., Hecker, J., Gauthier, S., Petit, H., Moller, H. J., Rogers, S. L. and Friedhoff, L. T. (1999). The effects of donepezil in Alzheimer's disease—results from a multinational trial. *Dementia and Geriatric Cognitive Disorders*, **10**, 237–44.

Chen, C. P., Alder, J. T., Bowen, D. M., Esiri, M. M., McDonald, B., Hope, T., Jobst, K. A. and Francis, P. T. (1996). Presynaptic serotonergic markers in community-acquired cases of Alzheimer's disease: correlations with depression and neuroleptic medication. *Journal of Neurochemistry*, **66**, 1592–8.

Cummings, J. L. and Back, C. (1998). The cholinergic hypothesis of neuropsychiatric symptoms in Alzheimer's disease. *American Journal of Geriatric Psychiatry*, **6** (Suppl. 1), S64–78.

Drugs and Therapeutics Bulletin (1999). Withdrawing patients from antidepressants. *Drugs and Therapeutics Bulletin*, **37**, 49–52.

Esiri, M. M. (1996). The basis for behavioural disturbances in dementia. *Journal of Neurology, Neurosurgery and Psychiatry*, **61**, 127–30.

Haddad, P. (1998). The SSRI discontinuation syndrome. *Journal of Psychopharmacology*, **12**, 305–13.

Liu, B. A., Mittmann, N., Knowles, S. R. and Shear, N. H. (1996). Hyponatremia and the syndrome of inappropriate secretion of antidiuretic hormone associated with the use of selective serotonin reuptake inhibitors: a review of spontaneous reports. *Canadian Medical Association Journal*, **155**, 519–27. [Erratum published in *Canadian Medical Association Journal*, **155**, 1043.].

Liu, B., Anderson, G., Mitmann, N., To, T., Axcell, T. and Shear, N. (1998). Use of selective serotonin-reuptake inhibitors of tricyclic antidepressants and risk of hip fractures in elderly people. *Lancet* **351**, 1303–7.

McKeith, I., Fairbairn, A., Perry, R., Thompson, P. and Perry, E. (1992). Neuroleptic sensitivity in patients with senile dementia of Lewy body type. *British Medical Journal*, **305**, 673–8.

McKeith, I. G., Ballard, C. G. and Harrison, R. W. S. (1995). Neuroleptic sensitivity to risperidone in Lewy body dementia. *Lancet*, **346**, 699.

McKeith, I. G., Galasko, D. *et al.* (1996). Consensus guidelines for the clinical and pathologic diagnosis of dementia with Lewy bodies (DLB): report of the consortium on DLB international workshop. *Neurology*, **47**, 1113–24.

McKeith, I. G., Piggott, M. A., Marshall, E. F., Ballard, C., Perry E. K., Thomas, N., Lloyd, S., Court, J. A., Jaros, E., Burn, D., Johnson, M. and Perry, R. H. (1999). Striatal dopaminergic markers in dementia with Lewy bodies, Alzheimer's and Parkinson's diseases: rostrocaudal distribution. *Brain*, **122**, 1449–68.

McShane, R., Keene, J., Gedling, K., Fairburn, C., Jacoby, R. and Hope, T. (1997). Do neuroleptic drugs hasten cognitive decline in dementia? Prospective study with necropsy follow up. *British Medical Journal*, **314**, 266–70.

Mustard, C. A. and Mayer, T. (1997). Case–control study of exposure to medication and the risk of injurious falls requiring hospitalization among nursing home residents. *American Journal of Epidemiology*, **145**, 738–45.

Perry, E. K., Johnson, M., Kerwin, J. M., Piggott, M. A., Court, J. A., Shaw, P. J., Ince, P. G., Brown, A. and Perry, R. H. (1992). Convergent cholinergic activities in aging and Alzheimer's disease. *Neurobiology of Aging*, **13**, 393–400.

Perry, E. K., Haroutunian, V., Davis, K. L., Levy, R., Lantos, P., Eagger, S., Honavar, M., Dean, A., Griffiths, M. and McKeith, I. G. (1994). Neocortical cholinergic activities differentiate Lewy body dementia from classical Alzheimer's disease. *Neuroreport*, **5**, 747–9.

Piggott, M. A., Marshall, E. F., Thomas, N., Lloyd, S., Court, J. A., Jaros, E., Costa, D., Perry, R. H. and Perry, E. K. (1999). Dopaminergic activities in the human striatum: rostrocaudal gradients of uptake sites and of D1 and D2 but not of D3 receptor binding or dopamine. *Neuroscience*, **90**, 433–45.

Pollock, B. (1998). Drug interactions. *Geriatric Psychopharmacology* (Nelson, J. C., ed.), pp. 43–60. Marcel Dekker, New York, NY.

Pollock, B. G. (1999). Adverse reactions of antidepressants in elderly patients. *Journal of Clinical Psychiatry*, **60** (Suppl. 20), 4–8.

Ray, W. A., Griffin, M. R., Schaffner, W., Baugh, D. K. and Melton, L. J. D. (1987). Psychotropic drug use and the risk of hip fracture. *New England Journal of Medicine*, **316**, 363–9.

Rogers, S. L. and Friedhoff, L. T. (1996). The efficacy and safety of donepezil in patients with Alzheimer's disease: results of a US multicentre, randomized, double-blind, placebo-controlled trial. The Donepezil Study Group. *Dementia, 7*, 293–303.

Rogers, S. L., Farlow, M. R., Doody, R. S., Mohs, R. and Friedhoff, L. T. (1998). A 24-week, double-blind, placebo-controlled trial of donepezil in patients with Alzheimer's disease. Donepezil Study Group. *Neurology*, **50**, 136–45.

Rosler, M., Anand, R., Cicin-Sain, A., Gaulthier, S., Agid, Y., Dal-Bianco, P., Stehelin, M. B., Hartman, R. and Gharabawi, M. (1999). Efficacy and safety of rivastigmine in patients with

Alzheimer's disease: international randomised controlled trial. *British Medical Journal*, **318**, 633–8.

Ruthazer, R. and Lipsitz, L. A. (1993). Antidepressants and falls among elderly people in long-term care. *American Journal of Public Health*, **83**, 746–9.

Sharma, H. and Pompei, P. (1996). Antidepressant-induced hyponatraemia in the aged. Avoidance and management strategies. *Drugs and Aging*, **8**, 430–5.

Tariot, P. N., Erb, R., Podgorski, C., Cox, C., Patel, S., Jakimovich, L. and Irvine, C. (1998). Efficacy and tolerability of carbamazepine for agitation and aggression in dementia. *American Journal of Psychiatry*, **155**, 54–61.

Tune, L. E., Steele, C. and Cooper, T. (1991). Neuroleptic drugs in the management of behavioral symptoms of Alzheimer's disease. *Psychiatric Clinics of North America*, **14**, 353–73.

Yip, Y. B. and Cumming, R. G. (1994). The association between medications and falls in Australian nursing-home residents. *Medical Journal of Australia*, **160**, 14–8.

16 Pharmacological treatment of psychosis

Introduction

This chapter focuses on the pharmacological management of psychotic symptoms in dementia. Issues are discussed to facilitate treatment decisions, such as whether a pharmacological treatment may be appropriate, and the evidence of efficacy from clinical trials for different pharmacological treatment is reviewed. This information is then summarized and illustrative vignettes are given to examine some potential clinical scenarios.

Does the problem require treatment?

The key parameters deciding whether treatment is necessary are:

- the distress experienced by the patient;
- the distress experienced by their carergivers;
- practical management problems specifically relating to the symptom;
- the frequency with which the symptom occurs;
- the natural course of the symptom.

Only a third of patients with dementia are distressed by their psychotic symptoms (Gilley *et al.* 1991, Ballard *et al.* 1995), so in many cases the symptom may be almost coincidental. In addition, although psychotic symptoms can create problematic situations (Rabins *et al.* 1982), there is relatively limited evidence that they predispose to psychiatric morbidity among caregivers, which is often associated with other behavioural and psychological signs in dementia (BPSD) such as aggression (Donaldson *et al.* 1998). Treatment should therefore only be considered if there is a substantial level of distress either to the person with dementia or to their caregiver in the particular individual circumstances.

An additional consideration is the frequency with which the symptom is experienced. Many people experience these symptoms on only a few occasions per week, with less than a quarter experiencing them more than once a day (Ballard *et al.*

1995). Even if distressing, a symptom that occurs on a very infrequent basis may not require treatment; a strategy based around offering practical support at the times when the symptoms tend to occur may be more profitable.

Yet another consideration relates to the natural course of psychotic symptoms. Follow-up studies suggest, for example, that almost 50% of these symptoms resolve spontaneously within 3 months (Ballard *et al.* 1997). The symptoms most likely to persist are those that have already been present for 3 months at the time of assessment. Hence, if one is presented with a newly occurring psychotic symptom of only a few weeks' duration, unless the symptom is especially distressing or problematic, the most pertinent course may be to monitor carefully for a few weeks or months, during which time it may well resolve spontaneously. This is especially important when taking into consideration that the optimal time for response to pharmacological interventions may be 6 weeks or longer. The high rate of spontaneous resolution is probably one of the key reasons for the very large placebo response rates that are seen in clinical trials (Schneider *et al.* 1990).

If a symptom is particularly distressing or problematic and the severity or frequency of the symptom is such that it is preferable for treatment to be instigated, a range of potential treatment options should be considered. In making this decision one should be mindful of the potentially hazardous effects of pharmacological treatment approaches, particularly neuroleptic agents. These are reviewed much more thoroughly in Chapter 15, and some of the potential longer-term effects are discussed later in this chapter. The main adverse effects in the short term include parkinsonian symptoms, drowsiness, anergia, akathasia and falls (Tune *et al.* 1991). In addition, as it can be difficult to make an accurate clinical differential diagnosis between Alzheimer's disease and dementia with Lewy bodies, particularly among people who are experiencing psychotic symptoms, one should also be very aware of the possibility of severe neuroleptic sensitivity reactions (McKeith *et al.* 1992, Ballard *et al.* 1998).

If treatment is indicated, a pharmaceutical approach may not necessarily be optimal. This is particularly true if symptoms are episodic, when providing additional support such as sitters or attendance at a day centre may be more helpful. Specific psychological intervention strategies, such as caregiver training or individually tailored behaviour therapy packages, may also be beneficial, either as an alternative to, or in combination with pharmacotherapy. These approaches are reviewed in more detail in Chapters 10,11 and 12.

If, having considered each stage of this 'management sieve' (summarized in Fig. 16.1), a pharmacological treatment approach is considered to be the only realistic management option, then a cautious trial should be instigated.

The evidence from clinical trials

The literature relating to the management of behavioural disorders in dementia is full of anecdotal reports and open studies, but there are very few placebo-controlled

(A) Is treatment necessary?

1   Is the person with dementia severely distressed by their psychotic symptoms?

2   Is the carer looking after the person with dementia severely distressed by the psychotic symptoms experienced by the dementia sufferer?

3   Do the psychotic symptoms result in any major practical management problems that are difficult to overcome without treatment of the psychosis?

4   Has the psychosis developed recently (in which case is it likely to resolve spontaneously within a short time)?

5   How frequently does the symptom occur? If it is intermittent, can the problem be tolerated or can it be managed by offering practical support at difficult times if these are predictable?

6   Has the person got any concurrent medical condition or are they taking any medication that might be responsible for the psychosis that they are experiencing?

(B) If all of these filters have been passed through and treatment is considered necessary, how should the problem be resolved?

1   Could the problem be managed by increased practical support to the caregiver or person with dementia?

2   Are there any specific psychosocial or non-pharmacological treatment strategies which may be appropriate in this particular situation?

3   If all of these filters have been passed through and a pharmaceutical treatment is considered to be the only realistic option, a cautious, closely monitored trial is indicated.

Fig. 16.1 A management sieve for treating psychotic symptoms in people with dementia.

double-blind trials. The latter group of studies are the focus of the current review, which will concentrate largely on Alzheimer's disease because of the lack of double-blind treatment trials pertaining to BPSD in other dementias.

In a landmark study, Schneider *et al.* (1990) demonstrated clearly the lack of data from double-blind trials regarding the effectiveness of neuroleptic agents in the treatment of BPSD. Still only 14 double-blind trials of neuroleptics have been published. Placebo response rates across trials for BPSD are approximately 40%, and are hence a very major consideration, with an additional effect size of <20% for neuroleptic drugs (Schneider *et al.* 1990).

These studies are illustrated in Table 16.1. Three of them are large, recent, multicentre studies with 'atypical' neuroleptic agents, which between them have included more than 1000 patients (De Deyn *et al.* 1999, Katz *et al.* 1999, Street *et al.* 1999). Subjects for each of these studies were selected on the basis of cut-off scores on standardized instruments for the assessment of BPSD. One of the studies, using olanzapine, failed to demonstrate a significant advantage over placebo. The other three studies, two using risperidone and one using olanzapine, demonstrated a significant advantage over placebo for the overall reduction in BPSD.

As each of these reports group together different BPSD, which are probably disparate, to give an overall composite score, it is difficult to estimate the effectiveness of these agents specifically for psychotic symptoms. Several of the reports, however, undertook a secondary analysis of psychosis scores. In two of the studies, the psychosis scores did not improve significantly more in the patients receiving active treatment

Table 16.1 Double-blind, placebo-controlled, randomized trials of neuroleptics for BPSD

Study	Active agent(s)	Duration weeks	Sample size	Mean age (years)	Assessment of outcome	% Significantly improved	Comments
Abse et al. (1960)	chlorpromazine	8	32	75	clinical observation	non-significant	proportions not specified
Hamilton and Bennett (1962)	trifluoperazine	8	27	71	BAS	22% vs 0%	all medically unwell
Hamilton and Bennett (1962)	acetophonazine	8	19	71	clinical observation	64% vs 20%	–
Sugarman et al. (1964)	haloperidol	6	18	72	unvalidated checklist	89% vs 67%	–
Cahn and Diestfeldt (1973)	penfluridol		36	81	BOP	non-significant	proportions not specified
Rada and Kellner (1976)	thiothixine		42	76	BPRS	59% vs 55%	–
Petrie et al. (1982)	haloperidol, loxepine	8	61	73	BPRS	65% vs 58% vs 36%	–
Barnes et al. (1982)	thioridozine, loxepine	8	53	83	BPRS	59% vs 68% vs 47%	–
Finkel et al. (1995)	thiothixene	11	33	85	CMAI	65% vs 19%	–
Katz et al. (1999)	risperidone	12	435	83	BEHAV-AD	68% vs 61%	overall difference only significant for risperidone 2 mg/day
De Deyn et al. (1999)	risperidone, haloperidol	12	344	81	BEHAV-AD	76% vs 69% vs 61%	–

BAS, Behavioural Assessment Scale; BOP, Beoordingsschaal Oudere Pattienten; BPRS, Brief Psychiatric Rating Scale; CMAI, Cohen-Mansfield Agitation Inventory. Only the CMAI and BEHAV-AD are specifically validated for use with dementia patients, additional active comparison and single-blind trials are reported in the literature.

compared with those taking placebo. In the other two studies (one on risperidone and one on olanzapine), psychosis scores were significantly reduced in people taking the active drug compared with those receiving placebo treatment. As these patients were not selected specifically on the basis of psychotic symptoms, it is unclear how many of the participants were actually experiencing a clinically significant psychotic condition, or what proportion of those people had a meaningful level of improvement.

The only study to specifically select participants suffering from dementia and clinically significant psychosis is a recently completed comparative, double-blind trial of quetiapine and haloperidol, which has not yet been published. The absence of a placebo control group is an important limitation; nevertheless, the trial is important as it is the only one to focus upon clinically significant psychosis. In this 6 week study, both delusions and hallucinations significantly reduced to an equivalent extent in these quetiapine- and haloperidol-treated patients, representing a mean decrease of approximately 50% in delusion and hallucination scores on the Neuropsychiatric Inventory.

A further issue of concern pertains to the short duration of treatment in the majority of studies; usually <3 months. Although, in this short time-frame, it appears that low doses of neuroleptic drugs, particularly the atypical agents, are well tolerated, the issues of longer-term efficacy and safety are not addressed. A number of the trials have indicated the possibility of a small drop in Mini-Mental State Examination score. Although the differences are only of the magnitude of one point, and do not reach significance in any individual studies, the same trend is observed in a number of different reports and may well be highly significant given the short duration of many pharmaceutical trials. It is particularly concerning in the context of work suggesting that neuroleptic agents might accelerate cognitive decline over longer-term follow-up (McShane *et al.* 1997). In addition, short-term efficacy does not necessarily indicate that these agents confer ongoing benefits. One naturalistic follow-up study found no difference in the persistence of psychotic symptoms over 1 year between people taking and not taking neuroleptic agents (Ballard *et al.* 1997). Similarly, the risks of many adverse events will become greater over time. This particularly applies to involuntary neuroleptic-induced movements, such as tardive dyskinesia, and falls. The problems of side effects are reviewed in considerably more detail in Chapter 15.

An additional clinical problem pertains to the discontinuation of neuroleptic agents which have been previously prescribed. There are very few data to inform practice regarding the ideal length of neuroleptic prescription. The discontinuation and crossover phase within one of the risperidone trials (De Deyn *et al.* 1999) did suggest that BPSD may worsen again in a substantial proportion of people when pharmacological intervention is discontinued after 3 months. The majority of relevant information has, however, been obtained from studies in nursing home environments, where long-term prescription of neuroleptic agents has been a major clinical problem, to such an extent that, in the USA, legislation has been introduced to restrict prescribing (Shorr *et al.* 1994). Within these settings a number of reports have suggested that neuroleptic agents can be stopped without any significant exacerbation of BPSD occurring (Bridges-Parlet *et al.* 1997). There is, however, a huge gulf between drugs that have been taken for 3 months, and long-term prescriptions which may have been taken for a number of years. The limited information available makes evidence-based practice guidelines impossible at the moment, and further studies are clearly needed. The issue is complicated even further by the fact that the studies that reported upon discontinuation of neuroleptic agents looked at the overall effects on BPSD rather than the specific effect upon psychosis.

Given the impact of neuroleptic agents upon quality of life and their detrimental side effects, it would appear reasonable to instigate a trial discontinuation period at least once every 3 months, for 2 weeks or longer. It may be helpful to combine this with an individually tailored psychosocial management strategy or a caregiver training programme, to help combat any recurrent BPSD.

One double-blind trial for the treatment of agitation has been undertaken with carbemazepine (Tariot *et al.* 1998), but there are no specific studies of psychosis *per se*. A number of other agents, including benzodiazepines and buspirone, have been evaluated in open or active comparative studies; there is no evidence that any of these agents have an antipsychotic effect in people with dementia.

Encouraging data are starting to emerge from secondary analysis of cholinesterase inhibitor trials, suggesting that 50% or more of patients with psychotic symptoms experience improvement or resolution of psychotic symptoms (Raskind *et al.* 1997, Morris *et al.* 1998). Similar evidence of potential 'antipsychotic activity' is apparent from studies with muscarinic agonists and modulators (Antuono 1995, Bodick *et al.* 1997). In these trials patients were not recruited because of clinically significant psychotic symptoms, so these studies do not constitute sufficient evidence of efficacy, but they do strongly indicate the need for specific treatment trials and may offer important opportunities for safer and more effective pharmacological therapies for psychosis.

A preliminary report (Shea *et al.* 1998) and a double-blind, placebo-controlled trial (McKeith 1999) also indicate that cholinesterase inhibitors may significantly improve psychosis in people suffering from dementia with Lewy bodies. In the McKeith study, BPSD symptoms were the primary outcome measure, hence this does constitute more convincing evidence of efficacy. In patients with dementia with Lewy bodies, given the marked risk of severe neuroleptic sensitivity reactions (Chapter 15; Ballard *et al.* 1998), cholinesterase inhibitors should probably be the treatment of choice if a pharmacological intervention is required.

Practical advice for the instigation of pharmaceutical treatments

If a pharmacological approach is considered necessary, the available evidence favours the two agents that have been tested in the largest, most rigorous clinical trials, namely risperidone and olanzapine. These also have a slightly preferable side-effect profile than some of the older typical agents, although side effects are still common and severe adverse neuroleptic sensitivity reactions have been reported (Ballard *et al.* 1998). These agents should be commenced at the lowest available dose and careful monitoring should be undertaken. Most severe neuroleptic sensitivity reactions occur in the first 2 weeks after a new treatment or dose change has been instigated and many occur within a few doses. Particular vigilance is therefore required during the initial period of prescribing. Although further recommendations are based largely upon clinical experience, the dose should be increased at no more than weekly intervals, again by the smallest increment. Eventual doses should be those used in the large multicentre trials, that is 1 mg/day of risperidone or 5 mg/day of olanzapine. If there is evidence of detrimental adverse side effects, the dose should be reduced or, preferably, the agent stopped. Where extrapyramidal symptoms are experienced, these are probably best managed by reducing the dose rather than prescribing an additional anticholinergic agent such as procyclidine, which might increase confusion.

The majority of treatment trials are for between 6 and 12 weeks. If a favourable therapeutic response is going to occur, it should happen within this period, but may take more than a few weeks. There is no evidence that doses higher than those used in the treatment studies are any more effective, and higher doses should be avoided. Neither is there any evidence to suggest that changing from one neuroleptic agent to another is likely to produce a beneficial treatment effect. If there is no therapeutic response within a 12 week period, the drug should be discontinued. Use of multiple drugs in this group of patients is to be strongly discouraged.

If the symptoms respond well to treatment, a carefully monitored period of discontinuation should be instigated after 3 months. If the symptoms do not improve with the neuroleptic treatment and remain at a severe and distressing level where further pharmacological therapy is considered necessary, there is very little evidence to support any specific strategy. It is therefore important to revisit the 'management

1 Start with the lowest available dose of one of the two newer atypical agents that have been shown to be effective in placebo-controlled clinical trials, i.e. risperidone or olanzapine.

2 Monitor the side effects, particularly closely over the first 2 weeks of treatment.

3 Increase the dose slowly, with the minimum available increment.

4 Aim for eventual doses of risperidone 1 mg/day or olanzapine 5 mg/day.

5 There is no evidence to suggest that higher doses than this should have more effect; higher doses should be avoided.

6 Treatment should be continued for up to 12 weeks to see whether effectiveness is demonstrated.

7 If not effective the treatment should be discontinued, polypharmacy should not be attempted.

8 If a successful response is seen to the treatment, a trial of discontinuation should be instigated after 3 months.

Fig. 16.2 Guidelines for prescription of neuroleptics in people with dementia.

sieve' to ensure that treatment is necessary and that a psychological treatment approach is not appropriate as a solo therapy in the individual circumstances. If this is the case, we would recommend that the original drug was discontinued and a drug from a different class tried. Potentially suitable agents might include carbamazepine, sodium valproate or trazadone. Each should be started at a modest dose and increased in small increments. Any new treatment should be tried for a realistic period of time as a single pharmaceutical strategy, and should be combined with psychosocial management approaches.

If the symptom does not settle and problems remain severe, then hospital admission is preferable to potentially dangerous use of multiple drugs.

There is insufficient evidence to recommend prescription of cholinesterase inhibitor therapies specifically for the management of psychotic symptoms in Alzheimer's disease. However, if a person with a clinical diagnosis of probable Alzheimer's disease, with cognitive deficits that are within the recommended range for therapy, has a psychotic symptom, a cholinesterase inhibitor may be an effective strategy to improve both cognitive and non-cognitive symptoms.

Theoretical justification for pharmacological approach to psychosis in dementia

The evidence relating to the biological basis of psychosis has been reviewed in Chapter 3. It is, however, useful at this point to reflect upon the evidence relating to some of the compounds that are used in clinical practice for the pharmacological treatment of psychosis and other BPSD. The main class of agents used in the treatment of psychosis are neuroleptics, which act mainly as dopamine antagonists, particularly at D2 receptors. Some of the newer 'atypical' neuroleptic agents have a less pronounced action at D2 receptors, but have a more varied neurochemical profile, which includes anatagonism of serotonin (5-hydroxytryptamine, or 5-HT) receptors. The selection of neuroleptic agents as a potential therapy for the psychosis of dementia is based largely upon the assumption that psychosis in dementia has a similar neurochemical basis to schizophrenia, where there is strong circumstantial evidence to implicate the dopaminergic system. The type of psychotic symptoms seen in people with dementia are, however, very different from those which arise in schizophrenia, and there is very limited evidence to support any involvement of dopaminergic systems in the psychotic phenomena of dementia (see Chapter 3). There is, therefore, very little theoretical rationale for the use of neuroleptic agents. While there is some evidence to suggest imbalances of 5-HT and norepinephrine, there is a paucity of placebo-controlled trials to test these hypotheses. Perhaps the clearest evidence from scientific studies relates to the relationship between cholinergic depletion and visual hallucinations. This offers a strong rationale for the potential value of cholinesterase inhibitors, or agents that work upon cholinergic receptors, as potential treatments for visual hallucinations.

Although there are few clinical data, it is important that we critically challenge the rationale for our pharmacological intervention strategies and use scientific hypotheses to identify agents which should be tested in placebo-controlled clinical trials.

Future directions

A great deal of additional emphasis needs to be placed upon rigorous trials of non-pharmacological intervention strategies and trials that combine pharmacotherapy with psychosocial management strategies for people with difficult or treatment-resistant problems. Clinical trials themselves need to focus upon specific, clinically significant and meaningful symptom clusters, such as psychosis rather than a disparate group of BPSD. In addition, given the highest spontaneous resolution rates mirrored by the high placebo response rates within clinical trials, a different type of trial design would be preferable. This would incorporate an initial period of monitoring for 4–6 weeks, possibly combined with a psychosocial management approach. People who continue to experience clinically significant psychotic symptoms could then be randomly assigned to active drug or placebo. This would be much more informative in terms of the actual dilemma with which we are faced in clinical practice.

A further area where we have very sparse information, and where rigorously controlled trials are required, is treatment discontinuation. Studies in this field need to address questions such as the optimal time for a trial of discontinuation, the speed with which discontinuation should be undertaken and the potential value of introducing psychosocial management strategies in conjunction with discontinuing the pharmacological management approach.

Pharmacogenetics may also offer us important opportunities both of predicting response to specific drugs and predicting who will be particularly vulnerable to adverse events. Studies that look at treatment outcome with a variety of agents examining various receptor polymorphisms and polymorphisms of enzymes involved in the metabolism of psychotropic drugs are likely to be particularly important in this regard.

Further scientific studies are required to identify the chemical systems and brain areas involved in the geneses of different psychotic symptoms, to help formulate specific hypotheses about treatment strategies which might be efficacious, and which can then inform the selection of agents for placebo controlled trials. Given the relative lack of efficacy of neuroleptic agents over placebo, this kind of more innovative science-led approach is imperative in order to achieve safer and more effective treatments. From the data so far available it is clear that specific placebo-controlled trials of cholinesterase inhibitors are indicated for people with clinically significant psychotic symptoms.

Summary

- Although psychotic symptoms are extremely common in people with dementia, many are mild, non-distressing or short lived and do not automatically require treatment.

- If treatment is indicated for psychosis in dementia, strategies for practical support, psychosocial interventions or other non-pharmacological approaches may be the least harmful and the most effective.

- If a pharmacological treatment strategy is felt to be the only practicable one, best evidence exists for two of the newer atypical neuroleptic agents, risperidone and olanzipine. Treatment should, however, be initiated cautiously and monitored carefully, with discontinuation after 3 months if the symptom resolves.

- Further work is needed to examine the potential value of cholinesterase inhibitors and anti-psychotic agents, and to develop scientific understanding of the basis of these symptoms to allow us to select patients for trials which can focus upon these symptoms more effectively.

Clinical vignettes dealing with some potential clinical dilemmas

> Mrs X has been experiencing visual hallucinations for the last 2 weeks. They occur one day a week, lasting for approximately 1 h. During this time, Mrs X is extremely distressed. She tends to see figures of children in the house in the late afternoon and then starts to become restless as she believes that she needs to pick up her own children from school. Her husband finds this situation very difficult to deal with as she repeatedly asks to leave the house and he feels the need to restrain her physically at this time to prevent her from going outside, where she would be at potential risk.

This is clearly a difficult situation, where a symptom is causing some distress and practical management problems but has been fairly short lived. Although it is very problematic when it does occur, it happens relatively infrequently. The situation should certainly be evaluated to see whether there is any possible precipitant, such as an acute medical condition (e.g. urinary tract infection) or environmental precipitant to explain the onset of the symptom, or whether any drugs could be exacerbating the symptom. Drugs with anticholinergic effects or antiparkinsonian treatments might, for example, precipitate or exacerbate visual hallucinations. If this is not the case, the situation will need careful consideration. Given the short duration of the symptom, however, it is likely that it will spontaneously remit over a fairly short period of time. In addition, because it only happens only about once per week and at a fairly predictable time of day, it may be possible to offer a helpful support package. This might revolve around a sitter coming for an hour each evening to help with the situation or to allow Mr X to leave the house and have a break from the situation. There may also be some potential for helping Mr X to learn new strategies to distract Mrs X without the practical management difficulties resulting in a direct conflict. Other approaches might be tried, such as taking Mrs X out for a walk. Taking a balanced view of the likely spontaneous remission of this symptom within a defined period against the potentially serious side effects of pharmaceutical treatment, there would be insufficient indication for a pharmacological approach in the first instance. The situation should, however, be carefully monitored and if the symptom becomes much more severe then the optimal approach could be reconsidered. If the symptom persists but the practical management strategies are effective in successfully dealing with the situation then there would appear to be little indication for a pharmacological intervention.

> Mr Y believes that his wife has been plotting against him with other family members. He thinks that she has been stealing his pension and having an affair with a stranger who he believes is living in the loft, and that she therefore wants him out of the house and 'put into a home'. He expresses these beliefs three or four times each day, sometimes for periods of longer than an hour. When he is exhibiting these views he can become extremely distressed and confrontational and on several occasions has been physically aggressive, slapping Mrs Y across the face. These symptoms have recently increased in frequency, although have been present for the last 6 months. Mrs Y feels at the end of her tether and feels that she can no longer cope with the situation.

This is clearly a much more persistent and severe problem which is causing enormous practical management difficulties. However, an immediate pharmacological approach is still not necessarily the best management strategy. Even if a pharmacological approach was to be undertaken in the home environment, it is likely that a marked therapeutic effect would take 4–6 weeks, and due to the current mental state of Mrs Y it is unlikely that she will be unable to cope successfully with the situation for that long. It might therefore appear that Mr and Mrs Y both need a break from the current situation. This could be achieved by respite admission, admission to a hospital unit or perhaps by arranging for Mr X to visit another family member for a period of time. This would then enable much more detailed monitoring to be undertaken. Assessment strategies such as Antecedent Behaviour Consequence diaries could be used to evaluate the severity of the problem and potential triggers/exacerbants. In addition, it would give the opportunity to look at ways of handling individual situations when the symptoms arise and how they can be defused most effectively. If successful approaches can be found, after a few days or weeks away from the situation, Mrs Y could be helped to learn the skills of some of these approaches in order to manage the situation more effectively. If through this period of monitoring the symptoms remain severe or intractable or cannot be substantially reduced by psychosocial intervention strategies, or if it is felt that Mrs Y will not be able to use these strategies successfully to help manage Mr Y's behaviour, pharmacological intervention strategy would probably then be optimal, using some of the guidelines suggested. It may, however, still be worth pursuing the psychosocial approaches to management in conjunction, as a pharmacological approach may improve but not resolve the symptoms. In addition, if Mrs Y is empowered to handle the situation more effectively, it might enable her to look after Mr Y at home for longer, might help them to maintain a caring relationship, and could also facilitate more effective discontinuation of the pharmacological therapy when the psychosis abates.

REFERENCES

Antuono, P. G. (1995). Effectiveness and safety of velnacrine for the treatment of Alzheimer's disease. A double blind, placebo controlled study. Mentane Study Group. *Archives of Internal Medicine*, **155**, 1766–72.

Ballard, C.G. and O'Brien, J. (1999) Pharmacological Treatment of Behavioural and Psychological Signs in Alzheimer's Disease. How good is the evidence for current Pharmacological treatment *BMJ* **319**, 138–9.

Ballard, C. G., Saad, K., Patel, A., Gahir, M., Solis, M., Coope, B. and Wilcock, G. (1995). The prevalence and phenomenology of psychotic symptoms in dementia sufferers. *International Journal of Geriatric Psychiatry*, **10**, 477–85.

Ballard, C., O'Brien, J., Coope, B., Fairbairn, A., Abid, F. and Wilcock, G. (1997). A prospective study of psychotic symptoms in dementia sufferers: psychosis in dementia. *International Psychogeriatrics*, **9**, 57–64.

Ballard, C., McKeith, I., Grace, J. and Holmes, C. (1998). Neuroleptic sensitivity in dementia with Lewy bodies and Alzheimer's disease. *Lancet*, **351**, 1032–3.

Bodick, N. C., Offen, W. W., Shannon, H. E., Satterwhite, J., Lucas, R., Van Lier, R. and Paul, S. M. (1997). The selective muscarinic agonist xanomeline improves both the cognitive deficits and behavioural symptoms of Alzheimer's disease. *Alzheimer Disease and Associated Disorders*, **11** (Suppl. 4), S16–22.

Bridges-Parlet, S., Knopman, D. and Steffes, S. (1997). Withdrawal of neuroleptic medications from institutionalized dementia patients, results of a double-blind baseline-treatment-controlled pilot study. *Journal of Geriatric Psychiatry and Neurology*, **10**, 119–26.

De Deyn, P. P., Rabheru, K., Rasmussen, A., Bocksberger, J. P., Dautzenberg, P.L., Eriksson, S. and Lawlor, B. A. (1999). A randomized trial of risperidone, placebo, and haloperidol for behavioral symptoms of dementia. *Neurology*, **53**, 946–55.

Donaldson, C., Tarrier, N. and Burns, A. (1998). Determinants of carer stress in Alzheimer's disease. *International Journal of Geriatric Psychiatry*, **13**, 248–56.

Gilley, D. W., Whalen, M. E., Wilson, R. S. and Bennett, D. A. (1991). Hallucinations and associated factors in Alzheimer's disease. *Journal of Neuropsychiatry*, **3**, 371–6.

Katz, I. R., Jeste, D. V., Mintzer, J. E., Clyde, C., Napolitano, J. and Brecher, M. (1999). Comparison of risperidone and placebo for psychosis and behavioral disturbances associated with dementia: a randomized, double-blind trial. Risperidone Study Group. *Journal of Clinical Psychiatry*, **60**, 107–15.

McKeith, I. G. Del San T, Anand R, Cicin-sain A, Ferrara R and Spiegel, R. (2000) Rivastigmine provides symptomatic benefit in dementia with lewy bodies: findings from a placebo controlled international multi-center study *Neurology* **54** supplement 3 A450 (Abstract)

McKeith, I. G., Fairbairn, A., Perry, R., Thompson, P. and Perry, E. (1992). Neuroleptic sensitivity in patients with senile dementia of Lewy body type. *British Medical Journal*, **305**, 673–8.

McShane, R., Keene, J., Gedling, K., Fairburn, C., Jacoby, R. and Hope, T. (1997). Do neuro-leptic drugs hasten cognitive decline in dementia: Prospective study with necropsy follow-up. *British Medical Journal*, **314**, 266–70.

Morris, J. C., Cyrus, P. A., Orazem, J., Mas, J., Bieber, F., Ruzicka, B. B. and Gulanski, B. (1998). Metrifonate benefits cognitive, behavioral and global function in patients with Alzheimer's disease. *Neurology*, **50**, 1222–30.

Rabins, P. V., Mace, N. L. and Lucas, M. J. (1982). The impact of dementia on the family. *Journal of the American Medical Society*, **248**, 333–5.

Raskind, M. A., Sadowsky, C. H., Sigmund, W. R., Beitler, P. J. and Austen, S. B. (1997). Effect of Tacrine on language, praxis and noncognitive behavioural problems in Alzheimer's disease. *Archives of Neurology*, **54**, 836–40.

Shea, C., MacKnight, C. and Rockwood, K. (1998). Donepezil for treatment of dementia with Lewy bodies: a case series of nine patients. *International Psychogeriatrics*, **10**, 229–38.

Schneider, L. S., Pollock, V. E. and Lyness, S. A. (1990). A metaanalysis of controlled trials of neuroleptic treatment in dementia. *Journal of the American Geriatric Society*, **38**, 553–63.

Shorr, R., Fought, R. L. and Ray, W. A. (1994). Changes in antipsychotic drug use in nursing homes during implementation of the OBRA-87 regulations. *Journal of the American Medical Association*, **271**, 358–62.

Street, J. S., Clark, W. S., Gannon, K. S., Mitan, S. J., Sanger, T. and Tollefson, G. D. (1999). Olanzapine reduces psychotic symptoms and behavioral disturbances associated with Alzheimer's disease Abstract presented at the Eleventh World Congress of Psychiatry, Hamburg, 6–11 August.

Tanist, P. W., Erb R, Podgorski C, Cox C, Patel S, Jakimovich M and Irvine C (1998) Efficacy and Tolerobility of Carbamazepine from agitation and aggression in dementia. *American Journal of Psychiatry* **155** 54–61.

Tune, L. E., Steele, C. and Cooper, T. (1991). Neuroleptic drugs in the management of behav-ioural symptoms of Alzheimer's disease. *Clinics of North America*, **14**, 353–73.

17 Pharmacotherapy of depression

Introduction

The focus of this chapter will be on the pharmacological management of depression in dementia. Even when a clear diagnosis of clinically significant depression has been made, similar caveats outlined in the previous chapter apply with regard to the need for pharmacological treatment. Careful assessment needs to be made of the distress experienced by the patient and the care givers, the time for which the symptom has been present, and the duration and past history (treated or otherwise) of similar episodes. We saw in Chapter 4 that longitudinal assessment of depression occurring in the context of dementia reveals that only one in five patients experience depression lasting longer than 6 months. While this is clearly a very long period to wait for remission, many studies support the finding of a high rate of spontaneous resolution of depression in patients with dementia (Reifler *et al.* 1989, Ballard *et al.* 1996). Therefore, it is often sensible to wait for a brief period before intervening to see if depressed mood spontaneously remits. Indications for immediate treatment would be a long past history (before referral), significant distress to patient or carer, any indication of intent to self-harm or the presence of a very severe illness (perhaps as indicated by the presence of psychotic features or associated with a significant decline in self-care).

In mild cases of depression, perhaps while one is awaiting the possibility of spontaneous remission, there may be simple social interventions that may help. It is a common clinical observation that patients with dementia become more depressed and anxious when alone than when in company. Simple psychosocial interventions, such as use of a befriender, day care and home care, may improve mood considerably. In extreme cases, a move to a more social environment (such as to a residential home) may prove beneficial, though this course of action needs to be undertaken only cautiously and after full and careful assessment. This is because when depression occurs in the context of dementia, self-care and cognitive function decline and patients naturally become more apathetic and negative. In this context, they may be far more willing to consider that residential care is the answer to their problems. However, upon remission of depression, when their functional and cognitive abilities improve they may well regret this decision and once again wish they were at home, leading to considerable distress if irreversible decisions (e.g. selling the home) have been taken in the meantime.

Antidepressant therapy

If it is decided that a trial of pharmacotherapy is warranted, then the immediate problem is which drug to select. There is an almost overwhelming choice of anti-depressants; as shown in Table 17.1, 29 drugs are currently listed as antidepressants in the *British National Formulary* (BNF 1999). Even in elderly patients without dementia, rational choice of antidepressant remains problematic and extremely con-troversial. There is a relative paucity of antidepressant studies in the elderly but the limited work to date, which very much parallels work in younger subjects, is that no single antidepressant has demonstrable superiority over another. In cognitively intact elderly subjects, studies have generally shown antidepressants to be more effective than placebo and, usually, shown newer drugs to be as effective as 'gold standard' (usually tricyclic) comparators, though never more so (Gerson *et al.* 1988, Anstey and Brodaty 1995). There is, however, always the problem of whether the newer compounds are really as effective as older tricyclics. Limited data question this by suggesting a superiority for tricyclics over selective serotonin re-uptake inhibitors (SSRIs) when considering melancholic depression in younger cognitively intact patients (Perry 1996). It has also rightly been pointed out that extreme cau-tion is necessary in interpreting results of studies showing no differences between newer drugs and tricyclics, as studies have almost always been underpowered to allow sufficient confidence to conclude definitively that no real differences exist. This important issue will be considered in more detail later.

Pharmacokinetic changes and side effects

Pharmacokinetic changes are covered in Chapter 15. Of particular relevance is the increase during ageing of the proportion of fat to water in the body and a decrease in serum albumin, reducing the capacity for protein binding. Most antidepressants are highly (80–90%) protein bound, an exception being venlafaxine which is only 30% bound. Overall, steady-state plasma concentrations of tricyclic antidepressants are considerably higher in older patients than in younger ones. Of much more impor-tance is an increase with age in variability between individual, such that the plasma concentrations of a tricyclic following a standard oral dose can vary 30-fold between subjects. This makes it extremely difficult to predict a dose that is likely to be thera-peutic for any particular subject. In addition, SSRIs differ considerably in how they are influenced by age. For example, the plasma half-lives of fluvoxamine and fluox-etine are relatively unaffected by age, while the half-lives of paroxetine and the major metabolites of sertraline and citalopram are longer in the elderly than in younger people. Some SSRIs, for example fluoxetine and paroxetine, inhibit the P450 enzyme

Table 17.1 Antidepressants available in the UK as of September 1999

Tricyclic antidepressants	amitriptyline hydrochloride (Lentizol, Tryptizol), amoxapine (Asendis), clomipramine hydrochloride (Anafranil), dothiepin hydrochloride (Prothiaden), doxepin (Sinequan), imipramine hydrochloride (Tofranil), lofepramine (Gamanil), nortriptyline (Allegron), protriptyline hydrochloride (Concordin), trimipramine (Surmontil)
Selective serotonin reuptake inhibitors	fluoxetine (Prozac), citalopram (Cipramil), fluvoxamine maleate (Faverin), paroxetine (Seroxat), sertraline (Lustral)
Selective noradrenergic and serotonergic reuptake inhibitor	venlafaxine (Efexor)
Selective noradrenergic reuptake inhibitor	reboxetine (Edronax)
Related antidipressants	maprotiline hydrochloride (Ludiomil), mianserin hydrochloride (Mianserin), trazodone hydrochloride (Molipaxin), viloxazine hydrochloride (Vivalan)
Other antidepressant drugs	flupenthixol (Fluanxol), tryptophan (Optimax), mirtazepine (Zispin), nefazodone hydrochloride (Dutonin)
Monoamine-oxidase inhibitors	phenelzine (Nardil), isocarboxazid, tranylcypromine (Parnate)
Reversible monoamine-oxidase inhibitors	moclobemide (Manerix)

system, which is responsible for their own metabolism. This leads to non-linear kinetics with increasing drug dose (an increased dose leading to blood concentrations that are even higher than expected).

Arguably the most troublesome side effects of antidepressants in patients with dementia are their antimuscarinic effects, which can exacerbate cognitive impairment and precipitate delirium, and their anti-adrenergic effects, which can cause postural hypotension, potentially leading to falls and fractures (see Chapter 14). As a rule, it is nearly always sensible to avoid compounds with these particular effects (for example, the older tricyclics) in patients with dementia.

Evidence from clinical trials

The important questions are: what is the evidence for efficacy of antidepressants in this particular group, and which drugs have the best evidence to support their prescription in clinical practice? Given the above comments regarding the paucity of double-blind studies in cognitively intact elderly depressed patients, it is hardly surprising that there are even fewer studies of antidepressants in elderly patients with dementia and co-existent depression. Studies that have been published are shown in Table 17.2.

As can be seen, the evidence base is extremely limited. The earliest study was that of Reifler *et al.* (1989), which showed no difference between imipramine and placebo but a very high rate of spontaneous remission, reinforcing the importance of not rushing into pharmacotherapy of patients with dementia. Petracca *et al.* (1996) showed a clear benefit of clomipramine, whilst Nyth and Gottfries (1990) and Nyth

Table 17.2 Double blind controlled studies of depression in patients with dementia

Study	Subjects	Drug	Length of treatment	Result
Reifler et al. 1989	61 subjects with primary degenerative dementia of Alzheimer type, with or without depression	placebo or imipramine to maximum tolerated dose	8 weeks	no significant differences between treatments; there was a high rate of spontaneous remission with both placebo and imipramine; imipramine had a deleterious effect on functional abilities
Nyth and Gottfries 1990	96 with primary degenerative dementia and multi-infarct dementia	placebo or 20 mg of citalopram	1–4 weeks	no significant differences for patients with vascular dementia; for Alzheimer's disease patients, there was no significant difference on MADRAS, though ratings of irritability and depressed mood were significantly improved in patients receiving citalopram
Nyth et al. 1992	149 mild to moderate dementia	placebo or citalopram ≤30 mg/day	6 weeks	citalopram was significantly more effective than placebo with response rates of 50–60% compared with 30%
Olafsson et al. 1992	46 with primary degenerative dementia or multi-infarct dementia	placebo or fluoxetine ≤150 mg/day	6 weeks	no significant effect on a scale of emotional functioning, though a validated depression scale was not used
Fuchs et al. 1993	127 with primary degenerative dementia	placebo or maprotiline ≤75 mg/day	8 weeks	no significant differences between treatments
Roth et al. 1996	694 with DSM-III dementia with or without depression	placebo or 400 mg moclobemide	42 days	moclobemide was significantly better than placebo; there were no difference in side effects between the two groups
Petracca et al. 1996	24 with probable Alzheimer's disease	clomipramine ≤100 mg/day or placebo	6 weeks	remission rates were 30% with placebo and 82% with clomipramine, but 70% of those on clomipramine experienced side effects; few dropped out of the study
Taragano et al. 1997	24 with probable Alzheimer's disease	fluoxetine 10 mg/day or amitriptyline 25 mg/day	45 days	fluoxetine and amitriptyline were equally effective in improving depression in patients with Alzheimer's disease, though fewer patients on amitriptyline (42%) completed the study compared with fluoxetine (78%).
Katona et al 1998	198 with DSM-IIIR dementia	Paroxetine (≤40 mg or imipramine (≤100 mg)	8 weeks	there was no significant difference in efficacy between paroxetine and imipramine; at weeks 4 and 8 (but not end point) reduction in Cornell Depression Scales scores favoured paroxetine

et al. (1992) showed the efficacy of citalopram. In the few studies that have directly compared SSRIs with tricyclics, similar efficacy for both compounds has been demonstrated, but the SSRI were better tolerated. This is particularly the case in the study of Taragano *et al.* (1997), which, despite its limitations (it used small sample sizes), showed that the drop-out rate in the amitriptyline-treated group (58%) was almost three times that in the fluoxetine-treated group (22%). The largest study to date is by Roth *et al.* (1996), who investigated moclobemide and found clear evidence for efficacy and good tolerability for the drug. They also demonstrated a significant improvement in cognitive function of people taking this drug, though of course this is likely to be accounted for by the improvement in depression rather than a specific cognitive enhancing effect of moclobemide.

Rational choice of antidepressant for patients with dementia

How then, should clinicians approach the choice of which drug should be prescribed for elderly patients with dementia who develop a clinically significant depression? As with cognitively intact elderly patients, there is no universal consensus on this issue. If one accepts that no single antidepressant has demonstrable superiority over another in terms of efficacy, then the choice of a first-line agent will always remain a difficult, controversial and often idiosyncratic one. In patients with dementia, because of the dangers of antimuscarinic, cardiotoxic and hypertensive effects, it is very unwise to prescribe tricyclics and these drugs should generally be avoided. This is particularly important since there are often extreme cost pressures to prescribe older drugs. These are illustrated in Table 17.3, which shows that the cost of treating a patient for 30 days with an antidepressant varies 18-fold from £2.43 for 150 mg of amitriptyline to £42.83 for 150 mg of venlafaxine (BNF 1999). The issue of drug costs, however, is not the same as that of cost effectiveness and, although no work has specifically been done in patients with dementia, the notion that newer drugs are more expensive overall has been challenged by several economic analyses. These analyses take account of all underlying costs of treating depression, rather than simply drug costs; generally they show either similar costs overall or even an economic advantage of newer compounds over older drugs. For example, Jonsson and Bebbington (1994) found that the cost per successfully treated patient (in this case cognitively intact younger subjects) was lower for paroxetine (£824) than for imipramine (£1024), while Montgomery *et al.* (1996) found that overall annual costs were lower for nefazodone (£219) than for imipramine (£254). The main reason for these, at first surprising, findings are that the greater costs of newer compounds are offset by higher costs of 'treatment failure' because of higher dropout rates from older drugs. Costs of treatment failure include not only the cost of switching to another antidepressant but also specialist referral, hospital admission for some patients and further expensive treatments (e.g. ECT) in some cases with the continued expense of remaining ill. In addition, the cost of overdose with older tricyclics has been shown to be up to four times greater than that with newer

Table 17.3 Cost of treating depression for 30 days with selected antidepressants using a typical daily dose

Drug name	Dose (mg)	Cost (UK£)
Amitriptyline	150	2.43
Citalopram	20	17.99
Dothiepin	150	6.02
Fluoxetine	20	20.77
Lofepramine	210	15.81
Mirtazapine	30	25.71
Moclobemide	300	21.00
Nefazadone	400	18.00
Paroxetine	20	20.77
Reboxetine	8	19.80
Sertraline	50 or 100	28.40
Venlafaxine	75	21.41
	150	42.83

Costs listed are taken from the British National Formulary (BNF 1999).

drugs, largely because of a longer hospital stay. These economic analyses can certainly be criticized and, most importantly, have not been conducted in elderly depressed patients and certainly not in elderly patients with dementia and co-existent depression. However, it is an important point to note that drugs that are more expensive at first sight do not necessarily lead to greater healthcare costs overall.

When considering cognitively intact patients, Porter and O'Brien (1998) have argued that rational choice of antidepressant can be made after consideration of several factors as shown in Table 17.4. Similar principles are applicable to patients with dementia. If a subject has had a previous episode of depression which responded well to a particular agent, and which the patient could tolerate, there would seem to be no good reason not to prescribe the same drug again unless some clinical change has occurred to influence drug prescribing (for example the development of cardiac disease, worsening cognitive impairment or concurrent medication). Similarly, if a patient has been shown to be intolerant of a particular drug, there would be little point in trying this again unless, for example, the cause of the intolerance was clear (e.g. injudicious use of a particularly high starting dose). Concurrent physical illness and concurrent medication and possible interactions will be important factors in determining choice of compounds. For example, for patients on warfarin it may be sensible to avoid drugs such as fluvoxamine and, in patients who insist on continuing to drink large quantities of alcohol, drugs that have relatively few interactions (e.g. citalopram) may be preferable. Compliance is clearly an important issue and drugs with once-a-day dosing may have major advantages in patients with cognitive impairment. Toxicity in overdose is also a consideration in patients who present with suicidal intent.

Overall, from the results of the few studies conducted in patients with dementia (Table 17.2), it would seem possible to draw broad conclusions. Firstly, despite the

Table 17.4 Factors to consider when selecting an antidepressant drug for an elderly subject (after Porter and O'Brien 1998)

- history of response of previous episode to a particular agent
- history of tolerance (or intolerance) to particular drugs
- type of depression (agitated/retarded)
- concomitant drug treatment and possible drug interactions
- compliance
- concurrent physical illness
- liability to particular side-effects, such as hypotension, cognitive impairment and sedation

high placebo response, there is evidence that tricyclic, SSRIs and moclobemide are all effective in elderly patients with depression and dementia. Secondly, no particular drug has demonstrable superiority in terms of efficacy, though SSRIs and moclobemide are better tolerated than older tricyclics. Evidence to date seems to favour SSRIs (particularly citalopram, fluoxetine and paroxetine) and moclobemide, so it is suggested that these agents should be the drugs of first choice in the pharmacotherapy of patients with dementia. After due consideration of concurrent physical illnesses, concomitant drug therapy and associated factors, antidepressants should be started at the lowest recommended dose for the elderly and titrated cautiously against both clinical response and side-effect profile. Elderly patients with dementia may sometimes respond to low doses of drug, but, because of the large variability between subjects in plasma concentration of a drug after a single oral dose, some patients may require much higher doses. While one must be cautious with dose adjustment, it is equally important not to undertreat patients.

Treatment of resistant depression

In cognitively intact subjects, several strategies have been suggested for the management of depressed patients who do not respond to the usual dose of a single antidepressant given for an adequate length of time (usually 6–8 weeks in the elderly). These include:

- augmentation with lithium, T3 or anticonvulsants;
- changing to another antidepressant;
- giving an SSRI in addition to a tricyclic (which is not recommended when compounds such as venlafaxine exist);
- the use of ECT and other agents including pindolol, buspirone and amphetamine.

A comprehensive review of evidence in younger patients (Schweitzer *et al.* 1997) concluded that solid evidence in the form of well conducted double-blind studies was only available for augmentation with lithium, T3 and ECT. In cognitively intact patients, lithium augmentation leads to response in 20–60% of elderly treatment-resistant patients (Zimmer *et al.* 1991, Flint and Rifat 1994, Reynolds *et al.* 1996).

There have been no studies of treatment-resistant depression in patients with dementia. If patients do not respond to a full dose of a single antidepressant, then it would be reasonable to change to another class of drug (for example, changing from an SSRI to moclobemide). However, any further intervention or augmentation strategies will undoubtedly require specialist referral.

Maintenance treatment

Again, there is no evidence as to how long antidepressants should be continued in patients with dementia who have suffered a depressive episode severe enough to warrant treatment. Experience from cognitively intact elderly subjects shows that continuing full-dose antidepressants for ≥2 years after recovery reduces relapse rates by about 50% (OADIG 1993, Reynolds 1998, Reynolds *et al.* 1999). Direct extrapolation to patients with dementia is fraught with difficulties, not least because ongoing neurodegenerative processes may alter neurotransmitter balances over time but also because high spontaneous resolution rates may make maintenance therapy both less necessary and less effective. Conversely, in patients with what is effectively a terminal illness, optimizing quality of life is extremely important. The simple prescription of a relatively safe and well tolerated medication could prevent several months of misery because of a depressive relapse which may represent a significant portion of the patient's remaining life. On balance, in patients with dementia who respond to pharmacotherapy it would seem prudent to recommend maintenance at a full dose for at least 6–12 months, after which the need for continued medication should be reassessed. If patients have been entirely well, then withdrawal may considered, though it should be accompanied by careful advice for carers to be vigilant with regard to the early signs and symptoms of possible relapse. Given the problems with withdrawal reactions to all classes of antidepressants (see Chapter 14), gradual reduction over a 4–8 week period is recommended, particularly for patients who have been on antidepressants for several months.

Clinical vignettes

Mrs X, an 84 year old widow with dementia, has had intermittent depressive symptoms for about 3 weeks. Her daughter is concerned about her low mood and is seeking advice and possible treatment. Further enquiry reveals that Mrs X has always been a sociable lady and enjoyed the company of her large family. She adjusted poorly to the loss of her husband 5 years ago even before the onset of Alzheimer's disease, which began some 2 years later and is now of moderate severity. She has a home carer who visits three times a week. Her daughter calls twice a week and reports that her mother brightens up considerably in company, but can be quite distressed on the phone when she is on her own. There are no biological features of depression or suicidal ideation.

This is a mild depression of short duration. Given the reactivity of the mood, and the short duration of the history, immediate treatment with antidepressants would not be warranted. The suggestion that much of the low mood is situational and better in company, in a lady who has previously always been sociable, would indicate that social interventions should be tried in the first instance. These may include attendance at a day centre and perhaps increased home care or the use of a befriender. The need for antidepressant therapy should be reviewed in 4–6 weeks but in such a case it is highly likely that, in the face of psychosocial interventions, antidepressant therapy will not be needed after this period.

> Mr X is a 68 year old married man with vascular dementia which started with a stroke about 18 months previously. He walks with a frame and is prone to falls. Over the last 2 months he has become increasingly depressed; his wife describes him as having almost persistent low mood and tearfulness, which is worse in the mornings. On occasions he has even said that he does not believe life to be worth living. His appetite has declined and he has refused to go to his usual day centre, saying that he does not like it any more. From his past history, it is clear that he suffered a depressive episode 8 years previously after his retirement, though this responded well to a 6 month course of amitriptyline (100 mg once daily). His current medication is aspirin 75 mg once daily and warfarin.

This man has a more severe and persistent depression. In the face of the past history of good response to an antidepressant, it would be prudent to treat sooner rather than later with pharmacotherapy. The previous episode responded well to amitriptyline. At first sight, this would seem the first-choice drug to use now. However, since this time Mr X has had strokes and developed a vascular dementia. He would now be quite prone to the deleterious effects of the antimuscarinic profile of amitriptyline in terms of cognitive deterioration and, because of his walking difficulties, may be more prone to postural hypotensive effects, so the danger of a serious fall, with subsequent hip fracture, would be high. It would, therefore, probably be more appropriate to treat Mr X with one of the SSRIs or with moclobemide. As he is also on warfarin, it may be sensible to avoid fluvoxamine, fluoxetine and sertraline, which inhibit the P450 system responsible for its metabolism and paroxetine, citalopram or moclobemide would be suitable alternatives.

Mr X was subsequently started on citalopram 20 mg per day for 3 weeks with no effect. The dose was then increased to 40 mg, but after a further 3 weeks Mr X remains depressed. He has now been on citalopram for 6 weeks, though only 3 weeks at the higher dose. Given that response to antidepressants is often delayed in elderly subjects, it may be worth persisting for another few weeks. However, if no response is seen, then It might be worth trying another agent of a different class, such as moclobemide. Because of the possibility of interactions, at least a week must be left between ceasing the citalopram and starting moclobemide (see Chapter 15). If no response to the depression is seen after 3–4 weeks of moclobemide treatment, then specialist referral should be sought. Specialist referral may also be necessary at an earlier stage during treatment for a number of reasons, which would include:

worsening severity of depression, psychotic features, carer stress, definite suicidal ideation, severe weight loss or reduced fluid intake.

REFERENCES

Anstey, K. and Brodaty, H. (1995). Antidepressants and the elderly: double-blind trials 1987–1992. *International Journal of Geriatric Psychiatry*, **10**, 265–79.

Ballard, C. G., Patel, A., Solis, M., Lowe, K. and Wilcock, G. (1996). A one-year follow-up study of depression in dementia sufferers. *British Journal of Psychiatry*, **168**, 287–91.

BNF (1999): *British National Formulary*. Pharmaceutical Press, Wallingford.

Flint, A. J. and Rifat, S. L. (1994). A prospective study of lithium augmentation in antidepressant-resistant geriatric depression. *Journal of Clinical Psychopharmacology*, **14**, 353–6.

Fuchs, A., Hehnke, U., Erhart, C., Schell, C., Pramshohler, B., Danniinger, B. and Schautzer, R. *et al.* (1993). Video rating analysis of effect of maprotiline in patients with dementia and depression. *Pharmacopsychiatry*, **26**, 37–41.

Gerson, S. C., Plotkin, D. A. and Jarvik, L. F. (1988). Antidepressant drug studies, 1964 to 1986: empirical evidence for aging patients. *Journal of Clinical Psychopharmacology*, **8**, 311–22.

Jonsson, B. and Bebbington, P. E. (1994). What price depression? The cost of depression and the cost-effectiveness of pharmacological treatment. *British Journal of Psychiatry*, **164**, 665–73.

Katona, C. L., Hunter, B. and Bray, J. (1998). A double-blind comparison of the efficacy and safely of paroxetine and imipramine in the treatment of depression with dementia. *International Journal of Geriatric Psychiatry*, **13**, 100–8.

Montgomery, S. A., Brown, R. E. and Clark, M. (1996). Economic analysis of treating depression with nefazodone v. imipramine. *British Journal of Psychiatry*, **168**, 768–71.

Nyth, A. L. and Gottfries, C. G. (1990). The clinical efficacy of citalopram in treatment of emotional disturbances in dementia disorders. A Nordic multicentre study. *British Journal of Psychiatry*, **157**, 894–901.

Nyth, A. L., Gottfries, C. G., Lyby, K., Smedegaard-Andersen, L., Gylding-Sobroe, J., Kristensen, M., Retsum, H. E., Ofsti, E., Eriksson, S. and Syversen, S. *et al.* (1992). A controlled multicenter clinical study of citalopram and placebo in elderly depressed patients with and without concomitant dementia. *Acta Psychiatrica Scandinavica*, **86**, 138–45.

Old Age Depression Interest Group (OADIG) (1993): How long should the elderly take antidepressants? A double blind placebo-controlled study of continuation/prophylaxis therapy with dothiepin. *British Journal of Psychiatry*, **162**, 175–182.

Olafsson, K., Jorgensen, S., Jensen, H. V., Bille, A., Arup, P. and Andersen, J. (1992). Fluvoxamine in the treatment of demented elderly patients: a double-blind, placebo-controlled study. *Acta Psychiatrica Scandinavica*, **85**, 453–6.

Perry, P. J. (1996). Pharmacotherapy for major depression with melancholic features: relative efficacy of tricyclic versus selective serotonin reuptake inhibitor antidepressants. *Journal of Affective Disorders*, **39**, 1–6.

Petracca, G., Teson, A., Chemerinski, E., Leiguarda, R. and Starkstein, S. E. (1996). A double-blind placebo-controlled study of clomipramine in depressed patients with Alzheimer's disease. *Journal of Neuropsychiatry and Clinical Neurosciences*, **8**, 270–5.

Porter, R. J. and O'Brien, J. T. (1998). SSRIs may well be best treatment for elderly depressed subjects. *British Medical Journal*, **316**, 631.

Reifler, B. V., Teri, L., Raskind, M., Veith, R., Barnes, R., White, E. and McLean, P. *et al.* (1989). Double-blind trial of imipramine in Alzheimer's disease patients with and without depression. *American Journal of Psychiatry*, **146**, 45–9.

Reynolds, C. (1998). Maintenance therapies for late-life recurrent depression:research and review circa 1996. In *Geriatric Psychopharmacology* (Nelson, J., ed.), pp 127–39. Marcel Decker, New York.

Reynolds, C. F. III, Frank, E., Perel, J. M., Mazumdar, S., Drew, M. A., Begley, A., Houck, P. R., Hall, M., Hulsant, B., Shear, M. K., Miller, H. D., Cornes, C. and Kupfer, D. J. (1996). High relapse rate after discontinuation of adjunctive medication for elderly patients with recurrent major depression. *American Journal of Psychiatry*, **153**, 1418–22.

Reynolds, C. F. III, Frank, E., Perel, J. M., Imber, S. D., Cornes, C., Miller M. D., Mazumdar, S., Houch, P. R., Drew, M. D., Stack, J. A., Pollock, B. G. and Kupfer, D. J. (1999). Nortriptyline and interpersonal psychotherapy as maintenance therapies for recurrent major depression: a randomized controlled trial in patients older than 59 years. *Journal of the American Medical Association*, **281**, 39–45.

Roth, M., Mountjoy, C. Q. and Amrein, R. (1996). Moclobemide in elderly patients with cognitive decline and depression: an international double-blind, placebo-controlled trial. *British Journal of Psychiatry*, **168**, 149–57.

Schweitzer, I., Tuckwell, V. and Johnson, G. (1997). A review of the use of augmentation therapy for the treatment of resistant depression: implications for the clinician. *Australian and New Zealand Journal of Psychiatry*, **31**, 340–52. [Erratum: *Australian and New Zealand Journal of Psychiatry*, **31**, 787.]

Taragano, F. E., Lyketsos, C. G., Mangone, C. A., Allegri, R. F. and Comesana-Diaz, E. (1997). A double-blind, randomized, fixed-dose trial of fluoxetine vs. amitriptyline in the treatment of major depression complicating Alzheimer's disease. *Psychosomatics*, **38**, 246–52.

Zimmer, B., Rosen, J., Thornton, J. E., Perel, J. M. and Reynolds, C. F. (1991). Adjunctive lithium carbonate in nortriptyline-resistant elderly depressed patients. *Journal of Clinical Psychopharmacology*, **11**, 254–6.

18 Pharmacotherapy of agitation, aggression and restlessness

Introduction

The majority of treatment trials have grouped together different behavioural and psychological symptoms in dementia (BPSD), as discussed in Chapter 3. As the trials of neuroleptics are covered in detail in that chapter, the focus of this chapter will be mainly on the use of non-neuroleptic drug treatments. The use of varying and overlapping terminologies makes it difficult on occasion to pull the literature together in a meaningful way. Most studies combine different BPSD syndromes, whilst others focus upon symptom clusters such as agitation. Others evaluate the treatment of specific symptoms, such as aggression or restlessness. Practical principles of psychotropic prescribing for the management of aggression and restlessness in the elderly with dementia will be outlined and a number of cases will be used to illustrate key points in clinical management.

One of the major difficulties in this area has been a tendency to regard BPSD as a homogeneous group of symptoms with similar underlying mechanisms. There is growing evidence that these symptoms may have a different neurobiological basis and are therefore likely to respond to different classes of drugs or different doses of the same medication. This issue was highlighted in a recent *British Medical Journal* editorial (Ballard and O'Brien 1999).

Clear evidence from the available literature is emerging slowly. The situation is compounded by a number of variables. There are relatively few double-blind placebo-controlled trials in this area and clinical trials have been mainly an open design. These trials have been small with insufficient numbers of patients to make reasonable power calculations. The tendency to cluster together groups of disparate symptoms in treatment trials continues to occur. A landmark review by Schneider and Sobin (1991) has been supplemented more recently by small double-blind control studies.

Neuroleptics

In-depth reviews of these compounds are given in Chapters 14 and 15. However, a brief overview will be given with an emphasis on the use of these drugs in aggression and restlessness. There are two broad categories:

(1)   Conventional or 'typical' neuroleptics, which are mainly dopamine D2 blockers and include such agents as haloperidol, thioridazine and trifluoperazine. These agents differ mainly in their side-effect profile, with extrapyramidal side effects being common.

(2)   'Atypical' neuroleptics are a range of newer drugs which are mainly 5-hydroxytryptamine (5-HT) 2A and dopamine D2 antagonists, and include risperidone, olanzapine and quetiapine. They have much a lower incidence of extrapyramidal side effects and are generally much better tolerated by elderly patients.

Conventional neuroleptics are the most commonly prescribed psychotropics to patients with dementia in nursing-home environments (Ray et al. 1980, Gilleard et al. 1983). Despite their widespread use, their beneficial effects are modest, with only 18% of patients responding more with active drug than with placebo (Schneider et al. 1990). The adverse side effects of these drugs are well known, and include extrapyramidal side effects and postural hypotension (secondary to D2 blockade and α-adrenergic blockade, respectively) and the problematic effects of anticholinergic blockade. Recently these drugs have been associated with worsening cognition and more rapid deterioration (McShane et al. 1997).

Conventional neuroleptics

Studies in randomized control trials have included chlorpromazine, trifluoperazine, acetophenazine, loxapine, thioridazine and thiothixene. In a highly significant recent study, Finkle et al. (1995), using thiothixene, specifically looked at aggressive behaviour in a double-blind trial. They reported a significant reduction in agitated behaviours including a significant reduction in verbal agitation and physically aggressive behaviours in the evening. In another recent study, Devanand et al. (1998) randomized patients to placebo, low-dose haloperidol (0.5–0.75 mg) or standard-dose haloperidol (2–3 mg). The Behavioural Syndrome Scale for Dementia (Devanand et al.1992) scores for physical aggression, agitation and physical aggression were measured together with other psychiatric symptoms. This study reported that low-dose haloperidol was comparable to placebo but that standard-dose haloperidol led to significant improvements in behavioural symptoms. However, a significant number of those receiving the standard dose experienced moderate to severe extrapyramidal side effects. There have been very few studies looking at depot antipsychotics for this group of patients. Several authors advocate the use of ultra-low-dose depot neuroleptics (Risse et al. 1987, Gotlieb et al. 1988). This author (Swann) has found the depot neuroleptic fluspiriline to be particularly well tolerated and efficacious in elderly patients in doses in the range 1–2 mg weekly. Fluspiriline is from the same phenothiazine group as trifluoperazine. It is the only depot neuroleptic that is water based, which has the advantage of allowing a rapid washout of drug should problematic side effects occur. Fluspirilene is no longer listed in the *British National Formulary* due to low demand, but is available on a named-patient basis.

Atypical' antipsychotics

These compounds, which were originally used for younger patients with schizophrenia to minimize troublesome side effects and target negative symptoms, have recently been studied in BPSD. The original 'atypical' antipsychotic, clozapine, was originally launched in the mid-1970s but was withdrawn because of leucopenia. In the late 1980s it was reintroduced on a named-patient basis with close haematological monitoring. Clozapine has limited application in the elderly because of its strong anticholingeric side effects. In a small study (Oberholzer *et al.* 1992), seven of 18 severely demented patients had a favourable response with low doses of clozapine (75 mg/day was the maximum dose). Currently the most extensive evidence base of any antipsychotic is for risperidone, with published data on 969 patients involved in two randomized double-blind placebo-controlled trials. (De Deyn *et al.* 1999, Katz *et al.* 1999). Although both trials clustered diverse behavioural and psychiatric symptoms, their size ensures their importance in the literature. The overall reduction in BPSD was significantly better with risperidone than with placebo. Secondary analysis showed reductions in psychosis and aggression. The studies suggest a dose of 1–1.5 mg/day. Doses of ≥2 mg result in significant extrapyramidal side effects. The studies therefore indicate a narrow therapeutic window for risperidone. The study by De Deyn *et al.* compared risperidone with haloperidol and found significantly greater severity of extrapyramidal side effects in patients on haloperidol.

The original 'atypical' neuroleptic, olanzapine, shows similar efficacy to risperidone (Street *et al.* 1999). This study, of 260 patients, has been published only in abstract form, and suffers from a drawback similar to those mentioned above, namely the clustering of disparate BPSD.

Anticonvulsants

Carbamazepine

This is a tricyclic compound that has been available since 1974. Primarily an anticonvulsant, its main action is as a postulated benzodiazepine receptor agonist located on the γ-amino butyric acid (GABA) receptor complex. Proposed mechanisms of action in aggression include an anti-kindling effect and an increase in firing from the locus ceruleus.

Carbamazepine is now used for a wide range of different clinical disorders, including seizure disorders, trigeminal neuralgia and chronic pain syndromes. In psy-

---

Box 18.1   Practical clinical aspects—'atypical' neuroleptics

---

Risperidone   available in liquid form
               doses as low as 0.25 mg can be given
               0.25 mg tablet is now available
               narrow therapeutic window (1–1.5 mg/day)
               more extrapyramidal side effects at doses of >2 mg/day
               causes less weight gain than other antipsychotics

Olanzapine   2.5 mg tablets now available
               causes more weight gain than other antipsychotics
               sedative medication
               theoretical anticholinergic properties

Quietapine   starting dose: 25 mg
               extrapyramidal side effects *rare*
               may be the preferred antipsychotic in Parkinson's disease
               higher effective antipsychotic dosage possible without extrapyrimidal side effects

---

chiatric practice it is indicated in prophylaxis of bipolar disorder, the treatment of rapid cycling disorder and acute mania.

There were early reports of its usefulness for treating agitation, irritability, aggression and impulsivity in schizophrenia and mild learning difficulties (Neppe 1983, Yassa and Du Pont 1983, McAllister 1985). There then followed a number of case reports describing significant improvement in agitated behaviour in patients with dementia (Anton *et al.* 1986, Essa 1986, Leibovici and Tariot 1988). There have also been two case reports of hypersexuality, rage and aggression being reduced in in patients with Kluver–Bucy syndrome when treated with carbamazepine (Hooshmand *et al.* 1974, Stewart 1985).

These were followed by some open studies with small numbers of patients who typically did not respond to conventional neuroleptics or were intolerant of these compounds (Patterson 1987, 1998, Marin and Greenwald 1989, Gleason and Schneider 1990). There are suggestions that carbamazepine may be useful where neuroleptics have been ineffective (Gleason and Schneider 1990, Lemke 1995). The first double-blind placebo-controlled crossover study (Chambers *et al.* 1982) reported no overall benefit of carbamazepine. In this paper, the 19 demented patients studied had mainly wandering behaviours with a minority showing aggression. The negative results of this study may be related to this initial low level of aggression or to the short duration of treatment (4 weeks). A preliminary placebo-controlled trial, involving 25 nursing home residents, did show significant reductions in physical agitation, anxiety and irritability during carbamazepine treatment (Tariot *et al.* 1994). The same group published the full results of their randomized, double-blind, placebo-controlled, parallel group study 4 years later, showing significant reductions in agitation and hostility with carbamazepine (Tariot *et al.* 1998). This well designed study targeted patients with specific behavioural problems. Patients were in the severely demented range (MMSE 6) and a modal dose of 300 mg carbamazepine was used. The study reported that women responded better than men and that there was a decrease in extra nursing time . In a further small placebo-controlled study, doses of ≤600 mg/day were tolerated by frail demented patients (Cooney *et al.* 1996).

Sodium valproate

Valproate is a carboxylic acid derivative that acts by reducing the catabolism of GABA. Its psychiatric indications include the prophylaxis of mood disorders and the treatment of acute mania. There have been a number of open trials using sodium valproate for the treatment of behavioural disorders in dementia in recent years

---

Box 18.2 Practical clinical aspects—carbamazepine

- start low (100 mg *nocte*); if necessary, increase in 100 mg steps every 2–3 weeks according to response
- maximum dose 300 mg *nocte*
- common side effects include sedation, transient leucopenia (10% in first 2 weeks), skin rashes (5%), Syndrome of Inappropriate AntiDiuretic Hormone, ataxia, diplopia (effects on central nervous system (CNS) are dose related)
- rare side effects include aplastic anaemia, hepatotoxicity (regularly check Full Blood Count and liver blood tests) cardiac conduction problems
- consider carbamazepine for episodic aggression and if the clinical picture suggests seizure disorder (see case vignette of Miss B); may be more effective in women and in manic-like symptoms
- may be less useful if psychosis or wandering is present
- common interactions with other drugs: avoid MAO inhibitors; increases CNS effects of lithium and neuroleptics; as carbamazepine is an enzyme inducer, must be cautious when giving it to people taking phenytoin etc.

(Lott *et al.* 1995). In a small study (Mellow *et al.* 1993), three out of four demented patients with behavioural problems improved on valproate. To date there have been no double-blind placebo-controlled trials. Early reports suggest similar indications to carbamazepine.

Trazodone

Trazodone is a triazolopyridine derivative that is pharmacologically distinct from other currently available antidepressants. It is often categorized as a specific serotonergic re-uptake inhibitor (SSRI), but it has other mechanisms including 5-HT 1a, 1c and 2 antagonism and 5-HT1 agonism. It also has actions on other neurotransmitter systems including α_1-adrenergic antagonism and H1 antihistamine properties (Haria *et al.* 1994).

The early literature on the use of trazodone in the management of agitated or aggressive behaviour in elderly patients with dementia consisted mainly of case reports (Greenwald 1986, O'Neil 1986, Simpson and Foster 1986, Tingle 1986, Pinner and Rich 1988, Schneider *et al.* 1989, Houlihan *et al.* 1994). In total these papers involved 55 patients, of whom 45 improved on trazodone. Trazodone compared favourably with buspirone in a placebo-controlled study (Lawlor *et al.* 1994). In a more recent study (Sultzer *et al.* 1997), a double-blind comparison of trazodone and haloperidol, repetitive, verbally, aggressive and oppositional behaviours responded preferentially to trazodone, while patients with psychotic symptoms, excessive motor activity and unwarranted accusations preferentially responded to haloperidol. Trazodone and haloperidol had similar overall efficacy, but there were significantly lower side effects in the trazodone group. The mechanism for this action of Trazodone remains uncertain, but there is no evidence that trazodone's known sedative properties are involved (Sultzer *et al.* 1997). Further support for a specific 5-HT neurotransmitter basis for aggressive behaviours in dementia comes from three case reports in which trazodone and tryphophan were combined

---

Box 18.3   Practical clinical aspects—sodium valproate

- usual dose range: 400–1000 mg/day
- may be better tolerated in frail elderly patients than carbamazepine
- reduced potential interactions with other drugs compared with carbamazepine (concentrations may be increased by aspirin; can displace highly protein-bound drugs; complex interactions with other anticonvulsants)
- side effects: sedation, diarrhoea, tremor, nausea, weight gain, abnormal liver function and (rarely) ataxia, anxiety and hepatitis

(Greenwald *et al.* 1986, O'Neil *et al.* 1986, Wilcock *et al.* 1987). It is postulated that alterations in serotonergic functioning are important in the pathophysiology of aggressive behaviours in people with dementia (Lawlor 1990). It must be emphasized that Trazodone has yet to be examined in a study with a placebo group.

Anxiolytics

Benzodiazepines

Benzodiazepines are commonly prescribed for patients with BPSD. In the UK, specialists tend to use them infrequently because of problems with physical dependence, over-sedation and worsening cognitive functioning. There are a number of placebo-controlled trials which show that benzodiazepines are superior to placebo and have a similar efficacy to neuroleptics (Chesrow *et al.* 1965, Kirven and Montero 1973). Most of these trials have been criticized as having shortcomings in their design (Class *et al.* 1997). There is evidence that longer-acting benzodiazepines should be avoided as there is increased risk of daytime drowsiness and falls with these compounds (Grad 1995, Patel and Tariot 1995). Most clinicians agree that

---

Box 18.4   Practical clinical aspects—trazodone

- starting dose: usually 50 mg *nocte*; this can be increased in 50 mg steps at fortnightly intervals
- effective dose range is usually 100–150 mg/day, but doses up to 300 mg daily can be used if the drug is cautiously increased
- also available as a liquid preparation, which allows doses as low as 25 mg to be given if patient has had previous intolerance of psychotropics (50 mg per 5 ml)
- common side effects: over-sedation and postural hypotension (the latter due to α-adrenergic blockade); over-sedation can be minimized by slow increase in dose as tolerance to the sedative properties of the drug occurs within 5 days
- this author (Swann) has experience of patients rarely developing a paradoxical manic-like syndrome of over-excitement and motor over-activity on trazodone
- main clinical indications: previous intolerance to conventional and atypical neuroleptics, verbal aggression, repetitive and oppositional behaviours; where aggression is in combination with sleep disturbance.

treatment with benzodiazepines should be short-term. However, a small minority of patients may require long-term treatment if other classes of drugs are not tolerated or are ineffectual.

Buspirone

The apparent clinical efficacy of serotonergic agents such as trazodone in BPSD led to some investigators using buspirone, a novel 5-HT 1a partial agonist. A number of case reports and open studies are in the literature (Colenda 1988, Tiller *et al.* 1988). In one placebo-controlled study comparing buspirone and trazodone, buspirone was well tolerated, but had no beneficial effects on agitation (Lawlor *et al.* 1994). Buspirone does reduce anxiety and, given its relatively good tolerability, it may have a useful place in the long-term management of mild anxiety.

Miscellaneous drug classes

Beta-blockers

These drugs have been found to be effective in younger patients with behavioural problems secondary to brain damage. The only controlled studies with propranolol and pindolol have been in brain-injured patients (Greendyke *et al.* 1989). There have been two uncontrolled reports using these drugs in dementia (Petrie and Ban 1981, Weiler *et al.* 1986). Treatment with beta-blockers can be limited in the elderly because of the frequency of side effects (hypotension and bradycardia).

Box 18.5   Practical clinical aspects—benzodiazepines

- use compounds with short half-lives, e.g. lorazepam and oxazapam
- short-term treatment is preferred; if treatment is for >4 weeks, discontinuation must be slow
- target symptoms: anxiety, irritability and insomnia
- common side effects: over-sedation, ataxia, worsening cognitive impairment and increased risk of falls
- there are occasional paradoxical reactions where marked disinhibition occurs (clinicians tend to avoid their use in disinhibited patients or patients with prominent frontal lobe deficits)
- if intramuscular administration is required, the only compound with reliable intramuscular absorption is lorazepam

---

Selegiline

Selegiline is an irreversible inhibitor of monoamine oxidase B (MAO-B) and is used mainly in the management of Parkinson's disease. A study examined the effects of a low dose (10 mg) of selegiline, which only has MAO-B effects, compared with a high dose (40 mg), which inhibits both MAO-A and MAO-B. Selective improvements in the Brief Psychiatric Rating Scale for the lower dose group was reported (Tariot *et al.* 1987). This suggests that MAO-B may be involved in behavioural disturbances in dementia. In a small single-blind trial using selegiline 10 mg/day, significant improvements were described in cognition, carer stress, psychotic symptoms and activity disturbances (Goad *et al.* 1992). However, the largest and most recent placebo-controlled study showed no effect of selegiline treatment (Burke *et al.* 1993). A criticism of the study was that the patients selected did not exhibit psychiatric or behavioural symptoms.

Sex hormones

It has been suggested in animal studies that physical aggression in males may be linked to testosterone. This can be reduced by giving oestrogens or anti-androgen drugs. There are some case reports in the literature describing the use of oestrogen, which was found to decrease physically aggressive behaviour in demented elderly men (Kyomen *et al.* 1991). Another case report suggests the use of intramuscular medroxyprogesterone acetate (MPA) every 2 weeks. These three patients exhibited inappropriate hypersexual activity, which improved significantly when they were given MPA (Weiner *et al.* 1992).

Cholinesterase inhibitors

Possibly the most exciting advance in the drug treatment of BPSD is the unexpected success in the amelioration of these symptoms in patients treated with cholinesterase inhibitors for cognitive enhancement. The therapeutic effects of these compounds in the treatment of psychosis is described in Chapter 15. Tacrine, the first cholinesterase inhibitor to receive a licence in the USA (it has not been licensed in the UK) has been shown to significantly reduce apathy and aberrant motor activity (Kaufer *et al.* 1996). Patients with moderate dementia (MMSE 11–20) had improvements in behaviour while those in the more severe range (MMSE <10) became less apathetic (Kaufer *et al.* 1998b). Donepezil, which was licensed in the UK in 1997, has similar effects (Kaufer *et al.* 1998a), with overall reductions in the Neuropsychiatric Inventory (Cummings *et al.* 1994). Initial analysis of rivastigmine in dementia with Lewy bodies significantly reduced apathy, delusions and visual hallucinations (McKeith *et al.* 2000).

General principles of prescribing for aggression

These are illustrated in Figure 18.1.

Is treatment necessary?

- is the patient suffering or distressed?
- are the caregivers distressed?
- are there major management problems?
- have the symptoms developed recently? (they may resolve soon)
- are the symptoms intermittent?
- 'inappropriate behaviour'—inappropriate for whom?

If treatement is necessary—is drug treatment required?

- could the situation be managed by increased practical support to caregiver or patient?
- are there specific psychosocial interventions which may be appropriate?

If the above filters have been passed through, a careful choice and monitored trial of medication is indicated.

Basic principles of drug treatment in the elderly

- 'start low and go slow'
- use the smallest effective dose
- have a clear treatment aim
- discontinue if there is no discernible benefit
- avoid polypharmacy

Case vignettes

> Mrs A is an 80 year old widow who is living alone in sheltered accommodation. She has a diagnosis of Alzheimer's disease, which had been present for 3 years. Mrs A was accusing her main carer—her daughter—of stealing money from her and altering her medication in order to poison her. She also believed that the rest of the family were colluding with this daughter. There have been some episodes where she had left the house in the small hours of the morning and had been found by the police. Because of the degree of risk she was placed in residential care. The first few days went well, but Mrs A was becoming verbally and physically aggressive towards the care staff and towards also members of the family if they visited. Most of the time she would appear reasonably content, but suddenly she would become distressed, demand to go home and physically assault other residents and the care staff. It was not possible to distract her during these episodes. The home requested that the GP referred her to the Old Age Psychiatry Service, saying that they were no longer able to manage her and wished her to be transferred to another home.

Assessment of Mrs A revealed evidence of fluctuating paranoid beliefs regarding her family, irritable mood and a number of preoccupations. One such preoccupation was with her overcoat. Upon being admitted to the home, her family had bought her a new coat and taken away her old one. Unfortunately she did not recognize the new coat as her own. She also believed that the care staff were trying to harm her and were keeping her prisoner. When the care staff looked at precipitating factors to these behaviours it was clear that the episodes usually occurred after the family had visited (often in large groups, of four or five members). The family agreed to limit their visits to one or two people once a week to allow Mrs A to settle into her new home. They also brought her old coat back and took away the new one. Mrs A was started on risperidone 0.5 mg *nocte*, which was slowly increased to 0.5 mg *mane* and 1 mg *nocte*. Over the course of 3 weeks, Mrs A's suspiciousness, irritability and paranoid beliefs diminished. She was able to tolerate the visits from her family without these precipitating aggressive outbursts. The family were able to increase the frequency of their visits slowly, and this was well tolerated. Three months after Mrs A had started taking the risperidone, it was slowly decreased, but Mrs A's paranoid beliefs regarding the carers and her physical aggression returned. Risperidone was therefore continued at a dose of 0.5 mg *mane*, 1 mg *nocte*.

> Miss B, a 75 year old woman with learning difficulties living with her sister was referred to the Old Age Psychiatry Service as her sister was finding it increasingly stressful looking after her. Over the past 2 years, Miss B had become increasingly dependent on her sister and was now no longer able to dress herself and would frequently misidentify her sister. The situation was further compounded by unpredictable episodes of verbal and physical aggression, which seemed to occur mainly at night. Assessment showed clinical evidence of a mild dementia syndrome superimposed on Miss B's learning difficulties. Her GP had started her on a low dose of haloperidol, which had caused some extrapyramidal side effects but had not altered her aggressive behaviour.

Miss B's sister was helped to produce an antecedents, behaviour and consequences (ABC) diary, which revealed some useful information. The episodes of verbal and physical aggression occurred mainly at night and could be directed at any person or objects in the vicinity. They were frequently preceded by some unusual ritualistic behaviour, such as ripping up pieces of paper into increasingly smaller pieces or staring into space in a trance-like manner. After these episodes, which generally lasted 30 min, Miss B often had a deep sleep, from which it was very difficult to rouse her. Her sister would attempt to waken her for her breakfast the next day but she would frequently not rise until mid-morning. Upon wakening she would appear more disorientated than usual and slightly drowsy.

From the ABC diary there were no obvious triggers. A clinical diagnosis of complex partial seizures was made. The paper-ripping ritual was thought to be an automatism and the profoundly deep sleep a post-ictal phenomenon. Miss B was initially given carbamazepine 100 mg *nocte*. The frequency of the episodes reduced. Four weeks later the carbamazepine was increased to 200 mg *nocte* with the virtual elimination of the episodes of bizarre and aggressive behaviour.

> Mr C was a 71 year old man with a known diagnosis of a vascular dementia after a stroke 2 years previously. He had been admitted to the nursing home 2 months before referral. Since his admission to the nursing home, his mood was described as irritable. He needed nursing assistance with his personal hygiene and toileting. During these periods of intimate care he would become verbally and physically aggressive towards his carers. He also had broken sleep and would waken several times during the night and go into other residents' rooms. He commonly became physically aggressive to the care staff when they redirected him to his own room. His GP has been called in and prescribed thioridiazine, which made him more confused and drowsy. He then had a trial of haloperidol, which caused marked extrapyramidal side effects.

On examination of Mr C there was evidence of an old right hemiplegia, a mild expressive dysphasia and significant receptive dysphasia. Mr C was able to understand one-stage commands but not more complex two- or three-stage commands. He was also quite deaf—his hearing aid had been lost when he moved into the nursing home and he had not obtained a replacement. The nursing home was fairly new and had relatively unskilled and untrained care assistants.

The initial management was to improve communication by replacing Mr C's hearing aid. The carers were given brief training on the nature of Mr C's difficulties. Advice was given on communication using clear, unambiguous statements, particularly when carers needed to attend to his personal care. Following these interventions the situation improved slightly, but Mr C still had a pervasive irritability, which could easily escalate into severe aggression when he required nursing interventions. He continued to have broken sleep and episodes of physical aggressive behaviour towards the night staff when they were directing him back towards his room. He was started on trazodone liquid, 25 mg *nocte*, which gradually increased in 25 mg steps on a weekly basis. Mr C tolerated this well. Three weeks later, on 25 mg *mane*, 50 mg *nocte*, his irritable mood and broken sleep had improved. The trazodone was slowly reduced 3 months later, but Mr C's broken sleep and nocturnal aggressive behaviours returned. Trazodone was therefore reintroduced at night; Mr C is currently maintained on trazodone 50 mg *nocte*.

REFERENCES

Aisen, P. S., Johannsen, D. J. and Marin, D. B. (1993). Trazodone for behavioural disturbance in dementia. *American Journal of Geriatric Psychiatry*, **1**, 349–50.

Anton, R. F., Waid, L. R., Fossey, M. and AuBuchan, P. (1986). Case report of carbamazepine treatment of organic brain syndrome with psychotic features. *Journal of Clinical Psychopharmacology*, **6**, 232–34.

Ballard, C. and O'Brien, J. T. (1999). Pharmacological treatment of behavioural and psycho-logical signs in Alzheimer's disease: how good is the evidence for current pharmacological treatments? *British Medical Journal*, **319**, 138–9.

Burke, W. J., Ranno, A. E., Roccaforte, W. H., Wengol, S. P., Bayer, B. L. and Wilcockson, W. K. L. (1993). Deprenyl in the treatment of mild dementia of Alzheimer type: preliminary results. *Journal of the American Geriatrics Society*, **41**, 367–70.

Chambers, C. A., Bain, J., Rosbottom, R., Ballinger, B. R. and McLaren, S. (1982). Carbamazepine in senile dementia and over-activity—a placebo controlled double-blind trial. *IRCS Medical Science*, **10**, 505–6.

Class, C. A.., Schneider, L. and Farlow, M. R. (1997). Optimal management of behavioural dis-orders associated with dementia. *Drugs and Aging*, **10**, 95–106.

Chesrow, E. J., Kaplitz, S. E., Vetra, A., Bernstein, M., Breme, T. T. and Marquardt, G. H. (1965). A double-blind study of oxazepam in the management of geriatric patients with behavioural problems. *Clinical Medicine*, **72**, 1001–5.

Colenda, C. C. (1988). Buspirone in the treatment of an agitated demented patient. *Lancet, ii*, 1169.

Cooney, C., Mortimer, A. and Smith, A. (1996). Carbamazepine in aggressive behaviour associated with senile dementia. *International Journal of Geriatric Psychiatry*, **11**, 901–5.

Cummings, J. L., Mega, M., Gray, K., Rosenberg-Thompson, S., Carusi, D. A. and Gornbein, J. (1994). The Neuropsychiatric Inventory: comprehensive assessment in psychopathology in dementia. *Neurology*, **44**, 2308–14.

De Deyn, P. P., Rabheru, K., Rasmusseu, A., Bocksberger, J. P., Dautzenberg, P. L. J., Erickson, S. and Lawlor, B. A. (1999). A randomised trial of risperidone, placebo, and haloperidol for behavioural symptoms of dementia. *Neurology*, **53**, 946–55.

Devanand, D.P., Brockingham, C.D., Moody, B.J., Brown, R.R.P., Mayeux, R., Eendicott, J. and Sachein, H.A. (1992). Behavioural Syndromes in Alzheimer's Disease. International Psychogeratics, **4** (Suppl. 2), 161–89.

Devanand, D. P., Marder, K., Michaels, K. S., Sackeim, H. A., Bell, K., Sullivan, M. A., Cooper, T. B., Pelton, G. H. and Mayeux, R. (1998). A randomised, placebo-controlled dose-comparison trial of haloperidol for psychosis and disruptive behaviours in Alzheimer's disease. *American Journal of Psychiatry*, **155**, 1512–20.

Essa, M. (1986). Carbamazepine in dementia. *Journal of Clinical Psychopharmacology*, **6**, 234–6.

Finkle, S. L., Lyons, J. S., Anderson, R. L., Sherrell, K., Davis, J., Cohen-Mansfield, J., Schwartz, A., Gandy, J. and Schnieder, L. S. (1995). A randomised placebo-controlled trial of thiothixene in agitated demented nursing home patients. *International Journal of Geriatric Psychiatry*, **10**, 129–36.

Gilleard, C. J., Morgan, K. and Wade, B. T. (1983). A pattern of neuroleptic use among the institutionalised elderly. *Acta Psychiatrica Scandinavica*, **68**, 403–23.

Gleason, R. P. and Schneider, L. S. (1990). Carbamazepine treatment of agitation in Alzheimer's outpatient refractory to neuroleptics. *Journal of Clinical Psychiatry*, **51**, 115–8.

Goad, D., Davis, C., Liem, D., Fuselier, C. and McCormack, J. (1992). The use of selegiline in Alzheimer's patients with behavioural problems. *Journal of Clinical Psychiatry*, **52**, 342–45.

Gottlieb, G. L., McAlister, T. W. and Gur, R. C. (1988). Depot neuroleptics in the treatment of behavioural disorders in patients with Alzheimer's disease. *Journal of the American Geriatrics Society*, **36**, 619–21.

Grad, R. (1995) Benzodiazepines for insomnia in community dwelling elderly; a review of benefits and risks. *Journal of Family Practice*, **41**, 473–481.

Greendyke, R. M., Berkner, J. P., Webster, J. C. and Gulya, A. (1989). Treatment of behavioural problems with pindolol. *Psychosomatics*, **30**, 161–5.

Greenwald, B. S., Marin, D. B. and Silverman, S. M. (1986). Serotonergic treatment of screaming and banging in dementia. *Lancet, ii*, 1464–5.

Haria, M., Fitton, A. and McTavish, D. (1994). Trazodone a review of its pharmacology, therapeutic use in depression, and therapeutic potential in other disorders. *Drugs and Aging*, **4**, 331–5.

Hooshmand, H., Sepdham, T. and Vries, J. K. (1974). Kluver–Bucy syndrome: successful treatment with carbamazepine. *Journal of the American Medical Association*, **229**, 1782.

Houlihan, D. J., Mulsant, B. H. and Sweet, R. A. (1994). A naturalistic study of trazodone in the treatment of behavioural complications of dementia. *American Journal of Geriatric Psychiatry*, **2**, 78–85.

Katz, I. R., Jeste, D. V., Mintzer, J. E., Clyde, C., Napolitino, J. and Brecher, M. (1999). Comparison of risperidone and placebo for psychosis and behavioural disturbance associated with dementia; a randomised double-blind trial. *Journal of Clinical Psychiatry*, **60**, 107–15.

Kaufer, D. I., Cummings, J. L. and Christie, D. (1996). The effect of tacrine on behavioural symptoms in Alzheimer's disease: an open labelled study. *Journal of Geriatric Psychiatry and Neurology*, **9**, 1–6.

Kaufer, D. I., Catt, K., Pollick, B., Lopez, O. and DeKosky, S. (1998a). Donepezil in Alzheimer's disease: relative cognitive and neuropsychiatric responses and impact on caregiver distress (abstract). *Neurology*, **50**, A89.

Kaufer, D. I., Cummings, J. L. and Christie, D. (1998b). The differential neuropsychiatric symptom responses to tacrine in Alzheimer's disease: relationship to dementia severity. *Journal of Neuropsychiatry and Clinical Neuroscience*, **10**, 55–63.

Kyomen, H. H., Noble, K. W. and Wei, J. Y. (1991). The use of oestrogen to decrease aggressive behaviour in elderly men with dementia. *Journal of the American Geriatrics Society*, **39**, 1110–12.

Kirven, L. E. and Montero, E. F. (1973). Comparison of thioridazine and diazepam in the control of non-psychotic symptoms associated with senility: a double-blind study. *Journal of the American Geriatrics Society*, **21**, 546–51.

Lawlor, B. A. (1990). Serotonin in Alzheimer's disease. *Psychiatric Annals*, **20**, 567–70.

Lawlor, B. A., Radcliffe, J. and Molchan, S. E. (1994). A pilot placebo controlled study of trazodone and buspirone in Alzheimer's disease. *International Journal of Geriatric Psychiatry*, **9**, 55–9.

Leibovici, A. and Tariot, P. N. (1988). Carbamazepine treatment of agitation associated with dementia. *Journal of Geriatric Neuropsychiatry and Neurology*, **1**, 110–12.

Lemke, M. R. (1995). Effects of carbamazepine on agitation in Alzheimer's inpatients refractory to neuroleptics. *Journal of Clinical Psychiatry*, **56**, 354–7.

Lott, A. D., McElroy, S. L. and Keys, M. A. (1995). Valproate in the treatment of behavioural agitation in elderly patients with dementia. *Journal of Neuropsychiatry and Clinical Neuroscience*, **6**, 205–9.

Marin, D. B. (1993). Trazodone for behavioural disturbance in dementia. *American Journal of Geriatric Psychiatry*, **1**, 349–50.

Marin, D. B. and Greenwald, B. S. (1989). Carbamazepine for aggressive agitation in demented patients during nursing care. *American Journal of Psychiatry*, **146**, 805.

Mellow, A. M., Salano-Lopez, C. and Davis, S. (1993). Sodium valproate in the treatment of behavioural disturbance in dementia. *Journal of Geriatric Psychiatry and Neurology*, **6**, 205–9.

McAllister, T. W. (1985). Carbamazepine in mixed frontal lobe and psychiatric disorders. *Journal of Clinical Psychiatry*, **46**, 393–4.

McKeith, I. G., Daniel, S., Ballard, C. G., Swann, A., Fairbairn, A. F. and Perry, E. K. (2000). Recent advances in therapy in dementia with Lewy bodies. Abstract presented at the International Psychogeriatric Association and Royal College of Psychiatrists Faculty of Old Age Conference, Newcastle, UK.

McShane, R., Keene, J. and Fairburn, C. (1997). Issues in the drug treatment for Alzheimer's disease. *Lancet*, **350**, 886–7.

Nair, N. P. V., Ban, T. A., Hontela, S. and Clarke, M. A. (1973). Trazodone in the treatment of organic brain syndromes with special reference to psychogeriatrics. *Current Therapeutic Research*, **15** (Suppl. 10), 769–75.

Neppe, V. M. (1983). Carbamazepine as an adjunctive treatment in nonepileptic chronic inpatients with EEG temporal lobe abnormalities. *Journal of Clinical Psychiatry*, **44**, 326–31.

O'Neil, M., Page, M. and Adkins, W. N. (1986). Tryptophan–trazodone treatment of aggressive behaviour. *Lancet*, **ii**, 859–60.

Oberholzer, A., Hendricksen, C., Monsch, A., Heierli, B. and Stahelin, H. (1992). Safety and effectiveness of low dose clozapine in psychogeriatric inpatients. *International Psychogeriatrics*, **4**, 187–95.

Patel, S. and Tariot, P. N. (1995). Use of benzodiazepines in behavioural disturbed patients: risk:benefit ratio. In *Behavioural Complications in Alzheimer's Disease* (Lawlor, B.A., ed.), pp.153–70. Americian Press, Washington, DC.

Patterson, J. F. (1987). Carbamazepine for assaultative patients with organic brain disease. *Psychosomatics*, **28**, 579–81.

Patterson, J. F. (1998). A preliminary study of carbamazepine in the treatment of assaultative patients with dementia. *Journal of Geriatric Psychiatry and Neurology*, **1**, 21–3.

Petrie, W. M. and Ban, T. A. (1981) Propanolol in organic agitation. *Lancet*, *i*, 324.

Pinner, E. and Rich, C. (1988). Effects of trazodone in aggressive behaviour on seven patients with organic mental disorders. *American Journal of Psychiatry*, **145**, 1295–6.

Ray, W. A., Federspeil, C. F. and Schaffner, W. A. (1980). A study of antipsychotic drug use in nursing homes. Epidemiological evidence suggesting misuse. *American Journal of Public Health*, **70**, 485–91.

Risse, S. C., Lampe, T. H. and Cubberley, L. (1987). Very low dose neuroleptic treatment in two patients with agitation associated with Alzheimer's disease. *Journal of Clinical Psychiatry*, **48**, 208.

Schneider, L. S. and Sobin, P. B. (1991). Non-neuroleptic medications in the management of agitation in Alzheimer's disease and other dementias: a selective review. *International Journal of Geriatric Psychiatry*, **6**, 691–708.

Schneider, L. S., Gleeson, R. P. and Chui, H. C. (1989). Progressive supranuclear palsy with agitation; response to trazodone but not to thiothixine or carbamazepine. *Journal of Geriatric Psychiatry and Neurology*, **2**, 109–12.

Schneider, L. S., Pollock, V. E. and Lyness, S. A. (1990). A meta-analysis of controlled trials of neuroleptic treatment in dementia. *Journal of the American Geriatrics Society*, **38**, 553–63.

Simpson, D. M. and Foster, D. (1986). Improvement in organically disturbed behaviour with trazodone treatment. *Journal of Clinical Psychiatry*, **47**, 191–3.

Stewart, J. T. (1985). Carbamazepine treatment of the patient with Kluver–Bucy syndrome. *Journal of Clinical Psychiatry*, **46**, 496–7.

Street, J. J., Clarke, S. W., Gannon, K. S., Mitan, S. J., Sanger, T. and Tollefson, G. D. (1999). Olanzapine reduces psychotic symptoms and behavioural disturbances associated with Alzheimer's disease. Poster presented at the Twelfth Congress of the European College of Neuropsychopharmacology, London, UK, September 1999.

Sultzer, D. L., Gray, K. F., Gunay, I., Berisford, M. A. and Mahler, M. E. (1997). A double-blind comparison of trazodone and haloperidol in treatment of agitation in patients with dementia. *American Journal of Geriatric Psychiatry*, **5**, 60–69.

Tariot, P. N., Cohen, R. M., Sunderland, T., Newhouse, H. and Yount, D. (1987). L-Deprenyl in Alzheimer's disease. *Archives of General Psychiatry*, **44**, 427–33.

Tariot, P. N., Erb, R., Leibovici, A., Podgorski, C. A., Cox, C., Asnis, J., Kolassa, J. and Irvine, C. (1994). Carbamazepine in the treatment of agitation in nursing home patients with dementia: a preliminary study. *Journal of the American Geriatric Society*, **42**, 1160–66.

Tariot, P. N., Erb, R., Podgorski, C. A., Cox, C., Patel, S., Jakimovich, M. and Irvine, C. (1998). Efficiency and tolerability of carbamazepine for agitation and aggression in dementia. *American Journal of Psychiatry*, **155**, 54–61.

Tiller, J. W. G., Dakis, J. A. and Shaw, J. M. (1988). Short term buspirone treatment of disinhibition in dementia. *Lancet*, *ii*, 570.

Tingle, D. (1986). Trazodone in dementia. *Journal of Clinical Psychiatry*, **47**, 482.

Weiler, P. G., Mungas, D. and Bernick, C. (1986). Propanolol for the control of disruptive behaviour in senile dementia. *Journal of Geriatric Psychiatry and Neurology*, **1**, 226–30.

Weiner, M. F., Denke, M., Williams, K. and Guzman, R. (1992) Intramuscular medroxy-progestrogene acetate for sexual aggression in elderly men. *Lancet*, **339**, 1121–2.

Wilcock, G. K., Stevens, J. and Perkins, A. (1987). Trazodone/tryptophan for aggressive behaviour. *Lancet*, *i*, 929–30.

Yassa, R. and Dupont, D. (1983). Carbamazepine in the treatment of aggressive behaviour in schizophrenic patients: a case report. *Canadian Journal of Psychiatry*, **28**, 568–8.

19 Management of other behavioural and psychological symptoms in dementia

Introduction

As for all behavioural and psychological symptoms in dementia (BPSD), it is important to consider the management sieve (Chapter 3): is the problem severe enough and persistent enough to need intervention? If so can an augmentation of the support package or environment, or a specific psychological intervention, resolve or substantially improve the situation? If conservative measures and non-pharmacological interventions have not been successful, is the problem severe enough to merit a trial of pharmacotherapy? For most of the BPSD considered in this chapter, there is very little evidence pertaining to treatment intervention, other than some notable trials of non-pharmacological approaches for the treatment of abnormal vocalizations. The potential side effects and consequences of drug interventions, particularly with neuroleptic agents, have been highlighted elsewhere (Chapter 15), but are particularly important when considering the absence of any adequate clinical trials.

For any symptom, it is important to make a detailed evaluation of the severity and frequency of the problem and to obtain a detailed description of what the apparent BPSD constitutes. For example, one is often informed that a resident in a care facility is 'shouting constantly', whereas a more detailed assessment may reveal that the person is in fact only exhibiting this symptom for a relatively small portion of the day in specific circumstances. In addition, the volume and content of the 'shouting' are important considerations when making a decision regarding the clinical significance of the problem and the appropriate treatment approach.

Abnormal vocalizations

A detailed evaluation to determine the severity and nature of the problem is essential. This could be undertaken using a standard antecedent, behaviour, consequence (ABC) diary; although we would recommend the Typology of Vocalizations (Cohen-Mansfield and Werner 1997b), which is specifically tailored towards a dimensional assessment of abnormal vocalizations and facilitates the selection of appropriate therapeutic strategies.

There is evidence from preliminary studies to indicate the value of white noise (Burgio et al. 1996), simulated presence, particularly video tapes of family members (Lund et al. 1995), and video tapes that encourage conversation, singing or activities (Lund et al. 1995). Clinical experience also indicates that video tapes depicting things of interest to the individual, such as a football match for someone who has always had a strong interest in this particular sport, can be very effective. In the most comprehensive study, Cohen-Mansfield and Werner (1997a) using a controlled trial design, demonstrated that personalized music, social interaction therapy and simulated presence of family members on video tape all reduced abnormal vocalizations to a significantly greater extent than placebo. Although a standardized treatment approach was adopted, Cohen-Mansfield and Werner (1997a) highlighted the value of a detailed assessment. For example, specific triggers of abnormal vocalizations, such as pain or deafness, were identified for some people; whilst abnormal vocalizations could be triggered either by isolation or crowding in different individuals. Furthermore, vocalizations related to specific needs responded best to social interaction and people distressed by crowded environments obtained benefit from video tapes, while individuals for whom the abnormal vocalization seemed to serve the purpose of self-stimulation were not helped by any of the treatment interventions. Several series of case reports illustrate how individualized assessments can be used to develop specific intervention programmes tailored to the needs of a particular person (Meares and Draper 1999).

Only case studies of pharmacological interventions have been reported in the literature. Improvements have been described following a variety of interventions, including trazadone (Greenwald et al. 1986), L-Tryptophan (Pasion and Kirby 1993), risperidone (Kopala and Honer 1997) and ECT (Carlyle et al. 1991, Snowden et al. 1994). In some people experiencing abnormal vocalizations, an underlying depressive illness may be important (Cohen-Mansfield and Werner 1997), and it is perhaps these individuals who may have responded to antidepressant or ECT treatment. In general, given the extremely high rates of placebo response for most BPSD (Schneider et al. 1990, Ballard and O'Brien 1999), case reports, case series and open trials provide inadequate evidence of efficacy. In situations where the problem is severe and non-pharmacological approaches have been unsuccessful, a careful trial of pharmacotherapy may be indicated. It is important to measure the severity of the abnormal vocalizations carefully before commencing the treatment, so that an informed decision can be made about the benefit of the therapy in relation to its side effects. In this way treatment is only continued if there is clear evidence of efficacy. The sieve from Chapter 3 should be followed, starting with small doses, increasing very cautiously and giving an adequate period of treatment with a single agent. For most people, the first choice of pharmacological agent should probably be an atypical antipsychotic, although this recommendation is based more on experience than evidence. Trazadone may also be an option, particularly if depressive symptoms are identified. A pharmacological approach may be most relevant to people with severe abnormal vocalizations that seem to be motivated by self-stimulation and that have not responded to non-pharmacological treatment. This is certainly an area where current knowledge is inadequate, and placebo-controlled trials are needed.

Some of the early literature recommended differential reinforcement (Spayd and Smyer 1988) or reinforcement coupled with planned ignoring (Brink 1980). Although these behavioural techniques may have some potential value in skilled hands, they are often inappropriately planned in care environments and frequently result in unintentional exacerbation of the problem. Our advice would therefore be to avoid this type of approach and focus on interventions such as social interaction, music/white noise and video tapes, where there is clear evidence of efficacy.

Eating disturbances

It is fairly uncommon for eating disturbances other than loss of appetite to present to clinical services. Potentially dangerous situations can arise when people put non-food substances in their mouths, although this is relatively infrequent and is usually managed successfully by the kind of precautions that would be taken for a small child. Messy eating or drooling can occasionally cause distress to specific caregivers or individuals with dementia, but difficulties can usually be resolved by careful planning of mealtimes, menu selection and planning the type of assistance that is required. Overeating may occur, often because meals are forgotten, but this rarely presents as a clinically significant problem. For individuals with relatively mild cognitive impairment a meal chart or diary may be helpful, where in other circumstances careful planning of the shopping can attenuate the problem.

Poor food intake with subsequent loss of weight increases the risk of skin breakdown and injury, and can be life threatening, particularly if combined with poor fluid intake. As with all problems, a careful assessment is essential. Many people with reduced appetite in the context of dementia have depression (Cullen *et al.* 1997), and a careful evaluation of mood is helpful. If the eating disturbance is thought to be the consequence of a clinically significant depression, then an anti-depressant agent may be beneficial (Chapter 17). In other circumstances a change in food preference may be responsible. This might particularly occur in care facilities with a limited menu choice, and can often be resolved by offering the individual a greater proportion of sweet items. Being fed by another individual can be quite a traumatic experience, and for some people with dementia who require assistance with feeding, the interaction with the care worker or the way in which the feeding process is conducted may cause anxiety or frustration. This can usually be determind without much difficulty by observing interactions during a mealtime. Offering the person with dementia more finger foods or helping the care staff develop an approach to feeding that is more suitable for that individual are usually effective interventions. For people living in their own homes or those residing in care facilities, an unidentified practical problem may be responsible. For example, an individual living at home may have lost their ability to shop or cook, or a person living in a care environment may have lost the skill to cut or chew their food. Once identified, these problems can be addressed by a well planned care package. It should not be forgotten that poor appetite or loss of weight with an adequate appetite could be related to a serious underlying condition, such as a malignancy. Appropriate investigations should be organized if there are any clinical indications of a systemic problem.

Sexual difficulties

Many of the key issues have been summarized in Chapter 7. Most importantly, a detailed evaluation is needed to determine whether the problem is related to an abnormal sexual behaviour, or whether it could have an alternative goal, be an easily corrected misperception or be an expression of the need for affection (Chapter 7). Some of the key issues related to this are explored in the case examples. If a sexual behaviour is confirmed, a detailed assessment using an antecedent, behaviour, consequence (ABC) diary is helpful to determine the severity of the problem and to identify possible triggers or reinforcers. These factors can be very variable in different individual circumstances, and specific interventions should be planned on the basis of the evaluation. Particularly within care environments, if an individual has been expressing abnormal sexual behaviours, demeaning nicknames can sometimes arise. It is important to emphasize to care staff that this is inappropriate and may well have a detrimental impact. Some of the main issues related to assessment and intervention are highlighted in Figure 19.1. For the majority of situations, simple interventions—such as removing the trigger for sexual behaviours, deploying same gender or experienced care staff to assist with personal care tasks or working with care staff regarding a specific approach tailored to the individual situation—are effective. For people living at home with a partner or cared for by care workers in the community, the same principles apply. In unusual circumstances, particularly among people suffering from dementia of the frontal lobe type or those who have experienced frontal lobe injuries, severe sexual disinhibition can pose a threat to the community. In such circumstances compulsory admission for treatment in a hospital facility, and a long-term care plan that involves placement in an appropriate environment, may be necessary.

The above section is based entirely upon good principles of care. There is a very little evidence to inform practice in this area. This is particularly true for aversion therapy, behavioural interventions and pharmacological treatments. Benperidol is sometimes prescribed, although there are no trials specifically in people with dementia. Anti-testosterone agents are sometimes used to reduce sexual drive, although again the evidence in people with dementia is extremely limited, and there are serious ethical considerations regarding consent. There are case reports indicating that specific serotonin re-uptake inhibitors may be helpful (Stewart and Shin 1997).

Communication

1. Sexual expression is a basic human need; it is not necessarily inappropriate for adults of any age to want to express sexual feelings.

2. Discussion among those affected by inappropriate sexual behaviour may help identify the source, result and boundaries of the person's actions. Problems of this nature can be very distressing for all those concerned and additional support may be required.

3. It is important for carers to agree upon a consistent response to unwanted behaviour. If possible, demonstrate the agreed response to all those involved, to avoid misinterpretation. Carers' actions must not be punitive, but should be centred on helping people maintain their dignity and express themselves appropriately.

4. Be aware of the person's dignity when passing on information about incidents. Avoid the use of humour and labelling (for example, stating 'Randy Jane's been at it all morning'). Unkind comments are not only disrespectful to the person, but also fail to illuminate the reasons and extent of the problem.

5. Assess how visitors to the person's home understand the situation. If necessary, provide education and support to alleviate distress and embarrassment.

Organic

1. The person may be seeking to alleviate physical pain through sexual expression. Identification and treatment of physical problems may assist in reducing inappropriate sexual behaviour.

2. In residential care, most physical contact people receive is of a functional nature (for example, help with removal of clothing, assistance with toileting). Inappropriate sexual behaviour may be created by the desire for 'expressive' touch. Acceptable forms of expressive touch may include holding hands and hugging.

3. Therapies such as aromatherapy massage* by qualified carers may provide an alternative form of expressive touch.

4. Sexual contact that is mutually desired in both new and existing couples should be permissible. However, carers must consider the memory loss of the people involved and the effects this may have on their choices, values, judgements and ultimate safety.

Psychological

1. Carers may attempt to identify and, if possible, address the needs being expressed through sexual behaviour. The person may desire affection and closeness, both physical and non-physical. They may also be seeking to alleviate anxiety or depression through physical closeness.

2. It is helpful to consider whether the behaviour is really disruptive and problematic, or whether it is the attitude of staff/relatives that could be adjusted.

3. Private time free of interruptions can be agreed in residential settings.

Environment

1. For sexual behaviour to take place, the provision of private places for people is recommended.

2. Carers in residential settings should knock and wait before entering any person's private room.

3. People who masturbate in front of others should be helped to find their own bedroom area. However, this should be done quietly and compassionately, taking into account the difficulties a person experiences when confused and disorientated.

4. Consider seating arrangements: people who may potentially harrass others can be placed accordingly in order to minimize distress.

5. It may be necessary to keep those who present a particular threat to others within sight of carers.

Fig. 19.1 Inappropriate sexual behaviour. Reproduced with permission of Jason Fisher and Eleanor Cain.

Pharmacological intervention is very rarely indicated and, given the absence of evidence, should be limited to extreme situations.

Case examples

> Mr X lives in a care facility. He frequently walks into the main lounge and starts undoing his trousers. The staff ask him to stop doing this, but he has poor verbal comprehension skills. He is escorted to his room and lies on the bed. He seems restless and reluctant to stay, but is told that 'he has to remain in his room until he can go into the lounge without being randy'. When the care worker returns 30 min later, Mr X has been incontinent of urine. The care worker seems frustrated and informs Mr X that he is constant trouble.

Mr X is expressing a need to go to the toilet. Because he is unable to make a verbal request, this need has not been identified. The care staff, although understandably frustrated by the situation, have undermined Mr X and treated him in a derogatory fashion. A regular toileting programme, and an evaluation of his comprehension skills, to explore his ability to understand pictures and written material, would probably improve the problem.

> Mr Y has recently moved into a care facility. He is generally cheerful and well liked by the care staff. He requires some assistance to get dressed in the mornings, during which the staff banter with him. One morning, Mr Y pats one of the female care staff on the backside. She makes a joke of it and laughs. Over the next few days, Mr Y continues to touch care staff on the backside, and on one occasion puts his hand inside the dress of one of the care assistants. She is upset by this, and shouts at Mr Y.

Although it is excellent care practice to maintain friendly and cheerful interaction, it is important to respond kindly but clearly if a person has been touched in a way that could indicate sexual intent. A clear explanation at this stage is likely to prevent further or escalating problems and will probably correct the majority of misinterpretations, without harming the relationship between the person and the member of care staff.

> Mr Z lives alone in his own home. He suffers from a dementia of moderate severity and is visited by a care worker three times a day. Very frequently, particularly during the morning visit, Mr Z makes sexual comments, referring to a morning erection and suggesting a sexual liaison. On some occasions he tries to press his penis against the care worker while she is helping him to get dressed. She tends to become embarrassed, blushes and usually leaves the room to make a cup of tea, returning several minutes later. She finds attending to Mr Z particularly stressful.

There is little doubt that this is an example of an abnormal sexual behaviour. It is important within care teams that mutual support and supervision are provided to enable carers to manage the situation more effectively. In this situation the care worker found the situation particularly stressful and it was decided that a different, older care worker, who had experience in similar situations, should take over the care duties. The reasons for this change were clearly but politely explained to Mr Z. A clinical psychologist became involved and asked the care worker to keep an ABC diary, after explaining the objectives and the type of information that was needed. Over several weeks, it became evident that Mr Z immediately started to express sexual statements as soon as he heard the door open, but began to become distracted after a few minutes. The intensity of his behaviour increased if any response at all was given, including any requests to ask him to stop. It was decided that, when the care worker arrived, she would say hello without going into Mr Z's bedroom. After 5 min of housework duties, she would take him a cup of tea and then return to other jobs for a further 5 min. This approach worked well and by the time Mr Z had finished his tea, he was usually making only very occasional sexual remarks when helped to dress. When such remarks were made, the care worker carried on with other themes of conversation in a matter-of-fact way and did not acknowledge the sexually orientated statements. Over the next few months the sexual remarks diminished further.

Not all cases are as easily managed as this one, and the triggers and reinforcers vary from individual to individual. A careful assessment and well planned approach will, however, be successful in the majority of situations.

Anxiety

Although anxiety is frequent in people with dementia, there is almost no literature regarding treatment. Individual psychotherapies and anxiety management training have been used as therapeutic options for people with dementia, although they have not been systematically evaluated for the treatment of anxiety. Teri *et al.* (1997) demonstrated that cognitive behaviour therapy and an activity programme were both significantly better than placebo for the treatment of depression occurring in the context of dementia. This is a very important study and emphasizes the need for similar studies to examine the efficacy of these management approaches for people with anxiety.

In the absence of clear evidence, it is important to conduct a thorough assessment of the situation. To someone with dementia, many aspects of managing a day-to-day routine or coping with their environment can be stressful or anxiety provoking. A detailed assessment will highlight areas where intervention may be helpful. Examples might include helping someone to organize their bills through direct debit, a care plan to assist with shopping, clear signs to help someone find their room in a care facility or a planned programme of social interaction for someone who feels frightened when alone. Depending on the skills of particular individuals, some training to help them use a diary to plan their day, anxiety management training or some training in simple relaxation techniques, cognitive behaviour therapy or an activity programme may be helpful. Many people with dementia are able to learn new skills, such as relaxation techniques, with repeated practice. Sensory therapies such as aromatherapy, music or *Snoezelen* can be helpful for some people; and simulated presence therapy can be reassuring.

Fifty per cent of people with anxiety and dementia will have a clinically significant depression. These individuals may respond to antidepressant therapy. The evidence relating to the efficacy of antidepressant treatment in people with concurrent depression and dementia is reviewed in Chapter 17. Anxiety disorders in younger people can be successfully treated with antidepressant agents, even in the absence of depression. There is no current evidence to support this practice in people with dementia, although a carefully monitored trial of treatment with a selective serotonin re-uptake inhibitor may be worthwhile in cases of severe anxiety not responsive to more conservative measures. There is no systematic evidence from the literature pertaining to the use of benzodiazepines, neuroleptics or buspirone for the treatment of anxiety in dementia.

In practice, the most difficult situations tend to arise when people are frightened of being alone at night. In these circumstances it is not unusual for relatives or even emergency services such as the police or fire brigade to be telephoned 15 or 20 times a night. An individual in this situation probably needs a period of time in hospital, a care facility or an alternative environment with company, pending assessment and treatment.

REFERENCES

Ballard, C. G. and O'Brien, J. (1999). Pharmacological treatment of behavioural and psychological signs in Alzheimer's disease: how good is the evidence for current pharmacological treatments? *British Medical Journal*, **319**, 138–9.

Brink, C. (1980). Urinary continence/incontinence: assessing the problem *Geriatric Nursing*, **1**, 241–5.

Burgio, L., Scilley, K., Hardin, J. M., Hsu, D. and Yancey, J. (1996). Environmental 'white noise': an intervention for verbally agitated nursing home residents. *Journal of Gerontology*, **51B**, 364–73.

Carlyle, W., Killick, L. and Ancill, R. (1991). ECT: an effective treatment in the screaming demented patient. *Journal of the American Geriatric Society*, **39**, 637–9.

Cohen-Mansfield, J. and Werner, P. (1997a). Management of verbally disruptive behaviors in nursing home residents. *Journal of Gerontology*, **A52**, M369–77.

Cohen-Mansfield, J. and Werner, P. (1997b). Typology of disruptive vocalizations in older persons suffering from dementia. *International Journal of Geriatric Psychiatry*, **12**, 1079–91.

Cullen, P., Abid, F., Patel, A., Coope, B. and Ballard, C. G. (1997). Eating disorders in dementia. *International Journal of Geriatric Psychiatry*, **12**, 559–62.

Greenwald, B. S., Marin, D. B. and Silverman, S. M. (1986). Serotonergic treatment of screaming and banging in dementia. *Lancet*, **ii**, 1464–5.

Kopala, L. C. and Honer, W. G. (1997). The use of risperidone in severely demented patients with persistent vocalizations. *International Journal of Geriatric Psychiatry*, **12**, 73–7.

Lund, D. A., Hill, R. D., Caserta, M. S. and Wright, S. D. (1995). Video respite: an innovative resource for family, professional caregivers and persons with dementia. *Gerontologist*, **35**, 683–787.

Meares, S. and Draper, B. (1999). Treatment of vocally disruptive behaviour of multifactorial aetiology. *International Journal of Geriatric Psychiatry*, **14**, 285–90.

Pasion, R. C. and Kirby, S. G. (1993). Trazadone for screaming. *Lancet*, **341**, 970.

Schneider, L. S., Pollock, V. E. and Lyness, S. A. (1990). A metaanalysis of controlled trials of neuroleptic treatment in dementia. *Journal of the American Geriatric Society*, **38**, 553–63.

Snowden, T., Meehan, T. and Halpin, R. (1994). Case report—continuous screaming controlled by electroconvulsive therapy: a case study *International Journal of Geriatric Psychiatry*, **9**, 929–32.

Spayd, C. S. and Smyer, M.A. (1988). Interventions with agitated, disorientated or depressed residents. In *Mental Health Constitution in Nursing Homes* (Smyer, M. A., Cohn, M. D. and Brannon, D., eds), pp. 123–141. University Press, New York.

Stewart, J. T. and Shin, K. J. (1997). Paroxetine treatment of sexual disinhibition in dementia. *American Journal of Psychiatry*, **154**, 1474.

Teri, L., Logsdon, R. G., Uomoto, J. and McCurry, S. M. (1997). Behavioral treatment of depression in dementia patients: a controlled clinical trial. *Journal of Gerontology*, **B52**, 159–66.

20 Managing behavioural and psychological symptoms in residential and nursing home care

Background issues

The expanding elderly population inevitably means that the number of people with dementia will continue to increase well into the twenty-first century (Melzer *et al.* 1997), with enormous implications for care provision (Knapp *et al.* 1998). Residential and nursing homes form an integral part of the care network for these individuals, particularly during the later stages of the disease process (Bannister *et al.* 1998) or when concurrent psychiatric morbidity or behavioural problems arise (Steele *et al.* 1990).

Recommendations from the Department of Health and Social Security (1985) suggested the need for 25 local authority residential care places for every 1000 people over the age of 65. The majority of places are now provided within the private sector, with more than 1500 in Newcastle alone. This expansion of private-sector care provisions is reflected throughout the UK, with a six-fold increase over the last 14 years (Royal College of Physicians 1997). These facilities provide essential care to a large group of vulnerable individuals with complex mental health needs and limited ability to comment on the quality of care that they receive (Grimely Evans 1994, Brooker 1995).

Many residential and nursing homes have senior staff with limited experience in the specialized area of dementia care. In addition, almost all of the 'hands-on' care is provided by care assistants, a low-paid, mobile workforce without any formal training and often with limited experience of caring for patients with cognitive impairment. The introduction of National Vocational Qualifications has provided a framework for care assistants to acquire basic skills, but there are no statutory training requirements and often few incentives. Combined with the paucity of structured 'in-house' training programmes, this is a concerning situation.

As a consequence, in many residential and nursing homes, optimal enviromental design (Cohen and Day 1993), positive communication practices (Meddaugh 1990) and the skilful use of verbal and non-verbal communication (Ryden and Feldt 1992) are not implemented, with important implications for the quality of care and the frequency of behavioural and psychological symptoms in dementia (BPSD).

Prevalence of BPSD among people with dementia in care facilities

In the USA, >80% of residents in care facilities suffer from dementia (Rovner *et al.* 1990). In the UK, the proportion of residents with dementia is similar and the level of physical frailty of these residents is increasing (Stern *et al.* 1993). There have, however, been surprisingly few studies examining BPSD among residents with dementia in these settings, an important omission when considering that BPSD are an important trigger for admission to care facilities (Steele *et al.* 1990). Several large studies have included summary measures of behavioural problems (Jagger and Lindesay 1997), but are likely to have seriously underestimated the true prevalence, while the majority of other reports have focused upon specific symptoms such as:

- aggression, indicating a frequency of 30% in nursing home residents (Shah 2000);

- psychosis, suggesting a frequency of 25% (Cohen *et al.* 1998); or

- abnormal vocalizations, where frequencies of 11–30% have been reported (Ryan *et al.* 1988, Cohen-Mansfield *et al.* 1990, Cariaga *et al.* 1991).

A recent study from our group, evaluating 209 residents with dementia living in care facilities in Newcastle, UK, indicated an overall frequency of BPSD of 86% (Table 20.1), while Rovner *et al.* (1996) reported a frequency of 51% in a community nursing home in the USA. The most frequent individual symptoms in our cohort were agitation, irritability and motor restlessness, while the overall prevalence of psychosis was similar to that reported by Cohen *et al.* (1998). The symptom profile varied with dementia severity. Residents with milder dementia experienced higher

Table 20.1   Frequency of BPSD in residents of care environments

Symptom	Frequency of BPSD				
	overall ($n = 209$)	at CDR 0.5 ($n = 4$)	at CDR 1.0 ($n = 36$)	at CDR 2.0 ($n = 79$)	at CDR 3.0 ($n = 90$)
Irritability	81 (39%)	1 (25%)	15 (42%)	36 (46%)	29 (32%)
Disinhibition	45 (22%)	1 (25%)	6 (17%)	18 (23%)	20 (22%)
Apathy	58 (28%)	1 (25%)	10 (28%)	22 (28%)	25 (28%)
Euphoria	17 (8%)	0	4 (11%)	3 (4%)	10 (11%)
Anxiety	50 (24%)	2 (50%)	11 (31%)	17 (22%)	20 (22%)
Depression	72 (34%)	3 (75%)	18 (50%)	30 (38%)	21 (23%)
Agitation	117 (47%)	2 (50%)	17 (47%)	51 (65%)	48 (63%)
Hallucinations	13 (6%)	1 (25%)	2 (6%)	7 (9%)	3 (3%)
Delusions	46 (22%)	1 (25%)	13 (41%)	25 (32%)	7 (8%)
Aberrant motor behaviour	71 (34%)	0	12 (33%)	26 (33%)	33 (37%)
BPSD overall	179 (86%)	3 (75%)	29 (81%)	71 (90%)	76 (84%)

CDR – clinical dementia rating scale

frequencies of mood disorders, psychosis was most common in people with dementia of moderate severity and agitation increased with the severity of dementia (Table 20.1). The high prevalence of BPSD in these settings highlights their importance as a treatment priority. It is particularly difficult to provide good quality care for such people (Wilcocks *et al.* 1997), but <5% of these residents receive specialist mental health care input (Burns *et al.* 1993).

Prescription of psychotropic agents

Many (35–50%) of the dementia sufferers living in residential or nursing home care are prescribed neuroleptic drugs (Avorn *et al.* 1989, Buck 1989, McGrath and Jackson 1996, Thacker and Jones 1997, Ballard *et al.* 1999). These agents have limited efficacy (Ballard and O'Brien 1999) and are often given with little subsequent monitoring (Furniss *et al.* 1998). There is also evidence that they may often be prescribed inappropriately or indiscriminately (McGrath and Jackson 1996); for example, in our own recent study, there was no statistically significant relationship between psychotropic drug prescribing and the type of BPSD experienced by individual residents (Table 20.2).

The clinical importance of the problem is such that, in the USA, legislation has been successfully introduced to restrict prescribing of neuroleptics (Shorr *et al.* 1994). People with dementia are especially at risk of adverse events (e.g. parkinsonism, drowsiness, falls, accelerated cognitive decline or increasing mortality), with the Chief Medical Officer recommending particular caution when prescribing neuroleptics (Chief Medical Officer 1994).

In a recent study (Ballard *et al.* 2000), we have demonstrated that neuroleptic agents have a detrimental effect on key indicators of quality of life, including well-being, activities and social interaction (Table 20.3). It is hence evident that, while neuroleptic agents may be necessary, and are potentially beneficial for some residents with severe BPSD, the current level of over-prescribing is potentially harmful, and reduces the quality of life for many thousands of residents. Restricting prescriptions to situations where they are clinically necessary, and stopping unnecessary prescriptions, are clearly priorities.

The current section has focused primarily upon neuroleptic agents, as they are the

Table 20.2   Usage of psychotropic drugs and relationship to key BPSD

Drugs	Overall ($n = 209$)	Delusions ($n = 46$)	Agitation ($n = 117$)	Depression ($n = 72$)	Anxiety ($n = 50$)	Aberrant motor behaviour ($n = 71$)
Cognitive enhancers	4 (2%)	1 (2%)	2 (2%)	2 (3%)	1 (2%)	1 (1%)
Neuroleptics	87 (42%)	24 (52%)	59 (50%)	28 (39%)	3 (6%)	38 (54%)
Benzodiazepines	35 (17%)	7 (15%)	19 (16%)	12 (17%)	25 (50%)	15 (21%)
Antidepressants	40 (19%)	11 (24%)	11 (24%)	28 (39%)	12 (24%)	11 (16%)
Other psychotropics	7 (3%)	2 (4%)	3 (3%)	1 (1%)	3 (6%)	3 (4%)

Table 20.3 Psychotropic drugs: relationship with well-being, social withdrawal and activities

Drugs	Overall cohort (n = 112)	Ill-being	Time socially withdrawn (%)	Time engaged in activities (%)	Linear regression well-being		social withdrawal		engagement in activities	
					t	P	t	P	t	P
Neuroleptics	52 (46%)	9 (18%)	11.5	54.1	2.1	0.04	2.1	0.04	3.4	0.0009
Benzodiazepines	16 (14%)	2 (13%)	7.6	54.8	0.1	0.89	0.2	0.88	1.4	0.17
Antidepressants	21 (19%)	2 (10%)	10.0	64.6	0.45	0.65	0.5	0.65	0.6	0.53
Other psychotropics	5 (5%)	0 (0%)	10.1	49.2	0.21	0.84	0.2	0.84	0.9	0.33
No drugs	40 (36%)	0 (0%)	2.7	72.2						

From Ballard et al. 2000

most widely prescribed, and on the most potentially harmful of the psychotropic agents. However, all psychotropic agents are widely prescribed (Table 20.2) and have some important side effects, such as drowsiness and increased risk of falls. Caution should be exercised for each prescription of a psychotropic agent issued for someone with dementia.

Professional carers

Here we use the term 'professional carers' to refer to both trained nursing staff and untrained care staff within residential and nursing home facilities. Despite the very large number of untrained carers and their key role in delivering hands-on care, there has been very little research relating BPSD to staff burnout and psychiatric morbidity with this population (Jacques and Innes 1998). Exceptions to this include studies by Moniz-Cook et al. (1997) and Jenkins and Allen (1998). Moniz-Cook et al. examined 48 care staff from local authority homes and concluded that staff well-being was associated with lower instances of disruptive patient behaviour (e.g. aggression and uncooperative behaviour), environmental factors (e.g. the care environment) and organizational factors (e.g. shift patterns or career progress). Organizational issues were also found to be important by Jenkins and Allen (1998). They observed that positive behavioural interactions between staff and patients and lower staff burnout were associated with high degrees of perceived responsibility. In other words, lower levels of staff burnout were associated with high levels of perceived staff involvement in the decision-making process within the residential home.

The issues of staff responsibility and involvement are important. The experience of staff in the specialized area of looking after people with dementia varies widely. There are no statutory training requirements and few incentives to encourage completion. As a consequence, many staff are not taught the fundamental skills (e.g. effective verbal and non-verbal communication strategies (Meddaugh 1990, Ryden and Feldt 1992)) that can be used to minimize aggression and other forms of challenging behaviour. It is important to understand how these symptoms affect the morale and psychiatric morbidity of staff and whether they adversely interfere with the care process.

Some of these issues were explored by Innes (1998), who reviewed the process by which staff perceive and give meaning to patient behaviours. She explored the way in which care assistants categorize and label difficult behaviours and examined the various coping strategies employed by staff in line with their conceptual labels; for example, disruptive behaviours engaged in by residents labelled as 'easy' were coped with and tolerated more readily than similar behaviours engaged in by 'difficult' residents. It can clearly be seen how such attributions can occur, and, once established, they may play an important role in the establishment of cycles of negative interactions. Such interactions could create environments of 'malignant social psychology' (Kitwood 1993), which could further exacerbate the BPSD. Physical abuse is not uncommon in care environments (Pillemer and Moore 1989), and it possible that an adversive cycle of patient–carer interaction, related to escalating BPSD, could act as a trigger for abusive behaviour. The possible link between BPSD and physical abuse in care settings certainly merits study.

Recent service audit data from our own group suggest that professional carers do experience distress in response to BPSD. In a pilot cohort of 24 patients treated for BPSD, there were significant correlations between the severity of agitation ($r = 0.73$, $P < 0.0001$), delusions ($r = 0.82$, $P = 0.002$) and irritability ($r = 0.75$, $P < 0.0001$), respectively, and the level of distress experienced by the key worker. As an illustration, 33% of professional carers were moderately distressed and 38% were severely or very severely distressed as a consequence of patient agitation. This is clearly an area of priority for further work.

Treatment

Summary of the main issues

An understanding of the background issues gives some insight into the areas which could be fruitfully tackled in order to provide better quality care, to reduce the frequency of BPSD and to minimize unnecessary and potentially harmful prescriptions of psychotropic agents. The key areas include:

- better access to training and information;
- improved liaison from medical and specialist dementia care teams with regular review of residents with BPSD; and
- a statutory monitoring system that is more sensitive to the quality of the environment and the hands-on care.

Many of these problems have been highlighted in recent papers regarding strategies for improving the quality of care in residential and nursing home settings (Kitwood and Woods 1996, Leaper 1998), and they are also the focus of recent government papers (e.g. Department of Health 1998).

Management of BPSD in individual residents

Management of BPSD in individuals with dementia residing in care facilities should follow the same pathway as for other people with dementia. The procedures for assessment and management are described in detail elsewhere and rely upon developing a detailed profile of the particular individual in order to understand the precipitants of a particular problem. It is of note, however, that many of the studies reviewed in the sections on behavioural and alternative management strategies were conducted in nursing home environments; these included music therapy (Gerdner 1997), planned walks, simulated presence therapy (Allen-Burge et al. 1999), video-respite therapy (Allen-Burge et al. 1999), an enhanced environment for restlessness (Cohen-Mansfield and Werner 1998) and social interaction for verbally disruptive behaviour (Cohen-Mansfield et al. 1997).

Better monitoring

The system for monitoring the quality of care provided within residential and nursing home environments will vary from region to region and country to country (Department of Health and Human Services 1989). In the UK this function is undertaken by Joint Inspection Teams, acting within different local authorities, each setting their own standards, which depend on the size of the authority and the number of homes to be assessed. This inevitably leads to some inconsistencies at the national level. Perhaps more importantly, the evaluations do not involve any direct observation of resident–resident, or resident–staff communication or interaction, and perhaps fail to evaluate sensitively the parameters that are central in determining the quality of life of individual residents.

Measuring the quality of care received by dementia patients is not straightforward, however, particularly given the difficulties of reliable verbal feedback; direct observational methods are probably preferable. Observational approaches to evaluating the quality of care have been evaluated by Brooker (1995), who concluded that, overall, Dementia Care Mapping (DCM) was probably the most useful method within clinical care settings. DCM (Kitwood and Bredin 1994) is a direct, operationalized, observational method based upon the theoretical sociopsychological theory of personhood in dementia (Kitwood 1993). The method quantifies activities using behavioural category codes, which are recorded every 5 min, measuring key parameters such as well-being and personal detractors, achieving κ values for inter-rater reliability greater than +0.8 (Brooker *et al.* 1998). The development of DCM has been a major advance, making it easier to evaluate reliably the quality of care in facilities for patients with dementia and, hence, also providing the means to assess the value of interventions aimed at improving the quality of care in these environments. This kind of approach could provide a much more sensitive and meaningful evaluation of a particular care facility and could be completed by a team of trained 'care mappers' in a single day, as a supplement to other aspects of the evaluation.

Provided that adequate training programmes are made universally available, a statutory requirement for all staff to attend a specified number of training days over a specific period could be very helpful. Statutory requirements regarding specific aspects of environmental design, especially for new establishments in the planning stages, may also be beneficial.

Training and access to information

Well organized environments that facilitate walking, do not emphasize exits, arrange seating in a manner that encourages communication, with adequate but not over-bright lighting, appropriate levels of background music and a comfortable temperature can improve the quality of life for residents, and reduce BPSD (Lindesay *et al.* 1991, Ryden and Feldt 1992, Berg *et al.* 1998, Cohen-Mansfield and Werner 1998, Gerdner 1998). Many of these objectives can be achieved without spending money, but do require an adequate level of information. A number of pub-lications are available providing advice in these areas, but the development of local resource teams that could provide practical advice would be a major advantage. Although the potential benefits of many of these individual aspects of environ-mental design have been established, there is a paucity of research evidence regard-ing the value of more global improvements in the care environment, which is an important area for further work. The value of good staff–patient communication, particularly during highly stressful times such as personal care, is clear to those working in the field, although again it is an area where clear research evidence is lacking. In a pivotal study, Lindesay *et al.* (1991) were, however, able to demonstrate that a combination of high quality nursing care and good communication skills between staff and patients, in small, well-designed Domus-style units, improves the level of functioning of dementia sufferers and reduces their level of behavioural dis-turbance. Given that these units cost two and a half times more than nursing care, Domus-style units are not feasible as a general alternative to traditional care environments. The task is, therefore, to find a way of improving the quality of exist-ing care in a cost-effective manner.

While better training is clearly a necessity, the reports so far concentrating on staff training programmes within care facilities have been rather disappointing. Cohen-Mansfield *et al.* (1997), Moniz-Cooke (1998) and Shah and De (1998) were all able to demonstrate some short-term gains from a training programme. Improved staff knowledge (Cohen-Mansfield and Werner 1997, Moniz-Cooke *et al.* 1998), improvements of the way in which staff managed people experiencing BPSD (Cohen-Mansfield and Werner 1997) and a reduction in the level of aggression (Shah and De 1998) were all achieved by training, although there was no reduction in the frequency of BPSD among residents in two of the studies, and the benefits of training were short lived. More thought needs to be given to the structure of train-ing programmes and the way in which they are organized and delivered. For example, if any benefits are not sustained, would 'refresher sessions' be helpful, or could a dif-ferent model of training be used, whereby senior staff were trained to provide a rolling programme of education within their own facilities? Supervision models such as this have been demonstrated to benefit individuals at each step in the chain and to use senior staff time efficiently while disseminating benefit to a large target group (Milne and James 1998). It is also possible that training programmes have not paid sufficient attention to the areas that are important to care staff, such as the input of care workers into the planning of care, and the well-being of staff (Moniz-Cooke *et al.* 1997, Jenkins and Allen 1998). Although the provision of staff train-ing is essential, it is also important—given the limited established efficacy of these interventions—that programmes provided in individual settings are carefully evalu-ated to determine their benefit. In this way, resources will not be wasted upon ineffective interventions and knowledge about the optimal design of training programmes will grow and can then be adopted more widely.

DCM, described in Chapter 8, and referred to in the section regarding monitoring, has been used widely in clinical practice for audit and training. The detailed observational data provide a profile of the patterns of activities and interactions and can highlight areas of excellent care and areas in which care is less than optimal or is not 'person centred'. Following the evaluation, feedback is given to the staff of the environment that has been 'mapped', following standardized guidelines (Kitwood and Bredin 1997). An excellent study examining the impact of regular audit/feedback using DCM in an NHS trust demonstrated marked improvements in the quality of care over three annual cycles (Brooker *et al.* 1998). This process provides a training component through the feedback sessions and highlights areas that senior staff can address through further training and reorganization. While further evaluation studies of this kind are required, this cycle of assessment and feedback is a potentially exciting way of addressing some of the training needs within care facilities.

Better access to medical input and specialist dementia care teams

People with BPSD, in the context of cognitive impairment, often taking multiple drugs and frequently with additional medical problems, have high levels of need, but often have very poor access to specialist services. The benefits of better liaison include the opportunities for informal training relating to the management of individual patients, the instigation of a more thorough evaluation of medical and environmental precipitants for a particular problem and the availability of regular medication reviews. Many of these issues have been covered in previous chapters, but it is particularly pertinent to emphasize the potential importance of sensory impairments (Chapman *et al.* 1999) and of pain and delirium as triggers for BPSD, as these frequently go unrecognized in residential and nursing homes.

Several key studies have examined the value of a liaison service. Rovner *et al.* (1996), in a ground-breaking study, were able to demonstrate that, in a community nursing home with 118 residents, a comprehensive intervention of regular educational reviews, an activity programme and guidelines for the prescription of psychotropic agents halved the frequency of BPSD and halved the use of antipsychotic medication over a 6 month period. This work provides strong evidence for the value of a comprehensive, medically led, dementia care programme. In a second study, Proctor *et al.* (1999) evaluated the impact of a training programme and regular reviews from a community psychiatric nurse upon BPSD in 60 residents with marked behavioural problems. There was no overall improvement in BPSD, but depression scores did significantly improve. Although this intervention was of value, the effect was considerably less than that reported by Rovner *et al.* (1996). This could possibly be explained by the greater severity of BPSD in the study by Proctor *et al.*; alternatvely, more substantial improvements may require the more comprehensive approach adopted by Rovner *et al.*

Reducing neuroleptic usage

Neuroleptic usage can be reduced in two ways: by limiting new prescriptions and by stopping prescriptions that are no longer necessary. The first issue has been discussed extensively in Chapter 6, and requires some knowledge of the natural course of the symptoms and sufficient understanding of the issues to decide whether the severity of a symptom merits the prescription of a drug or whether other, non-pharmacological, approaches are likely to be efficacious. An experienced clinician, who is able to make a detailed evaluation of the particular situation, provide support and direction to the care staff and monitor progress carefully, will be able to avoid pharmacotherapy in the majority of instances. Discontinuing existing prescriptions can be more problematic, as there is an understandable reluctance to discontinue a neuroleptic agent when a resident is problem-free, because of fears that the original BPSD will recur. There is, however, accruing evidence that withdrawing neuroleptic drugs in people with dementia only leads to an exacerbation of BPSD in a small minority of people (Bridges-Parlet *et al.* 1997, Cohen-Mansfield *et al.* 1999), especially if psychological management strategies are introduced in parallel (Cohen-Mansfield *et al.* 1999). Certainly further work is needed to evaluate the impact of neuroleptic discontinuation upon quality of life and to develop better criteria for selecting people who are likely to benefit from this approach. At the current level of knowledge, discontinuation of neuroleptic drugs should be seriously considered in people who have been free of severe BPSD for ≥ 3 months. Although careful monitoring is required, clinicians should be aware of the 'inverse placebo effect', where care staff tend to attribute any minor difficulty to the discontinuation of neuroleptic drugs. Unless there is clear evidence of a major increase in BPSD, we would recommend a trial discontinuation of ≥ 1 month. From the research evidence, it is likely that 90% of people will not require the neuroleptics to be reinstated (Bridges-Parlet *et al.* 1997).

The studies considered in the previous paragraph have evaluated neuroleptic withdrawal for discrete cohorts and provide important evidence regarding the safety of discontinuing these agents. Studies of this kind will give some individual clinicians the confidence to stop longstanding prescriptions, but there are few formal studies to evaluate the impact upon practice of different approaches aimed at reducing unnecessary neuroleptic usage. Within the USA, legal requirements relating to the continued prescription of neuroleptic agents within care settings have reduced the number of residents receiving these agents by 30% (Shorr *et al.* 1994), while in individual studies, strict prescribing guidelines (Rovner *et al.* 1996) and formalized programmes of liaison and education (Avorn *et al.* 1992) have also had a significant effect. The development of widely available, evidence-based practice guidelines is imperative and seems the obvious way forward.

Conclusion

The aim of this chapter has been to summarize some of the key issues relating to BPSD in care facilities and to outline some of the major work regarding interventions. Although there is a general paucity of studies, there are encouraging data regarding the value of comprehensive liaison services, non-pharmacological interventions and the discontinuation of unnecessary neuroleptic agents. It is important to build upon this work with studies that include broader evaluation parameters and that develop a better understanding as to the nature of what constitutes an effective staff training programme. Recent papers regarding strategies for improving care in residential and nursing home facilities will provide an impetus to this work. It is also imperative that more of the practice-related research in this field is transferred into routine clinical practice.

Clinical example

Given the clear educational needs within residential and nursing home facilities, an NHS trust decides to develop a teaching programme. They ask one of the senior nurses working within the old age psychiatry team to convene a group to develop a training package. A working group is established with two senior nurses, a consultant old age psychiatrist, an occupational therapist and a clinical psychologist. A programme of six talks is devised, which covers a range of topics: (i) background information about dementia, (ii) the philosophy of person-centred care, (iii) assessment of problem behaviours, (iv) non-pharmacological strategies for improving problem behaviours, (v) the use of activities within care facilities and (vi) stress management techniques. The talks are given at the hospital on six sequential Wednesday evenings, each session lasting one hour, with refreshments provided. All staff members from each care facility in the area are invited. The working group acknowledges that it is important to obtain some feedback about the value of the training, so they develop a questionnaire asking participants whether they found various aspects of the programme helpful. Between 20 and 25 people attend each session, and the feedback forms indicate that those who attended found the presentations very helpful.

This is the type of educational package that is developed and presented within many healthcare delivery settings. In many ways it was carefully thought through, developing a considered content; it involved a substantial time commitment from a number of senior staff members. However, this type of programme has a number of major flaws:

(1)   Although attendance was quite good, only a very small proportion of the total number of staff attended.

(2)   There is very little evidence that didactic teaching packages are effective.

(3)   The effects of any training package have been shown to be short-lived without an ongoing programme of training or liaison that reinforces the educational material and allows staff to consolidate newly acquired knowledge and skills through their own practical, hands-on experience.

(4)   The system of feedback is inadequate. Those attending the teaching programmes usually feel obliged to give positive feedback, particularly if the forms are handed back to the course organizers. In this example, no attempt was made to assess whether the programme had improved the knowledge or skills of staff;

or whether it had made any practical difference to the care received by residents in the care facilities.

There are, unfortunately, no quick-fix solutions. The programmes that have been successful are usually resource intensive and have involved taking the training programme to the care facilities, where an interactive approach to teaching has allowed staff to apply their newly developed skills in practice, supported by an ongoing liaison programme. If more cost-effective options are attempted, it is important to monitor their effectiveness thoroughly, otherwise it becomes an expensive exercise in tokenism. DCM is a method that lends itself well to a rolling audit cycle and can be introduced in parallel with an ongoing educational programme.

REFERENCES

Allen-Burge, R., Stevens, A. B. and Burgio, L. D. (1999). Effective behavioural interventions for decreasing dementia-related challenging behaviour in nursing homes. *Journal of Geriatric Psychiatry*, **14**, 213–32.

Avorn, J., Dreyer, P., Connelly, K. and Soumerai, S. B. (1989). Use of psychoactive medications and the quality of care in rest homes; findings and policy implications of a statewide survey. *New England Journal of Medicine*, **320**, 227–32.

Avorn, J., Soumerai, S. B., Everitt, D. B., Ross-Degnan, D., Beers, M. H., Sherman, D., Salem-Schatz, S. R. and Fields, D. (1992). A randomized trial of a programme to reduce the use of psychoactive drugs in nursing homes. *New England Journal of Medicine*, **327**, 168–73.

Ballard, C. G. and O'Brien, J. (1999). Pharmacological treatment of behavioural and psychological signs in Alzheimer's disease: how good is the evidence for current pharmacological treatments? *British Medical Journal*, **319**, 138–9.

Ballard, C., O'Brien, J., James, I., Mynt, P., Lanam, Potkins, D., Reichelt, K., Lee, L., McKeith, I., Swann, A. and Fussey, J. (2000). Quality of life from people with dementia living in residential and nursing home care: the impact of dependency, behavioural and psychological symptoms, language skills and isychorropic drugs. *International Psychogeriatrics*, in press.

Bannister, C., Ballard, C., Lana, M., Fairbairn, A. and Wilcock, G. (1998). Placement of dementia sufferers in residential and nursing care. *Age and Aging*, **27**, 189–93.

Berg, A., Hallberg, I. R. and Norberg, A. (1988). Nurses' reflection about dementia care, the patients, the carers and themselves in their daily caregiving. *International Journal of Nursing Studies*, **35**, 271–82.

Bridges-Parlet, S., Knopman, D. and Steffes, S. (1997) Withdrawal of neuroleptic medications from institutionalized dementia patients, results of a double-blind baseline-treatment-controlled pilot study. *Journal of Geriatric Psychiatry and Neurology*, **10**, 119–26.

Brooker, D. (1995). Looking at them looking at me. A review of observational studies into the quality of institutional care for elderly people with dementia. *Journal of Mental Health*, **4**, 145–56.

Brooker, D., Foster, N., Banner, A., Payne, M. and Jackson, L. (1998). The efficacy of dementia care mapping as an audit tool: report of a 3-year British National Health Service evaluation. *Aging and Mental Health*, **2**, 60–70.

Buck, J. A. (1989). Psychotropic drug practice in nursing homes. *Journal of the American Geriatrics Society*, **36**, 409–18.

Burns, B. J., Wagner, H. R., Taibe, J. F., Magaziner, J., Permutt, T. and Landerman, L. R.(1993). Mental health service use by the elderly in nursing home: another perspective. *American Journal of Public Health*, **83**, 331–7.

Cariaga, J., Burgio, L., Flynn, W. and Martin, D. (1991). A controlled study of disruptive vocalizations among geriatric residents in nursing homes. *Journal of the American Geriatrics Society*, **39**, 501–7.

Chapman, F., Dickinson, J., McKeith, I. and Ballard, C. G. (1999). Visual acuity and visual hallucinations in Alzheimer's disease. *American Journal of Psychiatry*, **156**, 1983–1985.

Chief Medical Officer. (1994). Current problems in pharmacology. Committee on Safety of Medicines Update, May 20-6.

Cohen, V. and Day, K. (1993). *Contemporary Environments for People with Dementia*. Johns Hopkins University Press, Baltimore, MD.

Cohen, C. I., Hyland, K. and Magai, C. (1998). Inter-racial and intra-racial differences in neuropsychiatric symptoms, sociodemography and treatment among nursing home patients with dementia. *Gerontologist*, **38**, 355–61.

Cohen-Mansfield, J. and Werner, P. (1997). Management of verbally disruptive behaviors in nursing home residents. *Journals of Gerontology*, **A52**, M369–77.

Cohen-Mansfield, J. and Werner, P. (1998). The effects of an enhanced environment on nursing home residents who pace. *Gerontologist*, **38**, 199–208.

Cohen-Mansfield, J., Werner, P. and Marx, M. S. (1990). Screaming in nursing home residents. *Journal of the American Geriatrics Society*, **38**, 785–92.

Cohen-Mansfield, J., Werner, P., Culpepper, W. J. II and Barkley, D. (1997). Evaluation of an in service training program on dementia and wandering. *Journal of Gerontological Nursing*, **23**, 40–47.

Cohen-Mansfield, J., Lipson, S., Werner, P., Billig, N., Taylor, L. and Woosley, R. (1999). Withdrawal of haloperidol, thioridazine, and lorazepam in the nursing home: a controlled, double-blind study. *Archives of Internal Medicine*, **159**, 1733–40.

Department of Health (1998). *Modernising Social Services*. Her Majesty's Stationery Office, London.

Department of Health and Human Services: Medicare and Medicaid (1989). Requirements for long-term care facilities final rule with request for comments. *Federal Register*, **54**, 5322.

Department of Health and Social Security (1985). *Government Response to the Second Report from the Social Services Committee 1984–1985 Session*. Community Care, London.

Furniss, L., Lloyd Craig, S. K. and Burns, A. (1998). Medication use in nursing homes for elderly. *International Journal of Geriatric Psychiatry*, **13**, 433–9.

Gerdner, L. (1997). An individualized music intervention for agitation. *Journal of the American Psychiatric Nurses Association*, **3**, 177–84.

Grimely Evans, J. (1994). Resuscitation of demented people. *Journal of Medical Ethics*, **20**, 53.

Innes, A. (1998). Behind labels: what makes behaviour 'difficult'. *Journal of Dementia Care*, **6**, 22–5.

Jacques, I. and Innes, A. (1998). Who cares about care assistant work? *Journal of Dementia Care*, **6**, 33–7.

Jagger, C. and Lindesay, J. (1997). Residential care for elderly people: the prevalence of cognitive impairment and behavioural problems. *Age and Ageing*, **26**, 475–80.

Jenkins, H. and Allen, C. (1998). The relationship between staff burnout/distress and interactions with residents in two residential homes for older people. *International Journal of Geriatric Psychiatry*, **13**, 466–72.

Kitwood, T. (1993). Person and process in dementia. *International Journal of Geriatric Psychiatry*, **8**, 541–6.

Kitwood, T. and Bredin, K. (1994). *Evaluating Dementia Care: the DCM Method*, 6th edn. Bradford Dementia Research Group, Bradford University, Bradford.

Kitwood, T. and Bredin, K. (1997). *Evaluating Dementia Care: the DCM Method*, 7th edn. Bradford Dementia Research Group, Bradford University, Bradford.

Kitwood, T. and Woods, B. (1996). *Training and Development Strategy for Dementia Care in Residential Settings*. Bradford Dementia Group, Bradford University, Bradford.

Knapp, M., Wilkinson, D. and Wigglesworth, R. (1998). The economic consequences of Alzheimer's disease in the context of new drug developments. *International Journal of Geriatric Psychiatry*, **13**, 531–43.

Leaper, R. (ed.) (1998). *Training and Qualifications for Work with Older People. Report of a National Conference with Recommendations for Action*. National Council on Ageing/Age Concern.

Lindesay, J., Briggs, K., Lowes, M., McDonald, A. and Herzberg, J. (1991). The Domus philosophy: a comparative evaluation of a new approach to residential care for the demented elderly. *International Journal of Geriatric Psychiatry*, **6**, 727–36.

McGrath, A. M. and Jackson, G. A. (1996). Survey of prescribing in residents of nursing homes in Glasgow. *British Medical Journal*, **314**, 611–12.

Meddaugh, D. I. (1990). Reactance: understanding aggressive behaviour in long term care. *Journal of Psychosocial Nursing and Mental Health Services*, **15**, 22–7.

Melzer, D., Ely, M. and Brayne, C. (1997). Cognitive impairment in elderly people: population based estimate of the future in England, Scotland and Wales. *British Medical Journal*, **315**, 462.

Moniz-Cook, E. (1998). Psychosocial approaches to 'challenging behaviour' in care homes. *Journal of Dementia Care*, **6**, 33–8.

Moniz-Cook, E., Millington, D. and Silver, M. (1997). Residential care for older people: job satisfaction and psychological health in care staff. *Health and Social Care in the Community*, **5**, 124–33.

Pillemer, K. and Moore, D. W. (1989). Abuse of patients in nursing homes: findings from a survey of staff. *Gerontologist*, **29**, 314–20.

Proctor, R., Burns, A., Powell, H. S., Tarrier, N., Faragher, B., Richardson, G., Davies, L. and South, B. (1999). Behavioural management in nursing and residential homes: a randomized controlled trial. *Lancet*, **354**, 26–9.

Rovner, B. W., German, P. S., Broadhead, J., Morriss, R. K., Brant, L. J., Blaustein, J. and Folstein, M. F. (1990). The prevalence and management of dementia and other psychiatric disorders in nursing homes. *International Psychogeriatrics*, **2**, 13–24.

Rovner, B. W., Steele, C., Shmuely, D. S. W. and Folstein, M. F. (1996). A randomised trial of dementia care in nursing homes. *Journal of the American Geriatric Society*, **44**, 7–13.

Royal College of Physicians (1997). *Medicine for Older People*. Royal College of Physicians, London.

Ryan, D. P., Tainsh, S. M. M., Kolodny, V., Lendrum, B. L. and Fisher, R. H. (1988). Noise making amongst the elderly in long term care. *Gerontologist*, **28**, 369–71.

Ryden, M. and Feldt, K. S, (1992). Goal directed care: caring for aggressive nursing home residents with dementia. *Journal of Gerontology Nursing*, **18**, 35–41.

Shah, A. (2000). Aggressive behaviour in the elderly. *International Journal of Psychiatry in Clinical Practice*, in press.

Shah, A. and De, T. (1998). The effect of an educational intervention package about aggressive behaviour directed at the nursing care staff on a continuing care psychogeriatric ward. *International Journal of Geriatric Psychiatry*, **13**, 35–40.

Shorr, R., Fought, R. L. and Ray, W. A. (1994). Changes in antipsychotic drug use in nursing homes during implementation of the OBRA-87 regulations. *Journal of the American Medical Association*, **271**, 358–62.

Steele, C., Rovner, B., Chase, G. A. and Folstein, M. (1990). Psychiatric symptoms and nursing home placement of patients with Alzheimer's disease. *American Journal of Psychiatry*, **147**, 1049–51.

Stern, M. C., Jagger, C., Clarke, M., Anderson, J., McGrother, C., Bettock, T. and McDonald, C. (1993). Residential care for elderly people: a decade of change. *British Medical Journal*, **306**, 827–30.

Thacker, S. and Jones, R. (1997). Neuroleptic prescribing to the community elderly in Nottingham. *International Journal of Geriatric Psychiatry*, **12**, 833–7.

Willcocks, D., Peace, S. and Kellehar, S. (1997). *Private Lives in Public Places*. Tavistock, London.

21 An integrated treatment approach

Introduction

The main aim of this chapter is to synthesize an approach to the management of behavioural and psychological symptoms in dementia (BPSD) using the principles and guidelines discussed in detail in the preceding chapters. From the outset, one must acknowledge the scanty evidence base for this integrated model: most of it comes from experience in clinical practice. It is a potentially risky venture to combine different paradigms in an all-encompassing integrated whole. It can be particularly problematic to combine an essentially psychosocial model as a cause for aggressive behaviour and, at the same time, equate the same behavioural problems with changes in neurotransmitter functioning. However, as clinicians, we strongly believe that these models are not mutually exclusive and that a careful, judicious combination of approaches can act synergistically. There are a number of central pillars to our proposed integrated approach:

(1) Problems need to be seen in an environmental context.

(2) Treatment should be person-centred (this also involves being staff-centred in terms of their skills and abilities).

(3) Drugs are often more effective if used in conjunction with other models of care.

(4) A comprehensive formulation is at the heart of good treatment.

This chapter will outline some basic principles in preventing BPSD and some guidelines on the initial assessment, involving principles of management based on a diagnostic formulation. A detailed case example will be given to help illustrate this management approach.

Prevention of BPSD

An appropriate environment and basic understanding of some common problems can substantially reduce the frequency of BPSD. For example, boredom and frustration are an important and understandable precipitant of restlessness and irritability. The lack of clear signs for important amenities, such as a toilet, can induce restlessness with specific problems such as inappropriate voiding of urine.

Facilitating interaction and appropriate engagement in activities can hence be extremely valuable. A relaxed environment, with a low level of suitable background music and sufficient but not over-bright lighting, is also helpful. The biggest single trigger of irritable and aggressive behaviour is personal care interventions. As an individual with dementia often has a limited understanding of the need for assistance, this can seem like an invasion of privacy, particularly if the person's comprehension is slightly impaired. The use of short, clear statements, calm tones of voice and reassuring non-verbal requests will minimize problems.

Clinical assessment

The broad principles of clinical assessment outlined in Chapter 17 will be briefly summarized here:

(1) Always take a collateral history, ideally from a relative or someone who has an in-depth knowledge of the patient.

(2) Get a clear description of the problematic behaviour. Seek clarification if terms such as 'agitated' or 'resistive' are used.

(3) Find out the frequency and duration of the behaviour, any triggers and if there is an emerging pattern.

(4) What event precipitated this referral?

(5) What is the impact of both the carer and the wider environment of the problematic behaviour?

(6) From a medical viewpoint is it helpful to rule out other primary causes for the problematic behaviour (which can be regarded as an epiphenomenon), for example, depression, psychosis, physical illness, constipation and pain.

Kitwood (1997) employed a conceptual model to facilitate the development of appropriate formulations designed to access the person's experience of dementia. This model has been adapted by one of the co-authors, Dr Ian James; the adapted model includes a mental health component, providing a more comprehensive framework (James 1999). According to this model, the factors one should consider when developing such a formulation are cognitive status, personality, history, physical status, environmental status and mental health status. This formulation helps one to obtain an insight into the experience of the whole person including their past and current perception of the illness. This enables the clinician to act in a manner that resolves acute difficulties (depression, paranoid psychosis, aggression behaviour), while simultaneously promoting the person's dignity and well being. The components of this model are described below:

> Cognitive status—some of the features displayed (behaviour, emotions) by the person with dementia reflect changes in brain pathology. Clearly, this must be taken into account when attempting to understand the individual. Because each form of dementia is associated with changes in different cortical and subcortical areas, each one tends to have its characteristic profile.

Personality—despite dementia being described as a process in which a person 'loses his personality', it is important to appreciate that a person's premorbid personality will be apparent throughout many aspects and phases of the condition. Indeed, it is common for an individual with even severe dementia to want to express lifestyle preferences (e.g. about accommodation, religious practices, food or sexual orientation). While some personality changes will be related to changes in brain pathology, others will be associated with psychological sequelae. For example, owing to an emerging sense of vulnerability, a person with dementia may become more emotional and seek more physical attention.

History—aspects of long-term and procedural memory remain relatively preserved in many of the dementias, so knowledge of a person's history is helpful in understanding their behaviour and communication. Information about the individual's life, relationships and roles will also be important. Indeed, it is common to observe historical themes (losses, traumas) re-emerging during the development of the dementing illness.

Physical health status—dementia tends to be an illness of old age, so it often occurs in a context of declining physical health. It is important to include health-related issues within the formulation.

Mental health status—the prevalence of mental health problems is high within older populations. Premorbid difficulties may well interact with current problems to produce psychiatric disorders. Changes in brain pathology may also result in the emergence of these disorders.

A management sieve for treating BPSD in a particular individual is shown in Figure 21.1.

An integrated treatment approach: case study

Mr X is a 76 year old widower who has been living in residential care for the past 3 months. He was admitted to residential care from the geriatric medical ward in the local District General Hospital. He had a chest infection complicating his chronic obstructive pulmonary disease (COPD) superimposed on a dementia syndrome. This was his fourth admission in 7 months and his family were concerned that it was no longer safe for him to live at home. During his chest infections, he became much more confused and aggressive and on several occasions he wandered out of the house in the small hours of the morning. Initially he settled in well to the residential home, but 7 weeks after admission a number of problems became evident. Firstly, he began to make sexually inappropriate remarks to the young female care staff and on a few recent occasions he has attempted to touch them inappropriately. Secondly, he had a further chest infection with resultant worsening of his confusion and nocturnal wandering. During this time he became preoccupied with the false belief that the home was being attacked by German soldiers, and barricaded himself into his room with his furniture. On a few occasions he physically assaulted members of staff when they tried to reassure him. Although his chest infection was treated, Mr X continued to have a false belief that the home was being attacked by an enemy army.

The assessment process will now be looked at in detail and a formulation developed. The initial assessment involved speaking to Mr X's family and to the staff at the residential home, and interviewing and clinically examining Mr X.

1. **Is treatment necessary?**
    - is the individual distressed?
    - is the problem causing severe distress to the caregiver or other people in the care situation?
    - is the problem self-limiting?
    - is anyone at risk?

2. **Can we support the caregiver?**
    - how often if the problem occurring?
    - are there particular demanding times and are these predictable?

3. **What kind of support package is feasible and will it address the needs of the person with dementia and their caregiver?**

4. **Can the problem be managed by improving the environment?**
    - space to walk
    - familiar layout
    - good signs for key areas and facilities
    - homely setting
    - relaxing background music
    - appropriate lighting

5. **Are there specific psychosocial interventions which may be appropriate?** The following examples have been shown to be effective in clinical trials:
    - a planned walk outside for relieving restlessness
    - a personalized music programme
    - a video message from a family member
    - aromatherapy
    - psychological treatments for depression in people with dementia

6. **Is medication necessary?**
    - is the patient or carer suffering severe distress, making medication an urgent requirement?
    - is there evidence of psychiatric symptomatology (depression or psychotic symptoms) making medication necessary?
    - is there significant risk to the person due to lack of sleep, retaliation from other residents, etc., making prescription for medicaton urgent?

7. **Which first-line medication should be used?**
    - 'typical' neuroleptics
    - 'atypical' neuroleptics
    - carbamazepine
    - trazodone
    - cholinesterase inhibitors
    - miscellaneous drug treatments

8. **Are the problems sufficiently complex to merit more elaborate interventions?**
    - involvement of Old Age Psychiatry multidisciplinary team is essential
    - a detailed multicomponent evaluation of the situation is required
    - specifically tailored intervention may be necessary

Fig. 21.1   Management sieve for treating BPSD in a particular individual.

Assessment

Background history

Mr X was born and bred in Newcastle and worked for most of his life in one of the heavy industry firms before retiring at the age of 58 due to ill health. He was the younger of two brothers; his brother died of a heart attack 10 years ago. He was in the army during the war and was a prisoner of war for 2 years; his family knew very little about his wartime experiences as he steadfastly refused to talk about them. His wife died 5 years ago. He has two sons, both of whom live locally and visit him regularly, and five grandchildren. Since retirement he enjoyed going to his local club four nights per week, where he drank beer and played cards with his male friends.

Personality

Mr X's sons described him as being shy and reserved with the family but a popular raconteur with his male friends in the club. One of his sons, who used to go with him to the club, described him as being 'a bit of a flirt' with the female bar staff.

Physical health

Mr X has had longstanding COPD, complicated by frequent infective exacerbations. Over the past year he has developed a short-stepped, wide-based gait and has had a few falls. He has also had some problems with urinary urgency. He has a past history of hypertension. His medications are salbutamol and becotide inhalers and bendrofluazide. His blood pressure is currently well controlled at 140/85 mm Hg.

Mental state

Mr X was engaging and co-operative at interview. There was no evidence of any depressed mood. There was evidence of persecutory beliefs: he falsely believed that the German army was trying to attack him. He firmly believed that he heard shooting and interpreted this as the army firing at him. Despite the seriousness of these beliefs he appeared mildly euphoric and fatuous. He misidentified one of his sons as his brother.

Cognitive state

There was no impaired level of consciousness. There was evidence of mild disorientation for time and significant disorientation for place (he falsely believed he was in his club). There was evidence of short-term verbal memory difficulties, which improved on cueing. Mr X's thinking processes seemed generally slowed down. His concentration was intact, although slower than normal. Overall, he scored 16/30 on a mini mental state examination (MMSE). On more detailed assessment of his frontal lobe functioning, he had poor verbal fluency and difficulties with abstract concepts, and was unable to do simple motor sequencing tests (Luria stages 2 and 3).

Neurologically, there was evidence of subtle cogwheel rigidity on a reinforcement test and generally brisk symmetrical reflexes. There was evidence of prominent pout reflex and bilateral palmomental reflexes. As mentioned above, his gait was wide based and short stepped. A subsequent computed tomography brain scan showed cerebral atrophy with marked ischaemic changes in the subcortical white matter, especially in the frontal horns of the lateral ventricles.

Environment

Mr X lived in a large 50-bedded purpose-built residential home. He spent most of his day sitting in one of the lounges, watching television in the company of other, mainly female, residents. A new wing was being built adjacent to this lounge, with frequent noises of hammering and loud voices from the workmen.

Staff assessment

The staff reported that Mr X had made sexually inappropriate remarks to them throughout his 3 month admission, but that this had worsened in recent weeks so that he was now touching female staff members inappropriately. This tended to happen while Mr X was in the lounge in front of the other residents. When cautioned about this, he would joke about it, making light of what had happened. This behaviour tended not to happen with older female members of the care staff or with male carers.

The staff believed that Mr X's paranoid beliefs first began at night when he was delirious as a result of a chest infection. His chest infection was now being treated but these beliefs have now caused him to be distressed and fearful during the day. The staff have noticed that the recent noises from the new building could be misinterpreted by Mr X as gunshots and would often trigger a period of preoccupation about being attacked.

Formulation

Mr X has a subcortical vascular dementia with prominent frontal lobe deficits. This is complicated by sexually inappropriate behaviour and a paranoid psychosis. He is prone to episodes of delirium secondary to infective exacerbations of his COPD. On looking at his problematic behaviours in more detail, it was noted that:

(1) The inappropriate sexual behaviour generally occurred in the main lounge area. Mr X misidentified the lounge as his old club. Given that his son described him as 'a bit of a flirt', it is hypothesized that he was misidentifying the young female care staff as barmaids. His mild frontal lobe syndrome further contributed to this disinhibited behaviour.

(2) Mr X's paranoid psychosis and resultant secondary aggressive behaviour were initially due to delirium. However, on resolution of the delirium, the paranoid psychosis remained encapsulated. The content of his paranoid beliefs is interesting given his prisoner-of-war status and his reluctance to discuss his wartime experiences with his family. He is clearly misinterpreting the noise from the new building work as gunfire and this is acting as a precipitating and perpetuating factor for his psychotic beliefs and resultant aggressive behaviour.

Interventions

Dealing with the abnormal sexual behaviour

(1) In order to deal with Mr X's inappropriate sexual behaviours, the above for-
     mulation was explained to the staff. It was suggested that, in any interventions
     with him, they introduced themselves as a care assistant and explained clearly
     what they needed to do. Where possible, the young female care staff were not
     involved in his care.

(2) Mr X's sons resumed their previous routine of taking him to his club on a weekly
     basis. This had the benefit of providing him with a valued connection with his
     old friends and also helped orientate him to the differences between his resi-
     dential home and the club.

(3) Mr X was introduced to other male residents who enjoyed playing cards and
     struck up a new friendship with these men.

Dealing with the psychosis and aggressive behaviour

(1) The building work was due to continue for a further 3 weeks. During this time,
     Mr X was moved to a different part of the residential home, as far away from
     the building activity and the resultant noise as possible.

(2) His visits out with his sons also helped to reduce his preoccupations about
     being attacked.

(3) Despite these simple measures, Mr X's false beliefs remained and there were still
     occasional episodes were he would barricade himself in his room. He was there-
     fore commenced on an antipsychotic agent. The atypical antipsychotic, risperi-
     done, was chosen, at a starting dose of 0.5 mg *nocte*. This was later increased
     to 1 mg *nocte* with positive results. If sleep disturbance had been more promi-
     nent, olanzapine could have been a possible alternative given its sedative prop-
     erties. Quetiapine could be considered if there were concerns of worsening
     extrapyramidal signs.

(4) Given Mr X's known COPD, his inhaler technique was assessed. This was not
     good mainly due to poor coordination. He was provided with a 'spacer'
     attachment for his inhaler, which improved his breathing. The staff were alerted
     to the early signs of an infective exacerbation of COPD. An arrangement was
     made with his general practitioner to give him nebulized salbutamol in the early
     stages of an attack. This resulted in significantly fewer episodes of infective
     exacerbations.

Outcome

Mr X's inappropriate sexual behaviour abated. He continued to enjoy regular outings to his club with his sons and to have regular contact with his male card-playing
friends at the residential home. He had fewer exacerbations of COPD and was less
confused at night. The paranoid psychosis responded well to risperidone 1 mg *nocte*.

This was reduced and stopped approximately 3 months later with no recurrence of the psychosis or aggressive behaviours.

Conclusion and future developments

BPSD vary considerably in intensity. Supporting the carer is of prime importance. It may be possible to plan a support package around the times of day when the symptoms tend to be particularly severe. If these periods are not predictable, the flexible availability of additional support may be helpful, e.g. flexible attendance at a day hospital or emergency respite care. Additional psychosocial interventions strategies that may be helpful include environmental modification, behaviour therapy and training carers to cope more effectively with BPSD problems. More complex individually tailored management programmes based on a behavioural evaluation (ABC) and an understanding of how an individual's personality and previous life experiences may be contributing to the problem will also significantly reduce BPSD. Such a programme will require the input from specialist clinicians with training in psychiatric disorders of old age.

Despite many recent advances in our understanding of these common problems, the available evidence for how to treat BPSD is modest. However, in recent years there have been significant advances, particularly in developing a person-centred approach to people with dementia. The late Tom Kitwood's work can be seen as a very useful platform to develop this approach further. There have also been developments in pharmacological approaches, particularly in the availability of drugs with more benign side effect profiles (e.g. 'atypical' neuroleptics). The emergence of new drug classes gives further opportunities. For example, clinical experience with cholinesterase inhibitors is in its infancy, but clinicians are already reporting remarkable improvements in difficult neuropsychiatric symptoms, improvements in patient's quality of life and reductions in carer stress. The need for education and training programmes directed at family and formal caregivers is undeniable. Trials would be helpful in clarifying the use of specific drug treatments, in particular behaviour syndromes and specific combinations of drug treatments and psychosocial interventions.

REFERENCES

James, I. A. (1999). A cognitive conceptualisation of distress in people with dementia. *Clinical Psychology Forum*, **134**, 21–5.
Kitwood, T. (1997). *Dementia Reconsidered*. Open University Press, Buckingham.

Index

Note: page numbers in bold refer to figures and tables